PANDEMIC SOCIETIES

PANDEMIC SOCIETIES

Edited by Jean-Louis Denis, Catherine Régis,
and Daniel Weinstock

with the collaboration of
Clara Champagne

Published by McGill-Queen's University Press
for the Katharine A. Pearson Chair in Civil Society and Public Policy,
McGill University, and Health Hub: Politics, Organizations, and Law,
Université de Montréal
Montreal & Kingston • London • Chicago

© McGill-Queen's University Press 2021

ISBN 978-0-2280-0904-7 (cloth)
ISBN 978-0-2280-0905-4 (paper)
ISBN 978-0-2280-1033-3 (ePDF)
ISBN 978-0-2280-1034-0 (ePUB)

Legal deposit fourth quarter 2021
Bibliothèque nationale du Québec

Printed in Canada on acid-free paper that is 100% ancient forest free (100% post-consumer recycled), processed chlorine free

Funded by the Government of Canada   Financé par le gouvernement du Canada   Canada Council for the Arts   Conseil des arts du Canada

We acknowledge the support of the Canada Council for the Arts.
Nous remercions le Conseil des arts du Canada de son soutien.

Library and Archives Canada Cataloguing in Publication

Title: Pandemic societies / edited by Jean-Louis Denis, Catherine Régis, and Daniel Weinstock; with the collaboration of Clara Champagne.
Names: Denis, Jean-Louis, editor. | Régis, Catherine, 1976– editor. | Weinstock, Daniel M., editor.
Description: Includes bibliographical references and index.
Identifiers: Canadiana (print) 20210240784 | Canadiana (ebook) 2021024092X
 | ISBN 9780228009047 (cloth) | ISBN 9780228009054 (paper) | ISBN 9780228010333 (ePDF) | ISBN 9780228010340 (ePUB)
Subjects: LCSH: COVID-19 Pandemic, 2020-—Social aspects.
Classification: LCC RA644.C67 P36 2021 | DDC 362.1962/414—dc23

This book was typeset in 10.5/13 Sabon.

Contents

Figures   ix

Introduction   3
Jean-Louis Denis, Catherine Régis, Daniel Weinstock, Clara Champagne

PART ONE | CULTURE, MASS EVENTS, AND SOCIABILITY IN A PANDEMIC

1 Nightlife in a Pandemic   9
   Will Straw and Jess Reia

2 "A Gateway between One World and the Next": Performance-based Arts in COVID Times   30
   Christos Carras and Eric Lewis

3 Can Sports Partisanship Survive in the Pandemic World?   54
   Daniel Weinstock

4 Getting Pandemic Education Outside of the Box   68
   Andrew Potter

5 The COVID-19 Pandemic and the Loss of the Urban   83
   Quill R Kukla

PART TWO | TRANSFORMING WORK AND RESTARTING THE ECONOMY IN A POST-PANDEMIC ERA

6 Technology and Globalization in the Post-COVID Economy   101
   Etienne Lalé and Sophie Osotimehin

7 Is Teleworking Here to Stay? Learning from the COVID-19
   Experimentation   117
   *Tania Saba, Gaëlle Cachat-Rosset, Kevin Daniel André Carillo,
   Alain Klarsfeld, Josianne Marsan*

8 Occupational Health and Safety Lessons Learned: Moving Forward
   after the Pandemic   135
   Katherine Lippel, Barbara Neis, Phil James

PART THREE | DEMOCRACY, LAW, AND POLITICS
IN PANDEMIC SOCIETIES

9 The Politics of Populism in an Era of Pandemics: Freedom and
   Contagion in Brazil   165
   Felix Rigoli

10 Borders and the Global Pandemic of COVID-19   182
   *Élisabeth Vallet, Mathilde Bourgeon, Laurence Brassard, Gabrielle Gagnon,
   Julie Renaud*

11 New Zealand's Scale-Free Response to a Scale-Free Pandemic   200
   Tim Tenbensel

PART FOUR | HEALTH, SCIENCE, AND PUBLIC POLICY DURING
AND AFTER COVID-19

12 Science and Public Policy in a Post-Pandemic World   219
   Nicholas B. King

13 Wise Government and Wise Science in Times of Crisis   228
   Jean-Louis Denis, Clara Champagne, Justin Waring

14 Rewriting the Story of How the World Developed COVID-19 Vaccines:
   A Work of Fiction on Responsible Health Innovation Path Creation   248
   *Pascale Lehoux, Renata Pozelli Sabio, Hassane Alami, Lysanne Rivard,
   Hudson Pacifico Silva*

PART FIVE | GLOBAL HEALTH AND INTERNATIONAL RELATIONS
IN A PANDEMIC CONTEXT

15 The Future of Health and Human Rights in Pandemic Societies   269
   Lisa Forman

16 A Stress Test for the World Health Organization (WHO) in a Pandemic World: What Can We Hope for the Future? 286
   Catherine Régis, Miriam Cohen, Pierre Larouche, Jean-Louis Denis, Stéphanie B.M. Cadeddu, Gaëlle Foucault

17 Fortress World: Refugee Protection during (and after) the COVID-19 Pandemic 308
   Y.Y. Brandon Chen

Contributors 331

Figures

7.1 Conceptual framework to analyze telework adjustment and intention to continue teleworking. 120

10.1 *Borne de signalisation contemporaine Mur de la Peste* (1721). Cabrières-d'Avignon, Département du Vaucluse (France). Photo by Michel Wal, 2009, under Creative Commons License. 186

10.2 "*Mur de la peste*," wall of dry stone, originally from 1720, in restoration since 1986. Photograph by Psycho Chicken, 2014, under Creative Commons License. 187

10.3 Mapping experiment: pandemic mobility restrictions in Canada. Map by Alex McPhee, https://twitter.com/ksituan/status/1251622724826542088, reproduced with permission. 188

11.1 Plotting COVID-19 health outcomes (deaths per million) against the stringency of policy responses. 208

11.2 A simple fractal structure. 211

14.1 The RIH value domains and attributes. 256

14.2 Key steps in vaccine development, production, and delivery. Adapted from WTO's infographic, "Developing and delivering COVID-19 vaccines around the world." 258

PANDEMIC SOCIETIES

Introduction

*Jean-Louis Denis, Catherine Régis,
Daniel Weinstock, Clara Champagne*

In early 2020, when the World Health Organization declared the novel coronavirus COVID-19 a global pandemic, few of us realized that this new virus would produce shockwaves across the world, and profoundly transform all aspects of our social, cultural, and political lives. It was possible to think, at first, that these changes would be fleeting. But evidence suggests that we will be operating in a context of moderate risk and living with the effects of this pandemic for some time to come. Moreover, it is also now widely recognized that there will be other pandemics to come, and that their effects will resonate through our highly interconnected world. "Pandemic society" will be with us for some time to come.

Our "new normality" reflects vulnerability, but it also bears witness to our adaptative capacities. At the outset of the pandemic, our capacity to face the disruptions that it swiftly brought about was lacking. Our world was destabilized in ways and to an extent we had not seen in decades. The virus has brought some of the most prosperous societies to their knees, forcing the realization that their perceived immunity from the upheavals that global public health crises might bring about rested on illusions. Our only option was to adopt a stance of humility and to recognize our interdependence in a globally connected world where viruses do not stop at borders. Photographs of lockdowns across the world reveal the scale of the retreat, and pictures of mass graves, overcrowded hospitals, and last moments caught on iPads reveal the scale of the catastrophe. At the time of this writing, over 4 million people had lost their lives to the virus. A cloud of grief hovers above each one of these deaths.

At this time, the pandemic is still active and variants threaten our hope for a return to normality. And yet, the Perseverance Rover landed on Mars in February. Humankind's scientific breakthroughs have always coexisted with our relative inability to adapt quickly enough to great challenges, including climate change. COVID-19 vaccines are being administered in many countries barely a year into the pandemic – an unprecedented achievement. Yet shortfalls in national capacities in many jurisdictions and fierce competition between countries, including between the richest and the poorest, to obtain doses illustrate discrepancies in our ability to achieve responsible scientific innovations and to truly transform institutions and societies. The pandemic is associated with scientific achievement, but also with the exacerbation of inequities and of violence of all kinds. In the light of the latter, it is easy to be pessimistic about our ability to respond collectively to the challenges that pandemic society confronts us with. But there are also clearly signs of our capacity to spring back, to adapt to a changed world – temporarily or permanently – in order to continue to live our lives and to pursue our individual and societal goals.

We decided to put this collection of essays together in order to take stock of the evolution of our new "pandemic societies." From telework and new family dynamics, to the way in which we interact with our fellow citizens in everyday contexts, to the more formal institutional contexts through which important societal goods such as law, health, and education are administered and delivered, it is hard to think of a single dimension of the existence of citizens that has not been disrupted, sometimes beyond recognition, in a matter of mere months.

In this volume, we bring together experts in a wide range of academic fields to analyze the ways in which their objects of academic expertise might be transformed in the context of pandemic society. The pandemic forces transformations of the ways in which global institutions, such as the World Health Organization, function, but it also reaches into our everyday lives, and forces changes in the ways in which we organize culture, performing arts, sports, tourism, cities, and the like. The contributors to this volume reflect on these transformations, and engage in prospective thinking about the ways in which we might reinvent institutions and practices that we have thus far thought of as intrinsically "face-to-face." We have chosen to organize the volume by starting off with ways in which the pandemic has altered people's everyday lives – the way they join together with others to play, to perform, to entertain themselves. Gradually, the volume pulls the lens back to take in the broader institutional and political contexts in which these quotidian activities are housed.

With this in mind, we have divided the volume into five sections. The first is concerned with how culture and sociability have been fundamentally shaken by the pandemic, and delves into the worlds of nightlife, performance arts, sports, and city living. We then turn to work and the economy, and explore themes such as globalization, "slowbalisation," digitalization, telework, and worker health and safety during the pandemic. The third section focuses on shocks to law and politics. These chapters reflect on populist politics in the time of COVID-19, pandemic border regimes and their potential "stickiness" post-pandemic, and the challenges of comparing pandemic experiences and responses between countries. The fourth section examines the interface between science, innovation, and public policy. These chapters contemplate the role of science during the pandemic, the intricacies of the relationship between science and government, and lessons to be learned from the development and distribution of COVID-19 vaccines on how to realign health innovation processes towards a more responsible innovation pathway. The fifth and last section probes into pan-national issues: challenges in international law relating to health and human rights; the legal framework that circumscribes the WHO's normative leadership capacities and how the pandemic proved to be a "stress test" for this structure; and refugee protection in a time of travel restrictions, border closures, and immobility. The hope is that the sections and chapters build upon one another to provide a sense of how these different levels interact in pandemic societies. The hope is also that we learn as much as possible from this pandemic so, next time, we will be prepared.

I

Culture, Mass Events, and Sociability in a Pandemic

I

Nightlife in a Pandemic

Will Straw and Jess Reia

The closing down of night culture was one of the first and most dramatic social effects of the COVID-19 pandemic's arrival in the West. On 10 March 2020, *Billboard*, the world's leading source of music industry news, reported on the shut-down of night clubs in Italy (Worden and Cantor-Navas 2020), wondering with alarm how far this might spread and how long it might last. By April, media around the world were already speculating about the ways in which night-life culture might be forever changed (Barrière-Brunet 2020). Over the next ten months, and in a busy environment for news, the crisis of nightlife became one of the most regularly reported features of the international pandemic.

In response, the nightlife sector itself bustled with activity. At the local, national, and international levels, nightlife actors formed new associations or lobbies, pushing for financial aid, issuing guides for the renovation of venues, and arguing for relaxed restrictions on life outside the home. Experiments of all sorts in reinventing the culture of the night – on-line film festivals, home concerts, theatre performances on Zoom, virtual night clubs, and discotheques whose patrons remained seated – arrived in rapid sequence. Some gained traction as possibly permanent innovations, while others quickly faded.

Before the imposition of new lock-downs in many countries in the autumn of 2020, resistance to this closing of the night largely took the form of widely-reported illicit nocturnal gatherings of young people, whose secret "raves" and other festive events fueled predictable headlines and moral panics (Berthet 2020). By year's end, however, as curfews were imposed in India, parts of Western Europe and, eventually, in Quebec, many were claiming more openly that the night had become a scapegoat for governments unwilling to acknowledge the failure of other measures in controlling the virus (Wood 2020). Even when these commentators saw the early closing rules imposed on night-time bars, clubs, and restaurants as necessary, the banning of all night-time movement outside the home stood for many as evidence of a resurgent nyctophobia, the age-old fear of the night (Van Praagh 2021).

This article charts the sequence of events, contexts, and arguments which has marked the fate of night-time culture during the pandemic thus far. While the cultural life of the night includes cinema-going, theatre, classical music, choirs, and a variety of other forms or activities, our principal focus here is the sector devoted to night-time entertainment and sociability – the world of bars, nightclubs, and night-time dining. This was the realm of night-time culture most dramatically affected by the restrictions, lockdowns, and curfews imposed around the world. It was also the cultural sector most marked by resistance to restrictions, by experimentation with new forms and formats, and by the development of organizational structures for sustaining and defending itself.

In the final section of this article, we will turn to the case study of a single city, Montreal. We will trace the ways in which a city criticized for lacking coherent tools or ideas for the governance of the night moved quickly, in the midst of the pandemic, to begin elaborating a new, comprehensive vision of what its nights might be.

BEFORE THE PANDEMIC: THE NIGHT AS OBJECT OF POLICY

The closing of nightlife around the world in February and March of 2020 followed a decade in which the nighttime of cities had emerged as a significant focus of interest from several quarters. These included city administrators and urban planners, activists in the cultural field, and scholars engaged in building a new interdisciplinary field called "night studies" (Straw, Gwiazdzinski, and Maggioli 2020). Beginning in the 1990s, a variety of actors had pushed cities to acknowledge the role of their "night-time economies" in fostering economic growth and attracting tourist spending. From 2000 on, cities seeking to develop their nights, or to resolve the conflicts (over noise and public order) which increasingly made the night a contentious time, had developed a range of governance instruments focused on the night. At first, these were well-meaning, ideally consensual statements of principle, reached through dialogue between all the social actors with stakes in the night. In French cities, for example, "Charters of Night Life" were drawn up and inter-sectorial "Night Councils" were established (Lyon 2019; Ville de Paris 2020).

In the 2010s, a number of cities began appointing (or recognizing) "Night Mayors," individuals with a mandate to protect and develop night-time cultural activity in their cities. Some of these "Night Mayors" (like Mirik Milan, who assumed the post in Amsterdam in 2012) came out of the night-time music and club sectors, and saw their role as one of sensitizing city administrators to the value of this sector. Typically, these figures worked with city officials to reduce violence, noise, and other sources of complaint. Others, like Amy Lamé, the Night Czar of London since 2016, were named by city government to oversee the culture of the night, often in the context of anxieties about that sector's economic decline. The first of these positions in Canada was that of Toronto's "Night Economy Ambassador," created and filled in November 2019 (Toronto 2019). By the end of 2019, as Seijas and Gelders have shown, more than forty cities around the world had some version of a "Night Mayor" (Seijas and Gelders 2020).

To this new focus by cities on something called a "night-time economy," and to the invention of new instruments of what has been called "nocturnal governance," we may add the tremendous proliferation of night-time and all-night cultural festivals around the world. Helsinki's Night of the Arts in 1989 is seen as the founding event in this recent history, but the significant explosion came after 2000, as *nuits blanches* art festivals, Museum Nights, Bookstore Nights and an array of other late-night events brought cultural forms (like literature), often associated with private consumption or solitary contemplation, into the sphere of night-time sociability. Many of these events took place in the cities of Latin America, where the holding of *Noches de museos* or *Noches de la librerias* in city centres was part of broader efforts to encourage city residents to remain in these districts, often considered dangerous or unsavoury, into the night.

Reading media coverage of night-time cultural initiatives from February 2020, one sees all of the tendencies just described continuing to unfold, with no sense of the calamities to come. In India, a flurry of interest in building a night-time economy spurred predictions that Mumbai might add billions to its economy by opening up its nights (Times of India 2020). The night-mayor of Groningen, in the Netherlands, told entertainment industry executives in Kingston, Jamaica, that his city's model of night-time governance, which avoided curfews, had made it a safer place (Small 2020). The French cities of Bordeaux, Paris, Nantes, and Liège released a jointly-authored document, "Politique publique de Vie Nocturne : Gouvernance et participation," which laid out principles for night-time governance developed by the national *Plateforme de la vie nocturne*, an association of people active in various kinds of night-time cultural activity (Lerivrain 2020)

All of these initiatives unfolded amidst an atmosphere of crisis, but that crisis had been gathering momentum prior to the arrival of the COVID-19 pandemic. Its most frequently diagnosed cause was the ongoing gentrification of cities. Gentrification stood more broadly for a wide range of transformations affecting urban cultural life over the previous decade: the rise of rents (which devastated bohemian residential districts and drove many music venues out of business), the growth of urban tourism, fueled by inexpensive air travel, transformations which saw many older sites of inner-city commerce and culture replaced by bars and nightclubs, and the spread of short-term rental systems like Airbnb, blamed for disrupting the rent structures and social ecologies of city neighbourhoods. Other effects of these changes included the economic migration of long-standing populations out of certain city neighbourhoods, and an intensification of conflicts over noise and perceived public disorder. While all of these developments had been noted since 2015 and 2016, they were felt most intensely in cities like Berlin, Mexico City, and Washington, DC, in the final months of 2019 and early days of 2020 (see, for example, Velasco 2020; Mock 2019).

While the COVID pandemic shut down night-time cultural activity in startling and unprecedented ways, it devastated a sector which was already confronting one of its most serious crises in decades. At the same time, however, COVID unfolded against the backdrop of unprecedented official recognition of the value of night-time culture to cities, in a context of high levels of organization and activism on the part of those committed to the preservation and growth of that culture. Thus, even as, in early 2021, the question of how night-life might recover from the pandemic remains an open one, the affected sector possesses more internal expertise and organizational infrastructure than ever before. Since March 2020, we have seen Montreal appoint its first municipal official charged with re-imagining the city's nights; we have seen organizations within the night-time cultural sector around the world release a stream of reports and manifestoes on ways to save night-life; and we have seen governments at all levels adopt (or reject) proposals to reimburse night-life institutions for their losses.

THE UNFOLDING CRISIS

In February 2020, two on-line news items from China captured the double dimensions of the Coronavirus' impact on night life. A blog post on *Hyperallergic*, on 13 February, spoke of Chinese punk bands "taking the Mosh Pit Online" – that is, live-streaming concerts from clubs emptied of patrons, or participating in networked "bedroom festivals" in which artists played from their homes. *Hyperallergic* spoke of this hasty emergence of an on-line musical culture in China as a "nationwide craze" (Raghav 2020). In the same month, the Xinhua News organization posted to YouTube a short video of public employees cleaning the streets of Luoyang. Against a jubilant keyboard soundtrack, we see battalions of trucks venturing along the empty streets of the night-time city, spraying disinfectant against a visual backdrop of lavishly illuminated buildings (New China TV 2020). Between them, these two reports mapped extremes in the early fate of the urban night under COVID: on the one hand, the quickly-evolved and rich inventiveness of on-line musical culture; on the other, a desolate void exemplified by empty downtown buildings and streets abandoned by all but the battalions of sanitization workers who laboured to make them virus-free.

On 11 March 2020, the day on which the World Health Association declared the COVID-19 crisis to be a pandemic, the music industry trade publication *Billboard* published a report with the headline, "No More Nightlife" (Worden and Cantor-Navas 2020). Indeed, "No more nightlife" was a phrase the Italian prime minister had used in an address to the nation, in which he told Italians to stay at home. In the week that followed, a steady stream of news from around the world signalled the uneven but ominous ways in which night-time culture was shutting down. Night clubs in Montreal, which for the moment could remain open with a maximum clientele of 250 persons, worried about the future, with larger venues complaining that such small crowds could not be profitable (Forster 2020).

In New Jersey, restaurants and bars began recording attendance, as part of the contact-tracing initiatives which would be applied in multiple places with limited consistency or uneven benefit (Hollan 2020). On 15 March, Manila, in the Philippines, instituted a night-time curfew as the pandemic-related death count rose to six (Reuters 2020). Hospitality industry representatives in the UK, on 18 March, warned that their industry was on the verge of ruin, and pleaded for government help (ITV 2020). Around the world, the final weeks of March saw night-time establishments adjusting to newly-imposed regulations but carrying on nonetheless, while organizations representing the night-time sector began publishing pandemic updates and elaborating demands for government assistance (Global Cities After Dark 2020).

The early rationales for shutting down the night were always multiple and of uneven credibility. In the most basic of these, night-time culture and entertainment were simply not essential services, and could easily be sacrificed in the pandemic's early days. Arguments made by the night-time sector since the 1990s – that the night possessed an economic and social force which belied its longstanding dismissal as a frivolous and secondary part of urban life – quickly lost their capacity to persuade.

Even when the culture of the night was not deemed non-essential it was seen, nevertheless, as difficult to control, as producing behaviours which, combining alcohol and a sense of nocturnal abandon, might threaten social-distancing guidelines on a massive scale. In May and June of 2020, the only tolerated collective expressions of festive sociability were the musical balcony tributes to commuting health-care workers, which would disappear as summer saw a lifting of restrictions in the global North and as political differences fractured the shared sentiments on which these tributes rested (Betts 2020). While they lasted, these charivari-like performances were recorded and scattered across social media platforms, producing some approximation of collective night-time effervescence outside the home (Straw 2020).

In April 2020, it was possible to point to a wave of inventiveness, by which the culture of the night was being re-imagined around the world, with results that offered at least momentary distraction. Even as police in Manchester, England, announced that they had closed down 660 Easter weekend parties – "some with DJs, fireworks and bouncy castles." (Forrest 2020), on-line versions of club events were proliferating, with experiments in one place covered by media elsewhere, as the global club music sector sought evidence of viable alternatives. In a rapidly-evolving commentary, virtual clubs, like the Zone in Los Angeles (which actually charged admission) were seen as superseding the simple streamed DJ sets which had been appearing since February. These clubs offered the possibility of unexpected encounters and multiple spaces more typical of a real-life club experience. Bloomberg Media's 15 April report on The Zone, fascinated by the fact that it offered sixteen virtual rooms, suggested that club owners were learning from the experiences of event planners and others engaged in on-line culture: "As nightlife appropriates technologies built for corporate conferencing and gaming, new party experiences are emerging to encourage interactivity and community, making the audience active participants rather than passive consumers" (Lhooq 2020).

More broadly we might point to the rapid transfer of hastily-acquired online skills between work and night-time entertainment in the early days of the pandemic. The experience of working or studying online quickly imparted the technical skills (and inspired the upgrades of in-home bandwidth and equipment) on which the consumption of on-line night-time entertainment depended. Zoom happy hours with friends mobilized skills recently learned during the work-day, just as screen-sharing in educational contexts trained people for collective evening film-viewing events.

POLICY AND SECTOR ORGANIZING

Across the spring and summer of 2020, we may point to a range of initiatives, from governments at all levels, intended to alleviate the pandemic's devastating effects on night-time entertainment. Already, in April, Sao Paulo had announced a new system of micro-credit to help night-time entertainment venues (São Paulo para. crianças 2020). Lisbon launched a program of "immediate aid" to the ailing Fado music sector (Noticas ao minuto 2020). In May, Texas politicians of both parties were urging the Federal Congress to provide aid to live music venues (Barber 2020b) and in Paris, France, a recovery plan laid out a series of measures intended to revitalize the nightlife sector, from direct aid to artists losing their livelihoods through new guidelines allowing restaurants and cafés to expand their use of outdoor space (Barber 2020a).

The Parisian initiatives in May offered an early glimpse of a broad rethinking of the recreational uses of public space. While these proposals were intended as temporary solutions to the problems of social distancing, it is this redesign of outdoor city space – rather than any significant movement of night-time culture online – which may be one of the pandemic's most durable legacies. Across the global North, the coming of summer and temporal decline of infection rates encouraged implementation of many of the features of what has been called the New Urbanism (Congress for the New Urbanism 2015): the closing of streets for pedestrian traffic, an expansion of bicycle paths and sidewalks, and the distribution of picnic tables, food trucks, and small-scale attractions throughout the city. To these were added some of the "emergency measures" deemed necessary if small-scale enterprises in the hospitality sector were to survive the pandemic: lighter regulation of alcohol sales, increased occupation by restaurants or bars of sidewalks and streets, the building of terrasses and so on.

These innovative moves offered significant relief for the hospitality industries (for restaurants and bars), but their direct impact on nightlife was uneven. Describing a daily itinerary which evoked Karl Marx's fantasy of daily life under socialism, Fredric Hocquard, deputy mayor of Paris in charge of nightlife, imagined a pandemic summer of 2020 filled with outdoor pleasures: "At ten o'clock, a sporting activity; at noon, a picnic; in the afternoon, a show (spectacle); and in the evening, a drink and a concert. If we can manage this in the summer for two months, it will be the 'Summer of Love'" (Carriat and Mayer 2020; translation by the authors).

Milder versions of this scenario were imagined in other places. The outdoor terrasse was certainly the urban form embraced with greatest enthusiasm as a solution to the problem of summer-time sociability under a pandemic. From Montreal to Barcelona to Manchester, outdoor tables were built and extended on a massive scale, made to bear the multiple burdens of restoring income to restaurant or bar owners and keeping patrons both sedentary and distanced from each other (CultMTL 2020; Sust 2020; Heward 2020). When they failed, this was often (as in Montreal) because early closing rules left people on the streets, in late evening, still desiring group sociability, or because (as in Paris), streets filled with such terrasses were the object of citizen complaints about noise, which limited the levels of festive nocturnal exuberance some might have expected (Syfuss-Arnaud 2020). The terrasse made possible a vestige of the sociability of pre-pandemic afternoons and evenings, but did little to salvage the culture of the night.

SCENARIOS FOR RECOVERY

On 23 July 2020, the first volume of a *Global Nighttime Recovery Plan* was released by the European group *nighttime.org* – an outgrowth of the VibeLab, an international consultancy established by Berlin Clubcommission's Lutz Leichsenring and the former Night Mayor of Amsterdam, Mirik Milan. Drawing on case studies of cities (Vilnius and Berlin) and the expertise of nighttime event organizers, this first of at least five volumes (some are still in preparation) bore the title "Open-Air Nightlife and COVID-19: Managing Outdoor Space & Sound" (Vibelab 2020). The document offers a comprehensive imagining of nighttime culture during the pandemic, with detailed plans for outdoor arrangements of festive space, the use of abandoned or unused sites, and an ongoing monitoring of risks to health and safety.

We may contrast the tone of this guidebook, which largely accepts the probability of continued restrictions on indoor nightlife, with that of another document, released a month later by the UK-based Night-Time Industries Association, which had commissioned it from an Institute of Occupational Medicine. In *Nightclub & Venue Reopening Strategy,* which set out "the case for a science-based, risk-assessed return to a COVID-secure opening of nightclubs and venues," we are offered a very different scenario: one of a tightly controlled and highly securitized nightlife happening indoors. In addition to following the same restrictions applied to retail outlets and restaurants, this report suggests, nightclubs might impose "thermal monitoring of guests on entry, restriction of capacity numbers overall and reduced numbers on dancefloors, and a requirement to wear faces masks while dancing – managed by security staff" (Night Time Industries Association 2020).

These two images of a pandemic nightlife – one re-imagining cities as series of festive outdoor spaces, the other re-opening nightclubs as profoundly controlled environments – have endured, with few new alternatives being offered, through the later months of 2020 and into early 2021. Further lockdowns and new curfews have dampened new thinking about the spaces and formats of nightlife. As we look ahead to the spring and summer of 2021, there is little to cheer beyond the occasional announcements that terrasses and pedestrianized streets, in cities like Montreal, will return.

MONTREAL: DESIGNING A NIGHTLIFE POLICY DURING A PANDEMIC

Montreal has a longstanding reputation as a festive city and place of vibrant nightlife. Over the previous century, the Canadian city had seen a boom in nightclubs and cabarets during the period of Prohibition in the United States, and again during World War II and the half-decade which followed. Montreal was known as the second liveliest city in the world for disco music in the 1970s (Straw 2014), and its underground music scenes and music festivals garnered significant international attention in the 2000s (Stahl 2001; Campbell 2013). The city's designation as "top student city in North America" in 2019 (QS 2019) rested in significant measure on a perception of its nightlife as youthful and creative.

Despite its exuberant nightlife, Montreal had been behind other major cities when it came to night-time policy and coherent tools or strategies for what is called "night-time governance." In the last decade, the city has seen an increase in complaints about night-time noise. The resulting conflicts, when combined with rising rents, would force well-established music venues like Le Cagibi (Dunlevy 2018) to move or, as were the cases with Le Divan Orange (Leavitt 2017) and Coop Katacombes (CBC News 2019), to close their doors permanently. The municipal government struggled to deal with growing discontent on the part of different stakeholders trying to navigate a complex administrative system and a less-than-ideal regulatory framework directed at the night.

While the provincial government of Quebec has long controlled the licensing of venues and events serving alcohol, the city and its many districts oversee and enforce legislation on noise, security, and city-wide public transportation. For example, noise complaints are enforced by the police, and event organizers need to obtain different types of permits from a variety of government departments. Even if the municipal government were willing to make changes related to night-time governance, it might bump up against provincial restrictions and regulatory bottlenecks. In 2014, when Montreal's mayor Denis Coderre decided to implement a pilot project to extend bars' opening hours, he faced opposition from Quebec's provincial bodies regulating the sale of alcohol (CBC News 2014).[1]

Two years later, in late 2016, the Quebec government granted Montreal the status of "metropolis," allowing the city to determine the opening hours of bars on its territory and to regulate other aspects of nightlife (Dion 2016).

In November 2017, *Projet Montréal* – a municipal party, led by Valérie Plante, espousing a progressive platform – was elected to govern Montreal, following a campaign that promised to address issues related to nightlife. In the early years of its mandate, besides drafting interesting action plans and holding consultations with music venues and bars' owners, the city government made little progress concerning the governance of the night. Indeed, small businesses of a cultural character, such as record stores, were still being fined weeks before the beginning of the COVID pandemic started, as a result of noise complaints or violation of business closing hour regulations (Harris 2019).

As had happened in so many other cities, the pandemic dramatically shut down night culture in Montreal. In March 2020, Quebec decided that bars, restaurants, and nightclubs would be closed until at least May, putting the province "on pause" (Forster 2020a). By May, Montreal had become Canada's COVID-19 "hotspot" and the seventh deadliest place in the world in terms of the virus' effects (Lindeman 2020). The city struggled to keep businesses afloat, including those in the cultural sector, and all three levels of government (federal, provincial, and municipal) offered financial aid. Not all small cultural venues were able to benefit from these measures, however (Harris 2020).

With summer quickly approaching and no perspective of recovery for the night-time economy in sight – despite a decline in COVID infections and deaths – the owners of cultural venues were forced to adapt to an easing of sanitary measures which, while welcome, did not allow for a full return to their pre-pandemic levels of activity. Many of these venues shapeshifted to adjust to changing rules. A repertory cinema began selling houseplants, while bars laboured to increase their sales of non-alcohol merchandise, like T-shirts. An emblematic example of adaptation was that of Casa del Popolo, one of Montreal's world-famous venues for independent music, which had existed since 2000. During the summer of 2020, faced with the impossibility of booking live concerts, the owners decided to turn a significant portion of the space into a retail store featuring in-house printed materials and locally crafted products.

The spring and summer of 2020 nevertheless saw significant developments for Montreal in the area of night-time governance and regulation. MTL 24/24, a non-profit organization advocating for the interests of various cultural players in Montreal's night culture, had been launched in 2017, the year of Valerie Plante's election to the mayor's office. In June 2020, MTL 24/24 launched the city's first *Conseil de Nuit* (Night Council), a multi-stakeholder body bringing together representatives of various organizations and sectors involved in the city's nightlife. MTL 24/24 voiced concerns over the city's longstanding treatment of the night and advocated for policies which would resolve this. The twelve members of the *Conseil de Nuit* are divided between four committees with specific mandates: "Health, Security, Diversity, and Inclusion"; "Nocturnal Lifestyle"; "Clubs, Cultural Bars and Venues"; and "Festivals and Events."

In June 2020, one of the first actions of this new body was to write an open letter to the mayor, offering strategies by which nightlife might be possible in the context of the pandemic, at least during the summer (Conseil de Nuit de MTL 24/24 2020). Recommendations included the use of industrial spaces for nocturnal socialization, permission to play music in certain public spaces, and the legalization of alcohol consumption in parks.

Somewhat unexpectedly, Montreal's city government began to elaborate a new, comprehensive nightlife policy in mid-2020. The first initiatives for night-time governance structures were announced, and, while these were not designed as a response to the pandemic itself, they included economic recovery plans for mitigating certain impacts of the ongoing pandemic. In June 2020, the city's Economic Development department appointed Deborah Delaunay as its first Commissioner of Noise and Night, after having advertised the position in February (Fournier 2020). With this appointment, Montreal had given itself the equivalent of the Night Mayors now found in over fifty cities worldwide.

Delaunay soon began regular consultations with MTL 24/24 and commissioned from them a *portrait diagnostique* of nightlife in Montreal. Throughout the month of August 2020, the new Commissioner organized working groups as the first step towards the reinvention of Montreal's nights. Within the framework of an economic recovery plan, the city decided to create a new nighttime economy policy based on four principles: recognizing, reconciling, promoting, and strengthening nightlife in Montreal. A steering committee was established, and various specialists and stakeholders were invited to contribute to four transversal working groups: (a) Nighttime economies; (b) Creative and cultural nights; (c) Health, security and diversity; and (d) Spaces and nocturnal mobilities. The working groups met four times between September and November 2020 to discuss night-related problems and to brainstorm solutions and recommendations.[2]

The next step involved a public consultation, which the City commissioned from MTL 24/24 in late 2020. This was intended to reach an understanding of the perceptions, needs, and desires of Montreal residents concerning a new night-time policy. While an international summit on the night was to have taken place in October 2020, ongoing travel restrictions and a rise in the number of COVID cases in the fall led to it being postponed. These activities unfolded against the backdrop of the second wave of the pandemic, which struck Quebec in early 2021. The provincial government reinstated lockdown measures and implemented a curfew from 8 p.m. to 5 a.m, thus altering the urban nightscape completely (Lalonde 2021, 2021a). The curfew, described as "shock therapy" by the premier of Quebec, François Legault (Kirkey 2021), was contested by many organizations, from those in the night culture sector through others advocating for the unhoused population in the city (since unhoused people were, at first, not made exempt from the curfew.)

The imminence of new municipal elections, in November 2021, has created uncertainty over the continuation of Montreal's new initiatives in the area of nighttime policy. According to the Economic Development department's timeline, a draft of the policy would normally be available for consultation and review by May 2021. However, the ever-changing constraints of the pandemic, combined with the challenges posed by the upcoming election, may have a significant impact on plans to develop a new regulatory framework for the night. At the same time, the lack of data about most night culture sectors in Montreal further complicates this scenario, since it makes it difficult to assess the economic damage of the pandemic or the potential for post-pandemic growth. Efforts by the Montreal Urban Innovation Lab (2020) to consolidate a Digital Data Charter could be a step in this direction, but conversations across municipal departments and with the public in a broad sense are needed.

CONCLUSION

In the last decade, we have seen the nighttime of cities become the principal site of political protests of all kinds. From Quebec's *printemps érable* through the Gezi park demonstrations in Istanbul in 2013, *Nuit debout* in France in 2016 and night-time rallies or occupations in Lebanon and the Sudan in late 2019, political protest in the night has taken over from the day-time marches down major city streets which typified political mobilizations in the twentieth century. If these nocturnal protests were rarely about the night, they made occupation of night-time space a significant feature of claims to social justice. The night-time demonstrations which followed the murder by police of George Floyd in May 2020 interwove all-encompassing claims for racial justice with specific reminders of how the policing of the night has been central to a racist social order, and not only in the United States. A "right to the night" has been a focus of recent feminist activism in India, whose hashtag #IWillGoOut rests in large measure on the claim to full and safe participation in the nightlife of cities (Taneja 2017).

Since the final months of 2020, we have seen, as well, a rise in claims that the culture of the night has been unjustly made the scapegoat for the pandemic's persistence (Geoffroy 2021). Some will base this claim on a demonstration of the ways in which curfews have a long history of suppression of the marginal, the radical, and the disadvantaged (Reverchon 2020). The curfews of early 2021 have generated claims, in Canada and elsewhere, that these new restrictions will disproportionately target and criminalize racialized populations (Lowrie 2021). Others will insist on the centrality of night-time sociability to mental health and social well-being, and suggest that these are being affected in disastrous ways by the curfews of early 2021 (Grossin 2020). The claim to the "right to party," tarnished in the United States context through its associations with right-wing pandemic-denying politicians like Florida Governor De Santis (The Alligator 2020) has assumed a more radical edge elsewhere, in countries like France, where "*le droit à la fête*" is increasingly advanced as a defence of culture itself (Roy 2021; Yumpu.com 2021).

Montreal is a good example of a city that has long remained behind other world cities in the development of nighttime governance mechanisms. The pandemic pushed the city to address long-standing issues concerning its night, and to respond to the new challenges that emerged throughout 2020. For the moment, there is reason to believe that the city is engaged in developing innovative policies whose result may well be a re-imagined, inclusive and participatory culture of the night. If so, these changes may endure long into the post-pandemic era.

NOTES

1 While an organization promoting the rights of bars – l'Association Québécoise de la vie nocturne – has existed in Quebec since the early 2010s, there are few signs that it is still active.
2 The authors participated in the working groups (b) and (d).

REFERENCES

Alligator (The). 2020. "The Right to Party? Gov. DeSantis Is on the Wrong Side of History – The Independent Florida Alligator." Editorial. *The Independent Florida Alligator*, 27 September 2020. https://www.alligator.org/article/2020/09/the-right-to-party-gov-desantis-is-on-the-wrong-side-of-history?ct=content_open&cv=cbox_featured.

Barber, Jess Dymond. 2020a. "Paris Installs Support Plan for the Economic, Voluntary and Cultural Sectors, Including Nightlife." NIGHTTIME.ORG, 19 May 2020. https://www.nighttime.org/update-paris-installs-a-support-plan-for-the-economic-voluntary-and-cultural-sectors-including-nightlife/.

– 2020b. "Surprisingly Bipartisan Effort out of Texas for US Congress to Include Live Event Venues in Future Relief Packages." NIGHTTIME.ORG, 26 May 2020. https://www.nighttime.org/surprisingly-bipartisan-effort-out-of-texas-for-us-congress-toinclude-live-event-venues-in-future-relief-packages/.

Barrière-Brunet, Sara. 2020. "Quel avenir pour la vie culturelle nocturne?" *Voir.ca*, 30 April 2020. https://voir.ca/musique/2020/04/30/quel-avenir-pour-la-vie-culturelle-nocturne/.

Berthet, Marie Avril. 2020. "Rave Culture Is Culture: Instead of Starting a Moral Panic, the Government Should Make Them Safe." *Novara Media*, 22 June 2020. https://novaramedia.com/2020/06/22/rave-culture-is-culture-instead-of-starting-a-moral-panic-the-government-should-make-raves-safe/.

Betts, Ty. 2020. "Why Humans Are Howling Every Night, and Why Wildlife Is Joining In." SOURCE, 28 April 2020. https://source.

colostate.edu/why-humans-are-howling-every-night-and-why-wildlife-is-joining-in/.

Campbell, Miranda. 2013. *Out of the Basement: Youth Cultural Production in Practice and in Policy*. Montreal: McGill-Queen's University Press.

Carriat, Julie, and Claire Mayer. 2020. "La terrasse, planche de salut des restaurateurs et cafetiers déconfinés." *Le Monde.fr*, 30 May 2020. https://www.lemonde.fr/societe/article/2020/05/30/la-terrasse-planche-de-salut-des-restaurateurs-et-cafetiers-deconfines_6041280_3224.html.

CBC News. 2014. "Denis Coderre Faces Some Opposition to Extended Bar Hours." *CBC News*, 26 May 2014. https://www.cbc.ca/news/canada/montreal/denis-coderre-faces-some-opposition-to-extended-bar-hours-1.2654610

– 2019. "Montreal Punk-Rock Venue Katacombes will Close for Good After Christmas." *CBC News*, 24 October 2019. https://www.cbc.ca/news/canada/montreal/katacombes-montreal-closing-music-venue-1.5334299.

Congress for the New Urbanism. 2015. "What Is New Urbanism?" *CNU*, 18 May 2015. https://www.cnu.org/resources/what-new-urbanism.

Conseil de Nuit de MTL 24/24. 2020. "Montréal, une ville 'cool'?" *Le Devoir*, 18 June 2020. https://www.ledevoir.com/opinion/libre-opinion/580986/montreal-une-ville-i-cool-i.

CultMTL. 2020. "Casa Del Popolo Has Reopened with a Sweet New Terrasse." *Cult MTL*, 19 July 2020. https://cultmtl.com/2020/07/montreal-music-venue-bar-restaurant-casa-del-popolo-has-reopened-with-a-sweet-new-terrasse/.

Dion, Mathieu. 2016. "Montréal décidera des heures d'ouverture des bars, parmi ses nouveaux pouvoirs." *ICI Radio-Canada*, 8 December 2016. https://ici.radio-canada.ca/nouvelle/1004645/montreal-statut-metropole-quebec

Dunlevy, T'Cha. 2018. "Le Cagibi settling into Little Italy, after being forced out of Mile End." *Montreal Gazette*, 31 July 2018. https://montrealgazette.com/news/local-news/le-cagibi-is-dead-long-live-the-new-co-op-le-cagibi.

Forrest, Adam. 2020. "Greater Manchester Police Issue Easter Warning after 660 Parties Shut Down." *The Independent*, 9 April 2020. https://www.independent.co.uk/news/uk/home-news/coronavirus-lockdown-parties-easter-manchester-police-marcus-rashford-a9457026.html.

Forster, Tim. 2020. "Some Montreal Nightclubs Are Closing Due to Coronavirus – But Not All." *Montreal Eater*, 13 March 2020. https://

montreal.eater.com/2020/3/13/21178171/montreal-covid-19-nightclub-closures-music-venues.

Fournier, Éloi. 2020. "Montréal compte maintenant une commissaire au bruit environnemental." *Journal des Voisins*, 2 September 2020. https://journaldesvoisins.com/montreal-compte-maintenant-une-commissaire-au-bruit-environnemental/.

Geoffroy, Romain. 2021. "Des fêtes condamnées à la clandestinité, faute d'alternatives légales et de propositions politiques." *Le Monde.fr*, 19 January 2021. https://www.lemonde.fr/societe/article/2021/01/19/faire-la-fete-un-enjeu-politique-en-temps-de-covid-19_6066738_3224.html.

Global Cities After Dark. 2020. "Coronavirus Latest News: Updated." *Global Cities After Dark*, 16 March 2020. https://www.globalcitiesafterdark.com/latest-corona-virus-news/.

Grossin, Benoit. 2020. "Covid-19 et couvre-feu: la vague de problèmes de santé mentale loin d'être retombée." *France Culture*, 18 October 2020. https://www.franceculture.fr/societe/covid-19-couvre-feu-la-vague-de-problemes-de-sante-mentale-loin-detre-retombee.

Harris, Colin. 2019. "Mile End Record Stores Uncertain About Future as They Face Fines Over Business Hours." *CBC News*, 11 December 2019. https://www.cbc.ca/news/canada/montreal/mile-end-record-stores-sonorama-phonopolis-fines-opening-hours-tourism-1.5393131.

– 2020. "Music Venues Work to Adapt to Pandemic as Government Aid Alone Won't Keep Them Afloat." *CBC News*, 7 August 2020. https://www.cbc.ca/news/canada/montreal/music-venue-aid-covid-19-1.5676490.

Heward, Emily. 2020. "Manchester's Streets and Squares Could Be Opened up as Beer Gardens." *Manchester Evening News*, 8 June 2020. https://www.manchestereveningnews.co.uk/whats-on/food-drink-news/manchesters-streets-squares-could-opened-18381013.

Hollan, Michael. 2020. "Jersey City Asking Bars to Take Attendance in Proactive Step against Coronavirus." *Fox News*, 12 March 2020. https://www.foxnews.com/food-drink/jersey-city-bars-attendance-coronavirus.

ITV. 2020. "Hospitality Industry Facing Ruin as Leaders Demand State Help." *ITV News*, 17 March 2020. https://www.itv.com/news/2020-03-17/hospitality-industry-facing-ruin-as-leaders-demand-state-help.

Kirkey, Sharon. 2021. "Shock Therapy: Curfew to Curtail COVID-19 Spread Might Just Worsen Public Mental Health, Morale." *The Chronicle Herald*, 9 January 2021. https://www.thechronicleherald.ca/lifestyles/health/shock-therapy-curfew-to-curtail-covid-19-spread-might-just-worsen-public-mental-health-morale-539069/.

Lalonde, Catherine. 2021. "Une nuit sans feu ni flamme à Montréal." *Le Devoir*, 11 January 2021. https://www.ledevoir.com/societe/593084/carnets-de-nuit-sous-couvre-feu-1-4-une-nuit-sans-feu-ni-flamme-a-montreal.

– 2021a. "Les rêves interdits des nuits de couvre-feu." *Le Devoir*, 25 January 2021. https://www.ledevoir.com/societe/593948/carnets-de-nuit-sous-couvre-feu-les-reves-interdits.

Leavitt, Sarah. 2017. "Popular Music Venue Le Divan Orange to Close this Spring." CBC *News*, 27 November 2017. https://www.cbc.ca/news/canada/montreal/popular-music-venue-le-divan-orange-to-close-this-spring-1.4422248.

Lindeman, Tracey. 2020. "Why Are So Many People Getting Sick and Dying in Montreal from Covid-19?" *The Guardian*, 13 May 2020. https://www.theguardian.com/world/2020/may/13/coronavirus-montreal-canada-hit-hard

Lhooq, Michelle. 2020. "Virtual Nightlife Grows Past DJ Livestreams to Paid Zoom Clubs – Bloomberg." *Bloomberg*, 14 April 2020. https://www.bloomberg.com/news/articles/2020-04-14/virtual-nightlife-grows-past-dj-livestreams-to-paid-zoom-clubs.

Lowrie, Morgan. 2021. "Amid Worries about Curfew Policing, Montreal Police Try to Sound Reassuring Note." CTV *News Montreal*, 7 January 2021. https://montreal.ctvnews.ca/amid-worries-about-curfew-policing-montreal-police-try-to-sound-reassuring-note-1.5258035?cache=yesclipId104062.

Lyon (Ville). 2019. "Charte Pour La Qualité de La Vie Nocturne | Ville de Lyon."https://www.lyon.fr/cadre-de-vie/bruit/charte-pour-la-qualite-de-la-vie-nocturne.

Montreal Urban Innovation Lab. 2020. "Montréal's Digital Data Charter.» October 2020. https://laburbain.montreal.ca/sites/villeintelligente.montreal.ca/files/25817-charte_donnees_numeriques_ang.pdf.

Mock, Brentin. 2019. "Go-Go Is the Sound of Anti-Gentrification in D.C." *Bloomberg CityLab*, 18 November 2019. https://www.bloomberg.com/news/articles/2019-11-18/go-go-is-the-sound-of-anti-gentrification-in-d-c.

New China TV. 2020. *Coronavirus Fight: Hundreds of Trucks Spray Disinfectants in Luoyang*. https://www.youtube.com/watch?v=3-RqckJAulM.

Night Time Industries Association. 2020. "Nightclub & Venue Reopening Strategy: The Case for a Science-Based, Risk-Assessed Return to a Covid-Secure Opening of Nightclubs and Venues." London, UK: 25

August 2020. https://www.ntia.co.uk/wp-content/uploads/2020/08/Nightclubs-Venues-Strategy.pdf.

Noticas ao minuto. 2020. "Lisboa anuncia 'apoio imediato' de 200 mil euros ao setor fadista." *Notícias ao Minuto*, 17 April 2020. https://www.noticiasaominuto.com/cultura/1459753/lisboa-anuncia-apoio-imediato-de-200-mil-euros-ao-setor-fadista.

Paris (Ville). 2020. "Conseil de la Nuit." https://www.paris.fr/pages/le-conseil-de-la-nuit-3365.

Quacquarelli Symonds (QS) World University Rankings. 2019. "Best Student Cities 2019." *Top Universities*. https://www.topuniversities.com/city-rankings/2019.

Raghav, Krish. 2020. "Under Lockdown and Quarantine, China's Punk Rock Bands Are Taking the Mosh Pit Online." *Hyperallergic*, 13 February 2020. https://hyperallergic.com/542468/under-lockdown-and-quarantine-chinas-punk-rock-bands-are-taking-the-mosh-pit-online/.

Reuters. 2020. "Metro Manila to Start Curfews as Deaths Rise to Six." *The Star*, 15 March 2020. https://www.thestar.com.my/news/regional/2020/03/15/metro-manila-to-start-curfews-as-deaths-rise-to-six.

Reverchon, Antoine. 2020. "'Couvre-feu': des cheminées recouvertes pour éviter l'incendie au Moyen Age à la privation moderne de liberté." *Le Monde.fr*, 21 October 2020. https://www.lemonde.fr/idees/article/2020/10/21/le-couvre-feu-l-heure-ou-les-braises-sont-mises-sous-cloche_6056789_3232.html.

Roy, Tiphaine Le. 2021. "Manif de teufeurs à Nantes: 'Sous couvert du Covid, la culture et toutes les libertés sont bridées.'" *Libération.fr*, 16 January 2021. https://www.liberation.fr/france/2021/01/16/manif-de-teufeurs-a-nantes-sous-couvert-du-covid-la-culture-et-les-libertes-sont-bridees_1817805.

São Paulo para crianças. 2020. "Governo de SP cria linha de microcrédito para empresas do setor cultural durante pandemia do COVID-19; entenda." *São Paulo para crianças*, 27 April 2020. https://saopaulopracriancas.com.br/governo-de-sp-cria-linha-de-microcredito-para-empresas-do-setor-cultural-durante-pandemia-do-covid-19-entenda/.

Seijas, Andreina, and Mirik Milan Gelders. 2020. "Governing the Night-Time City: The Rise of Night Mayors as a New Form of Urban Governance after Dark." *Urban Studies*. https://doi.org/10.1177/0042098019895224.

Small, Kimberley. 2020. "No Curfew = Safer City – Netherlands Night Mayor Says His City's Model Could Work for Kingston." *The Gleaner*, 23 February 2020. http://Jamaica-gleaner.com/article/

entertainment/20200223/no-curfew-safer-city-netherlands-night-mayor-says-his-citys-model.

Stahl, Geoff. 2001. "Tracing Out an Anglo-Bohemia: Musicmaking and Myth in Montreal." *Public*: 22–3. https://public.journals.yorku.ca/index.php/public/article/view/30328.

Straw, Will. 2014. "How Montreal became Disco's Second City." *Redbull Music Academy*. https://daily.redbullmusicacademy.com/2014/08/montreal-disco-feature.

– 2020. "COVID Nights." *Mediapolis*, 24 August 2020. https://www.mediapolisjournal.com/2020/08/covid-nights/.

Straw, Will, Luc Gwiazdzinski, and Marco Maggioli. 2020. "The Emerging Field of 'Night Studies': Steps towards a Genealogy." In *Night Studies: Regards Croisés Sur Les Nouveaux Visages de La Nuit*, 1–26. Grenoble: Editions Elya.

Sust, Toni. 2020. "Barcelona sale en masa a tomarse una caña de noche." *elperiodico*, 28 May 2020. https://www.elperiodico.com/es/barcelona/20200528/barcelona-bares-desescalada-coronavirus-7978194.

Syfuss-Arnaud, Sabine. 2020. "A Paris, le bruit des 8.000 terrasses éphémères fait craquer les riverains." *Challenges*, 19 September 2020. https://www.challenges.fr/france/a-paris-le-bruit-des-8000-terrasses-ephemeres-fait-craquer-les-riverains_727981.

Taneja, Richa. 2017. "#IWillGoOut: Women In 30 Towns And Cities Demand Safe Public Space." *everylifecounts.ndtv.com*, 23 January 2017. https://everylifecounts.ndtv.com/iwillgoout-women-in-30-towns-and-cities-demand-safe-public-space-9385.

Times of India. 2020. "Mumbai 24x7 Could Add Billions to Its Economy." *The Times of India*, 12 February 2020. https://timesofindia.indiatimes.com/city/mumbai/mumbai-24x7-could-add-billions-to-its-economy/articleshow/73660353.cms.

Toronto (City of). 2019. "Deputy Mayor Michael Thompson Appointed as the City's Night Economy Ambassador to Strengthen Toronto's Nighttime Economy." http://wx.toronto.ca/inter/it/newsrel.nsf/11476e3d3711f56e85256616006b891f/9a87b01d0071e948852584aa0047c0c6?OpenDocument.

Van Praagh, Nathalie. 2021. "Covid-19 – Le Marché de La Nuit Frappé de Plein Fouet Par La Crise Sanitaire." *www.lamontagne.fr*, 25 January 2021. https://www.lamontagne.fr/paris-75000/actualites/le-marche-de-la-nuit-frappe-de-plein-fouet-par-la-crise-sanitaire_13907281/.

Velasco, Carolina. 2020. "La cultura de club en Berlín, contra las cuerdas por la gentrificación." *El Salto*, 16 February 2020. https://www.elsaltodiario.com/gentrificacion/cultura-club-musica-electronica-berlin-peligro-subida-alquiler.

Vibelab. 2020. "Global Nighttime Recovery Plan." https://www.nighttime.org/chapter-one-open-air-nightlife-and-covid-19-managing-outdoor-space-and-sound/.

Hélène Lerivrain. 2020. "Vie nocturne: un guide méthodologique pour penser une politique globale." *La Gazette des Communes*. https://www.lagazettedescommunes.com/664558/vie-nocturne-un-guide-methodologique-pour-penser-une-politique-globale/.

Wood, Alice. 2020. "The Slow, Cold Abandonment of Manchester Nightlife." *The Mancunion*, 3 December 2020. https://mancunion.com/2020/12/03/the-slow-cold-abandonment-of-manchester-nightlife/.

Worden, Mark, and Judy Cantor-Navas. 2020. "With Italy on Lockdown, Europe's Music Industry Enters 'Uncharted Water.'" *Billboard*, 10 January 2020. https://www.billboard.com/articles/news/international/9331795/europe-music-industry-coronavirus-impact-italy-france-live-sector/.

Yumpu.com. 2021. "Livre Blanc: Les Etats généraux du droit à la fête." www.yumpu.com/fr/document/read/65231364/livre-blanc-etats-generaux.

2

"A Gateway between One World and the Next": Performance-based Arts in COVID Times

Christos Carras and Eric Lewis

> Historically, pandemics have forced humans to break with the past and imagine their world anew. This one is no different. It is a portal, a gateway between one world and the next.
> Arundhati Roy, *Financial Times*, 3 April 2020.

The rapid spread of the COVID-virus impacted the culture sector immediately and demonstrated the global interconnectedness of cultural organizations, institutions and individual artists, groups, companies, and collectives. Even before a given national or subnational jurisdiction decided to shut down its cultural sector (closing theatres, performance spaces, concert halls, and small to medium mixed-use venues like bars with stages) such sites for the presentation of live performance had already faced cancellations and major disruptions to their programming and funding. Travel restrictions, mandatory quarantines, rapidly evolving health and workplace protocols, and fear levels, all resulted in global disruptions to the flow of culture almost immediately. As the culture sector struggled to make sense of the overlapping jurisdictional forces impacting their abilities to operate, they also suffered from the fact that cultural production, presentation, and dissemination was not deemed essential, and so were shut down immediately in almost all jurisdictions. At times there appeared to be little consideration not only of the number of people employed in the "culture industry," but little thought given to the role culture, and the arts in general, might play in addressing a number of pressing problems created by our forced pandemic society.[1]

The reaction in Europe, where states are less integrated within a federal structure than in Canada, needs to be analyzed differently. Early on, statements and recommendations, such as that by Sabine Verheyen, chair of the European Parliament Committee on Culture and Education, underlined the fragility of the sector and its need for immediate support (c.f. European Parliament 2020), and there was an immediate coordinated mobilisation of the sector pushing for action (see, for example, European Music Council 2020). Nevertheless, the end result so far has primarily been a delegation of the response to individual member states rather than a EU-wide strategy[2] and an ensuing disparity that reflects pre-existing strength or weakness with regard to national cultural policy.[3]

The cultural sector itself responded by underlining its role in "easing feelings of isolation and contributing to the mental and emotional health and well-being of people in these challenging times" (European Cultural Foundation 2020). However, as we move through this crisis and take stock of how a breach has opened in what is "normal" and what passes for "second nature," allowing us to see relationships in a new light, already existing dynamics realign in new ways. It could be, then, that having found itself involved at a global level in a common challenge (even if the means to address it are of course unevenly distributed) the cultural sector could not credibly continue with "business as usual" but was forced to confront a range of crucial political challenges that inevitably intersected with its own exacerbated fragility. If art and culture are indeed to defend their claims to support in terms of their importance for the well-being of people, then perhaps they must engage frontally with precisely those issues that have emerged even more forcefully as being critical: the climate crisis, systemic racism, growing inequality, and precarity, for example.

The pandemic has given the cultural sector an opportunity, and perhaps the requirement, to address more widely its role in confronting signal issues of the day. And in view of the way most institutions but also individual artists or collectives have been obliged to communicate with their audiences and communities by in effect primarily publishing or broadcasting content online, their mode of intervention in the public sphere has shifted closer to that of traditional media, albeit using different forms of discourse and content. Understanding that cultural organizations are increasingly also media organizations is important if we are to conceive of ways in which they can articulate their potential as critical agents and create spaces for challenging discourses. If performed art is just another digitally mediated media accessed via a URL, how can it cut through the noise of the WWW, and reassert its unique status as a mode of artistic presentation?

The impact of the pandemic on the cultural sector was immediate and profound – larger organizations had to cancel seasons as performance spaces went dark. Smaller venues, often reliant on food and alcohol sales to subsidize their associated venues, were often unable to serve either, and found themselves beholden to rules governing both cultural spaces and bars and restaurants. While discussing the broader implications of the search for new revenue streams and business models we will touch but not focus upon the ways in which cultural spaces and organizations have both fared and responded to the complex of economic, financial, legal, and moral issues around finding ways for them to remain active, and often simply to continue to exist.[4] Rather we will focus on the reimagining that has and continues to take place concerning what it means in a COVID society to present performance-based art; how have individual artists and organizations adapted to our COVID reality and experimented with new forms of digitally mediated presentation of performance? COVID, for all the ways it has negatively impacted the cultural sector, has also opened up new opportunities for rethinking what it means to present performance-based arts; what the role of an audience could, or should, be; how artistic collaborations might take place; and more generally what constitutes and animates an increasingly global artistic community.[5] On the flip side, so to speak, while much of what we lose when performances move from stages, concert halls, and back rooms in bars to computer screens and cell-phones is readily apparent, we will suggest there are some less obvious worries that emerge when performance becomes just another form of digital media, and so subservient to its modes of delivery and subject to its dominant economic model. We will also focus more narrowly on music, but much of what we say holds equally well of performance acts traditionally viewed in real time by an audience co-present with the performers, and now "consumed" digitally via computers and mobile devices.[6]

LIVE STREAMING

By far the most common and immediate response to the closure of performance spaces was the move to live streaming. By live streaming we mean the recording of (usually) both audio and video of an actual performance, and having this recording transmitted at the time of performance via digital streaming platforms allowing one to view it on a computer or mobile device. Both venues, organizations, and individual artists moved quickly to live streaming. This transformation was facilitated by the availability of free and easy to use software for live streaming, such as Skype, Zoom, and Facetime as well as more specialised platforms such as Twitch. These software packages were all originally designed both for ease of use, and for video conferencing, that is to say to allow for the relative synchronization of audio with video, but at low qualities and, crucially for their use for streaming artistic performance, prioritizing sound reproduction of the human speaking voice to the detriment of the accurate transmission of other sounds. Technical issues abound here, but it is important to know that such platforms often employ algorithms to foreground the speaking voice, while actually suppressing other parts of an audio signal. And more generally there is no attempt made to transmit audio or video at high qualities. The choice of which platform to use was often simply based on the familiarity of those live-streaming with a given platform – if you have been "Zooming" a lot you were likely to use Zoom. Many long social media threads exist discussing the pros and cons of assorted platforms, which themselves continue to evolve and add new features as their use has, due to COVID, morphed from fun and lo-fi means of communicating in "real time" with others to their use for on-line instruction and, crucially, live-streamed performance, often now with the expectation that folks will pay to view the stream. Some, concerned with the politics and economics behind these platforms (most are owned by large corporations, and have oft-cited questionable practices associated with them concerning data-mining, ad selling, privacy, and the like), have chosen to use open-source platforms such as Jitsi.[7]

All live streaming, or telematic performance as it is sometimes called, must deal with the issue of signal latency. This is the transmission delay which audio and video signals suffer from due both to simple laws of physics (it takes time for a signal to travel), the nature of signal processing, and the ways in which the internet routes data. These lags or delays, often of different durations between audio and video, are familiar to anyone who has participated in a telematic meeting. Much effort has been undertaken since the onset of the pandemic to attempt to minimize latency. Live streams are always held captive to the latency inherent in the internet as a function of the overall load on the web and its network of servers, the upload and download speeds of an individual's network provider, bandwidth issues, along with latency inherent to the equipment one happens to be using. A live stream by a particular artist or organization on day X may well differ in quality from a feed on day Y, and latency within a given live stream tends to be quite variable.

Organizations and arts presenters had a variety of primary concerns behind their decision to promote live-streaming, and accordingly have implemented live streaming based on a number of different models. Behind these different decisions often lie distinct philosophies and funding structures, allowing or forcing them to focus on certain aspects of their continued ability to present and promote performance over others. For example, the Chicago-based Experimental Sound Studio (ESS), a registered US nonprofit whose mission is dedicated "to artistic evolution and the creative exploration of sound," began in March 2020 presenting "The Quarantine Concerts" and has to date (16 October 2020) streamed over five hundred performances by experimental and improvising musicians, averaging over two live-streams a day.

ESS acts as a web-based platform for these streams (which are viewed via Twitch) and promotes them. It also encourages viewers to make donations to the performing artists via its website, and 100 per cent of the funds so collected go directly to the artists. This model prioritizes the quantity of performance activity (indeed far more performances have been live-streamed then ESS would present and promote under normal circumstances) and strives to pay musicians who have otherwise lost often 100 per cent of their income. What this model gives up is any real control over the quality and precise content of the feeds. Individual artists performing in the Quarantine Concerts perform from their homes or studios, using whatever technologies to capture both sound and image that they happen to have. Many are solo performances, some are screen-captures of telematic improvisations involving musicians spatially distributed, often time-zones distant from each other, with many technical imperfections and glitches. The philosophy of ESS is to keep the music happening, to continue to promote the performance of experimental music, even when this requires giving up control over the conditions and standards to which the performances adhere.

Yet here too COVID offers opportunities. Experimental musicians and performance artists Sara Zalek, Scott Rubin, and Cristal

Sabbagh performed in this series on 24 July 2020. In their performance, video screens freeze and pop in and out of view. At times you see not the video feed but the computer screens of the performers attempting to load media or deal with a glitch. Audio quality ranges from satisfactory to quite frankly awful, and at times you cannot tell if what you are hearing and seeing is intended or the product of things going wrong (perhaps the performance was intended to blur this distinction). Yet for all this the performers note how this series gave them a first opportunity to perform together which they had been attempting to do for a long time. In the discussion after their performance Cristal Sabbagh notes that they and others are "Discovering new ways to collaborate because of the pandemic."[8] Sara Zalek makes the point that before COVID it was often difficult to get documentation of improvised performances, but "now we will always have it, whether we like it or not!" Scott Rubin asks, "How do you make the medium [Zoom] part of your art form…. How do we make the best of this horrible situation?" These points come up again and again when talking with performers who have performed telematically during COVID; new collaborations have been engendered, there is now a vast archive of documented performances, and performing artists are discovering new ways to adapt to the performance conditions that telematics operate with, to use the conditions creatively and not just try to work around them.[9]

Telematic live stream performances often involve a discussion before and after with the performers, and the ability of the audience to ask questions or make comments via the chat-room feature most platforms incorporate. We believe that these functions play a crucial role in pandemic performance, helping build connections between artists and audiences, and create spatially dispersed communities of the type that live performances cannot. A spatially distanced and isolated fan of a particular performer can now "attend" a performance wherever they may be and interact with the performer and other fans. One often gets to see performers in their living rooms and gain a sense of intimacy and familiarity different from that of staged live performances. If you follow the chat-room feeds during performances you often discover that they supply background information about the performances, advertise future performances, and introduce individual fans to each other – you can witness community-in-formation, often while, almost in the background, a live streamed performance is taking place. When community formation comes to the fore, technical issues surrounding the performance streams themselves matter less.

Other organizations were more concerned with reproducing to some degree the performance conditions that they normally operate under, and wanted to offer the public something different than (to only lightly parody) the performer at home propping-up their iPhone on a book, pointing it at themselves, and streaming a living room performance. SALA is a Montreal-based nonprofit that presents the annual Suoni per il Popolo Festival, focusing on experimental music and music by and for marginalized communities. They decided to offer a series of live-streams, but curated these from their main concert hall, the Sala Rossa. Believing (perhaps rightly) that the pandemic will affect venues' ability to present live performances into the future they wanted to offer more than "the bedroom (streaming) experience" of the sort that ESS promoted. Yet at the same time they were hesitant to invest in the first instance in all the expensive equipment needed to produce high-quality live streams, preferring to view the live-streamed 2020 version of the Suoni Festival as a "proof of concept." And so the performances took place on the main stage, and were streamed using open-source platforms, and offered for free to the public. Crucially, SALA paid the performers, independently of any direct appeals to the public for donations, as the assorted levels of Canadian government that help underwrite the festival were more than happy to have the funds used in this manner. By reproducing (to a degree) the appearance of a "normal" performance space and experience, SALA was hoping to attract viewers to their streams and have them stand out from the crowd of home-produced live-streamed performances. There were the inevitable technical bugs as they learned to master the complex process, but it was successful enough to have them consider keeping a live-streaming element even once things return to normal, as a way to boost audience reach and (with luck) produce a new revenue stream.[10]

A third model was employed by the Improvisation Festival (IF) curated by Ajay Heble, founder and long-time artistic director of the Guelph Jazz Festival, in Guelph Ontario.[11] He saw an opportunity during COVID to curate a festival of improvised art. Over one hundred artists, all paid, were invited to contribute a video clip of themselves performing. These were almost always simply files of what were live at-home improvisations. These were all collected and sequenced by Professor Heble into a continuous twenty-four hour performance which was itself live-streamed for real-time viewing only. This produced a live-stream of sorts, but one which avoided the massive technological problems that would have resulted from moving between over one hundred distinct live-streams in real time. What was lost was the sense of co-presence that accompanies a truly live-stream, while one thing which was gained was the ability to sequence in an interesting and aesthetically challenging way a large series of improvised performances.

This hybrid live and produced model has also produced massive public participatory performances. A good example of this is Music on the Rebound's presentation of Pauline Oliveros' "The World-Wide Tuning Meditation" each Saturday from 28 March–25 April 2020. This live telematic participatory event attracted over 4,600 participants, close to one thousand for each performance, from over thirty countries. This piece for voice has simple performance instructions, and a general invitation went out over social media for participants. The performance stretched Zoom's capabilities to the maximum, with close to a thousand distinct voices sounding for approximately twenty minutes. There were two ways to experience this event. Live, one could listen to the feed, and the massed voices in real time, with a wide variety of individual signal qualities and relative dynamics. However, Music on the Rebound also subjected the whole feed to complex "reverb" processing, which one also could choose to listen to in relative real time, and this processed feed was also subjected to further signal processing and posted for listening as a recording or artifact of each live-streamed performance.[12]

This highly participatory performance was very much in keeping with Music on the Rebound's stated goal to invent "new ways for us to come together through music." Attracting both professional musicians and the interested public, it afforded opportunities for contact and community formation both different from, and impossible for, standard site-specific performances. And the success of this event was clearly evinced by the lively and very active chat-room, filled with statements by individuals stating that they finally have been able to perform a Pauline Oliveros' composition, or to "meet" someone they have long wanted to encounter. Feelings of solidarity and community were strong both immediately before, during and after the performances, and it was clear this series served, even if only temporarily, to mitigate the feelings of isolation and loneliness many were feeling. The post-production work that was done also allowed for the performance to serve as a more "standard" object for aesthetic contemplation and pleasure, by smoothing out its "rougher edges" and subjecting it to a more unified aesthetic vision.

It is worth thinking a bit more theoretically about latency, telematics, and community formation. Latency is built into all communication. If I speak to you from thirty feet away, there is an approximately thirty millisecond latency between when you see my lips move and hear the words I am saying. Yet we do not perceive this latency, as we neurologically adapt so as to synchronise the auditory and visual signals. As a result of this cognitive adaptation, we have no difficulty experiencing such an interaction as live, as taking place now in real-time. We view the conversation as something we are doing together, which may then have us develop bonds of affinity and affection, the building-blocks of community.

What is it about telematic events that either facilitates or problematizes this sense of sharedness, of community, grounded merely in the mutual witnessing of a performance ("I was there, wow, you were too!")? Experiencing togetherness is here crucial and it implies contemporaneously witnessing or participating, or both in something with others. We feel a greater sense of fellowship with someone who attended the same concert as us than we do with someone who saw the same movie as us, but on a different day, even though the experiences themselves may be very similar in both cases. Live streamed events attempt to engage the public by offering them this sense of a contemporaneous shared experience with others, only mediated by the internet, and a vast array of technologies.

Presenters of telematic performances therefore undertake great efforts to facilitate the sense of simultaneity and the sense of copresence which follows, believing that it is this idea of experiencing a live feed with others that might tempt one to ideally pay for the experience, as opposed to simply finding a document of the live stream the next day on YouTube. Scrolling through YouTube streams is paradigmatic of the solitary lonesome activity many of us would point to as characteristic of our isolation during the pandemic. How does a live-stream, so similar to this in many ways, somehow invert this experience and make it potentially community building and a shared experience?

For simultaneity and copresence are myths created by the discourse around telematics, and undermined not by latency itself but by latency drawing attention to itself, when it rears its ugly head by producing differential lags between audio and video streams, producing echoes (a sound out of synch with itself), or foregrounding the different temporalities each participant in a streamed event actually inhabits. A wonderful example of this is watching a hockey game in Montreal when the weather is good, and folks have their windows open. If the Montreal Canadiens (the Montreal NHL team) is playing, a very large percentage of households are watching the game, on TVs, computers, mobile devices, or listening via radio. Each household is receiving their feed via complex and different networks of digital transmission. What results from this is a cognitively dissonant phenomena – as you watch the game you suddenly hear, from distinct homes, at distinct and clearly not simultaneous times, a series of discrete group cheers when the Canadiens score a goal. You may not yet have witnessed the goal yourself, although you are watching the same game as others. The temporal lag between the assorted cheers, including your own (please, do not tell me you are a Bruins fan) may approach a full minute or more. Suddenly you realize that your sense of experiencing "together with others" the game has been skewed and is a fiction. Yet how out of synch do these experiences have to be before your sense of co-experience is undermined? It is not the time-lag or latency per se that matters, but how and if it is brought to your attention. A warm weather important game allows you to hear the many distinct temporalities everyone is inhabiting, otherwise you would never know. Similarly, it is when telematic latency in live-streamed performance draws attention to itself that you can no longer act as if the fiction of copresence and simultaneity is really at play. What, then, really is the difference between watching a so-called live feed, versus waiting until tomorrow to watch a documentation of the feed?

If acute awareness of latency shatters the myth of copresence and simultaneity, is anything left to attract one to live feeds as opposed to pre-recorded performances, which might reinvigorate the community-forming and interpersonal connections which copresence facilitates? The answer, at least according to many who both create and participate in live-streamed performances, is, as mentioned above, in the chat and waiting rooms which accompany these streams. If technical glitches related to latency depersonalize livestream experiences, chat rooms and waiting rooms, re-inscribe a sense of copresence and belonging. It is not too much of a stretch to claim that the actual content of performed streams often seems to fade into the background against the active, often overwhelming, communication taking place on the sidebars of such streams.

For musical communities whose sense of self is already strongly centered upon copresence as such, the chat rooms of live streams can be so active that you can hardly read individual comments as they fly by. One such community is that centered around the Grateful Dead and the constellation of tribute and jam-bands which configure themselves around the Grateful Dead's legacy. Since 1995 when the band ceased to exist due to the death of its main creative force, guitarist, singer, and songwriter Jerry Garcia, the close-knit community centered upon the band has configured itself around a potpourri of related bands, sometimes including original band members, which serve as sites for the community to gather, often with little regard per se to the quality or significance of the music. The pandemic put an end to such physical gatherings, which were crucial to the perpetuation of this extended community. Yet just as when these derivative performances were taking place, live members of the community would attend them to seek out old friends, renew bonds of affinity and intimacy, and perpetuate a collectively constructed sense of self – the music serving as a backdrop more so than a focus of these interpersonal connections. The regular high-quality live streams which have taken place often multiple times a week directed at this community have had chat-feeds with thousands of participants, often professing or confessing the importance of continued contact with their fellow community-members, with many comments simply asserting the survival of the community and its importance to the person commenting. Whether it is a stream of an archived Grateful Dead concert or a live feed from an aesthetically or culturally related jam band, both serve primarily as a catalyst for the community to reassert and reinvigorate its presence and heath, and this is done primarily via the chat feeds.[13]

FILMED AND PRE-RECORDED PERFORMANCE

A very fine line divides live-streamed performance practices from examples of performances that are filmed or pre-recorded and then uploaded. The situation is of course very similar to that of recorded improvisation sessions: the moment of real-time interaction, with its energy, risks, and collective creative osmosis remains with us through time as a fixed text which would not have existed without that moment, but which is thereafter objectified. In the same way, a recorded Zoom session that remains on-line becomes fixed. Nonetheless, the aesthetic qualities of the recording, the multiple windows perhaps, the objective performance conditions with possible latency, low audio or video quality, the subjective condition of the performers perhaps deterritorialized by the experience of being in their sitting room and interactively listening and playing with people across the globe, do result in a different kind of artefact, one that demands further research.

The pandemic stimulated artists, producers, and presenters to think in innovative ways. *Piece by Piece*[14] (presented by the Irish Arts Council-funded Improvised Music Company) ditches the pretense to a unified performance context and places the improvisers participating in the project in an unusual situation. *Piece by Piece* is like a musical game of Chinese Whispers: an improvised piece is passed on from one musician to the next, each one reacting to the previous installment. Each piece was presented "live" at a certain date and time (and remained available for streaming) and the introductory sound of a pre-recorded "audience" created a simulacrum of a situated performance. The actual recordings however are accompanied by video works which make the home-studio context clear. It is as though the project could not break loose from the pretense of physical performance whereas its originality lies precisely in the temporal and spatial dissociation of the improvisers and the act of sending a message. The unifying dimension is the playback on YouTube which brings the pieces together in a form of indiscriminate simultaneity. It goes without saying that the pieces can, in retrospect, be listened to in any order and this in theory at least allows each listener to discover new affinities and musical affiliations.

A very different approach to creating a musical community and sharing musical content was adopted by sound artist Claudia Molitor. At the very beginning of her lockdown experience, Molitor set up the *Hausmusik Kollektiv*, "A growing collection of A4 sheet paper pieces to create, experience or perform at home" (Molitor 2020). The project sets out to actively engage people in sonic creativity and not simply to provide sonic content for passive listening, to create a community of practice that is extremely open, since the initial intention was for no musical technique to be required. The pieces on the (evolving) project website vary considerably. Some, such as "Where Speech Meets Sound I & II" by Amina Abbas-Nazari are instruction-scores very much in the Fluxus tradition, others such as "Facetime Duo #2: Sonic Portrait" by Molitor herself integrate technology by turning the microphone on mobile devices into a tool for sharing sounds. Hausmusik is an interesting hybrid proposal: it emerges from the restrictions resulting from the pandemic, it relies on the internet for its distribution, some of the pieces are extremely low-tech or even analog whereas others innovatively subvert the technologies that we usually use passively and all depend on the participation of the recipients to be materialized. This last point is perhaps the most promising: if one of the principal problems we face in COVID times is the separation of artists and audiences and the mediation of their possible relationship through the screen and communication technologies, Hausmusik proposes a model for as direct an involvement as is possible given the circumstances of physical distancing.

For many artists, physical-digital hybridity is a promising route to follow in this regard. The New Together[15] is a project developed, curated, and produced by Nicoleta Chatzopoulou, a composer, viola da gamba performer, and researcher based in Athens, Greece. Chatzopoulou published an open call addressed to composers, musicians, artists, performers, directors, writers, and scientists to create collaborative works while being in separate places around the globe. The call was structured into three categories: Composers and Performers, Sound and Other Arts, and Open. The curator paired the participants who had no prior experience of working together. As the project developed, she decided to present the results in three stages in her studio space in Athens and subsequently document the submitted projects and make them available online. Some of the works, for example Tim Tsang and Noisebringers' work, "Don't touch my strings," will be livestreamed. Some of the completed projects (the Composers & Performers section at the time of writing in October 2020) fully integrate distance collaboration platforms into their form ("Don't touch my strings," for example) others follow more traditional formal routes, always however respecting the starting principle of bringing together artistic work without being in the same physical space. As is the case with many of the examples we have mentioned, Chatozopoulou points out this dual nature of COVID performativity at a distance: the world is both more shut off and more open. Likewise, it is interesting that as the project developed she decided to hybridize it by creating a physical installation in her studio space that (restricted) audiences may visit. There is, generally, a growing fatigue in relation to online content as well as a quantitative saturation that is almost neutralizing and therefore integrating a physical format, however limited in terms of audience numbers, seems to many artists to be a lifeline to forms of performativity and presence whose loss is worrying. Finally, the intermediality of the project is important: this seems to be a natural approach for works created through the net.

In conversation Chatzopoulou mentioned that this intermediality suggests that VR (virtual reality) applications might be the next terrain to be more widely explored and it is interesting to reflect on this intuition. Platforms such as Mozilla Hubs or gaming platforms that allow the interaction of visitors within a virtual space are already becoming more common. As these tools become more sophisticated, including at the level of the spatialization of sound within the virtual spaces or of the mixing of various sources and forms of content or even of the possibility of live-streaming the output of performers within them, new forms of performance could emerge that will surely require us to re-think established concepts. For example, virtual spaces are likely to spawn new forms of participatory art. It is important to note that participatory art is not the same thing as art that just involves some kind of interaction on the part of the spectator; it implies a far more radical political ambition. The distinction between interactivity and participation obliges us to reflect upon the role of mediating technologies and to question the ways in which they inflect the potential effects of participation. Irish composer, performer, improviser, and storyteller Jennifer Walshe, in an interview for this chapter, described how her experience with filmmaking was an integral element of the videorecording of her recent piece, "Imagining Ireland: a dataset" which was exclusively streamed online. Thinking about how the performance will be framed and applying a cinematic grammar to the writing of the work profoundly modifies the end result for the public and suggests that the element of intermediality is becoming fundamental in this period in which almost all music has become an audiovisual experience for the audience and requires new skills on the part of the artists. The music video is of course nothing new and the world of popular music has for decades invested in high production values. What is perhaps new is the extension of this practice to the world of more experimental, non-commercial music and the practice of composing or improvising with the audiovisual technologies. All this suggests a technological "thickening" and ways in which a platform aesthetics is becoming an element in today's performance language.

As experience grows, it seems likely that this thickening will become a principal locus for experimenting with online performance. Paola Prestini, composer, co-founder, and artistic director of the National Sawdust in Brooklyn NY, also stresses the importance of building up a hybrid creative toolkit for composers and performers. This was the objective of the first Digital Discovery Festival run by National Sawdust. Prestini, in an interview for this chapter, suggests that, after the initial phase of basic telematics and home-performance, the way forward is to pursue a much richer form of digitally mediated performance practice, creating forms of digital stages that allow for improvisatory approaches and a hybrid meshing of media and platforms offering a pallet of technologies, platforms, formats, and contexts. These could include live elements and simulcast content, live audience participation, and social media feeds with the aim of "pushing the ephemerality of performance into a digital sphere." In this context, the role of performer, improviser, or composer is rapidly evolving to become that of producer. Artists to some degree must undergo this evolution to make a mark in a more and more saturated and complex online environment with its multiple layers of production.

The examples we have been discussing illustrate strategies for taking the technological mediation imposed by the closure of physical spaces as a creative opportunity and not as a limitation. A common dimension is that all of them use various forms of mediation (essentially platforms and online environments) as an element in the elaboration of an aesthetic proposal. No doubt, because these forms of mediation are relatively new, there is a risk of not sufficiently interrogating them, especially since in other forms they are pervasive in our everyday experience, having become a kind of "second nature." The nineteenth-century concert hall is also a technological mediation of performance, but in time we came to understand that it is also a political mediation, and this understanding has led to a by now well-established set of practices that aim either to critique, subvert, or completely bypass this particular condition.

By definition, all practices based on the internet involve the transmission and reception of data. That most of us go through our daily lives searching, communicating, interacting, navigating, and buying in the digital domain should not blind us to the implications of these actions and to an awareness that our artistic practices are also subject to these implications. For years now, critical theorists and social scientists have been alerting us to the ways in which the data we generate is used for influence and control. This control can range from the directly repressive, since security apparatuses are even better at using social media networks to track, influence, and repress movements of contestation than those movements are themselves (see Morozov 2011) to the profiling that our data use enables. Taking this critical approach a step further, in *The Age of Surveillance Capitalism* Shoshana Zuboff convincingly analyzes the ever deepening "*rendition* of all aspects of human experience into behavioral data" (Zuboff 2019, 338), a process that aims to massively increase the volume of data that predictive algorithms are trained on. However, the most efficient way of predicting someone's actions, attitudes, and preferences is to influence them and as we have seen in practice (for example, in the case of Cambridge Analytica) the ultimate "service" provided by the aggregators of all this data to those with the means and desire to wield power is to enable influence over our choices. The COVID pandemic has very clearly radically accelerated the already profound movement of much of our life into the digital domain and hence deepened our embeddedness within this overall system of extraction and manipulation. What are we to make of performances that are intended to perhaps be politically "progressive," to build community, to fight against assorted forms of oppression and repression, that are operating via technological platforms which serve to atomize us as collections of preferences and other data, which sell this data, and which are often literally the very agents of the political, social, and cultural wrongs one is fighting against?

At another level, we need to reflect upon what one might call the biopolitics of the screen. It could be argued that the pandemic has led to one of the most extensive biopolitical experiments the world has ever experienced as the entire global population is integrated into new structures of control and intrusive governing. Being a response to a health crisis, the types of control, restriction, and reorganization of all dimensions of our lives, political, economic, social, cultural, and corporeal have not up until now been seriously contested. The screen has become our prime interface at all these levels, exacerbating a trend that was already well underway. The implications for performance are potentially profound; after all, performance is an embodied and situated practice. In telematic performance and its reception, experience of the performative moment is literally flattened and homogenized. Even in the case of live-streamed events when the performer might conceivably be in a space whose characteristics inflect the sense of the performance, reception remains fundamentally standardized and atomistic. If, as has been suggested above, being together in a performance space creates a special kind of bond and if we posit that this kind of bond is part of what it means to be part of a public or a counterpublic then it is reasonable to assume that the elimination or radical modification of this experience can have an effect on the constitution of publics and their interactions.

A third overarching concern relates to processes of inclusion or exclusion that an increase in the level of technological mediation engenders. These processes are manifested at several distinct levels. Although it is generally the case that access to broadband internet services is increasing in Europe, North America, and many other areas of the world, this trend is by no means uniform with significant disparities along class, age, and geographic lines. Likewise, though today it is generally very easy to upload audio-visual material, we know that this proliferation of available content means that a correspondingly greater investment is needed in order to attract any kind of attention, a factor that can likely exacerbate the disparity between well-endowed and financially challenged organizations. Furthermore, although barriers of space and physical access are potentially obviated on the internet, it would be important to understand whether this leads to a greater diversification of audiences or whether the attendance patterns of physical spaces are basically reproduced online. Finally, many cultural practitioners recognise that engaging new communities involves physically going to those communities in ways that create connections with experiences and issues that are of importance to them. Achieving this online is far more unlikely.

All this of course is not to say that we should avoid performative practices that are mediated in some way by digital communication platforms and technologies any more than one should never again perform in a concert hall. However, there is a need for awareness and a search for creative and performative strategies that problematize the interfaces that are used and integrates an understanding that not only are these interfaces not transparent and neutral but that their unchallenged use in fact reinforces modalities of control and extraction whose political implications are profound.

There are also important issues to discuss in relation to the implications of working in the cultural sector and to the consequences for artists' and institutions' business models. While it is the case that the new conditions for performance have led to solutions that keep creative and often critical practices going, it is also undeniable that the COVID pandemic revealed serious and structural problems in the status of cultural workers. The European Parliament 2019 think tank on Employment in the Cultural and Creative Sectors, pre-COVID, merely confirms what we all know already: "An analysis of labour market data for culture and arts professionals [...] points to frequent incidence of short-term contracts, part-time jobs and seasonal employment, two or more parallel jobs for people with university diplomas, and this employment situation is frequently qualified as precarious. [...] The number of cultural professionals and artists is growing steadily, while their employment conditions become more and more unstable" (Pasikowska-Schnass 2019). Within this context we should also bear in mind that, in many countries, cultural work often takes place within a grey area where contracts do not exist and there is no social security contribution and limited capacity to claim benefits, and also remember that these conditions do not only affect artists but all those involved in the production chain, such as technical crews.

As the precarity of work for significant sections of the workforce (and cultural workers in particular) became clear, and as more and more people started to worry about how the extension of the gig or platform economy's principles might affect the status of work in general, a discussion around radical ideas to address these issues got underway. Foremost among them was a rekindling of interest in the idea of a Universal Basic Income. This is a complex issue that we cannot go into in detail here. What we would like to underline in the context of this chapter is that the pandemic stimulated discussions on the radical re-thinking of the relationship between work and income, that this discussion was not limited to the left but also involved governments and their agencies and that the experience of cultural workers is a significant factor in this discussion.[16] If this discussion were to lead to substantial reforms in the way work and remuneration are understood this would be a significant and positive result of the pandemic experience, for cultural workers along with all the others.

In the meantime – which might be a long time – the limited opportunities for physical performances have obliged artists, performers, and composers (who have seen royalty payments related to live performances of their works dry up) to find other ways to get paid for their work and have put pressure on distribution platforms and collection agencies to (temporarily) restructure their payouts.[17] The crisis has also radically affected performance spaces. Artists and venues are therefore searching for alternative business models and a key thing to notice is that in most cases these models rely on recordings.

Bearing in mind that even a live stream needs an audiovisual recording set-up (even if the recording can in many cases be low-fi) in many ways "performing in COVID times" in effect means "recording in COVID times." Likewise, the possible routes to monetizing performances primarily pass through distribution and streaming channels. It is, for the moment, difficult to obtain reliable information on revenues generated by "tickets" sold for "live" events. Though these are certainly increasing, it seems that their importance for revenues is less than that of streaming or selling content online, especially for independent and more experimental music.[18] The "live" event certainly seems to be an important element in creating awareness within a potential audience, but revenues, such as they are, still come primarily from sales through platforms. In other words, whereas live performance could have generated revenue in a more local, community-focused context, the pandemic is steering musicians more and more towards platforms.[19]

Of course, some venues that have managed to create a tight community of patrons and supporters in pre-COVID times are now finding that this is perhaps the key to resilience. One example is Cafe Oto in London, a performance space that is synonymous with adventurous music programming. Survival here depends on a mix of revenue streams: membership fees, donations, sales from the shop, and a digital download service with recordings made at the venue as well as performances in the venue for limited audiences. All this implies a substantial expansion of the tasks that a relatively small organization needs to undertake if it is to survive as a performance space.

Nonetheless, for most artists and ensembles, digital platforms might seem to offer the best chances of ensuring some level of revenues raising interest in initiatives such as Resonate that promote a different, co-ownership based model for streaming platforms or more artist-centered platforms, notably Bandcamp that allows a great deal of control over what is made available and at what price. A variation on this is Patreon Music that functions as a crowd-funding platform for music projects. In both cases however, the onus on driving sales is with the musicians. Much as was the case with venues, musicians are increasingly having to master a broad range of marketing and communication techniques and use a range of platforms in order to reach potential audiences online. All this suggests that performing in COVID times has a greatly increased workload and the stress attached to it.

What is clear is that the potentials the pandemic offers for rethinking performance as it transforms into a digital medium, and the threats such a transformation raises, creates a situation as rife with the potential for new forms of control, surveillance, and censorship by state and non-state actors as it portends new and exciting forms of community formation which transcend barriers of space and time configured around aesthetic expression. It will take much collective imagination and action to confront the former, while realizing the latter. As Arundhati Roy ends her article which began this essay:

> We can choose to walk through it [the pandemic], dragging the carcasses of our prejudice and hatred, our avarice, our data banks and dead ideas, our dead rivers and smoky skies behind us. Or we can walk through lightly, with little luggage, ready to imagine another world. And ready to fight for it.

The authors would like to thank the following individuals who took the time to be interviewed for this chapter: Ajay Heble, Peter Burton, Marc Jacoby, Ayelet Rose Gottlieb, Jennifer Walshe, Brigitta Muntendorf, Nicoletta Chatzopoulou, Paola Prestini, Claudia Molitor, Giambattista Tofoni (European Jazz Network).

NOTES

1 This generalization needs to be nuanced by jurisdiction. Governmental departments with culture as their portfolio were often strong advocates for the culture sector, but often lack relative clout in federated systems. For example, in Canada federal, provincial, and municipal arts funding agencies were both sensitive to and proactive concerning the stresses on the

culture sector. Funding for festivals and performance series were generally not cut, and often increased, even though the festivals and performance series themselves were cancelled or had their status very much unclear. Operating funds were also not cut, and often paid out into the future to help ensure arts organizations would not fold.

2 For an overview of the EU Coronavirus Response in relation to culture see European Commission: Culture and Creativity (2020).
3 An ongoing review of EU member state policies can be found in Compendium of Cultural Policies and Trends (2020).
4 See, for example, the comprehensive study undertaken by performance venues in Toronto (Nordicity 2020), partially in response to the fact that by 8 October 2020 Toronto had lost eleven live music venues in its downtown core. For information on reactions to this situation in Europe see Live DMA (2020).
5 These new possibilities opened up by the pandemic and creative responses to it are not limited to new technologically mediated means of performance, but even result from funding models and cancellations of seasons. For example, many arts organizations whose focus is the presentation of an annual festival discovered that their funding for the 2020 festival season remained secure, but the festival itself was canceled. This has allowed many smaller arts organizations, who usually survive financially year to year, zeroing out their budgets every year after they present their festival, to have, for the first time, a financial cushion and contingency fund. While it is still too early to tell, this may well allow arts presenting organizations that survive the pandemic to be on sounder financial footing than prior to the pandemic.
6 Our focus will be on responses to the pandemic by performers and arts organizations based in North America and Europe. A more systematic survey of these issues needs to be live to the possibility that the performance arts in other places may have, and continue to have, different responses to the pandemic.
7 It is worth mentioning the Digital Stage platform that was initially developed through a hackathon funded by the German Federal government: https://digital-stage.org/?lang=en
8 Other artists echo the point that COVID has forced them to rethink all aspects of their performance lives, and that this is a positive thing. Ayelet Rose Gottlieb, a Montreal-based vocalist, composer, and improviser, talks about the opportunities COVID has in effect offered her. She talks about the opportunities COVID has created to think in new ways about spatially distributed performances, and to confront issues around culture, difference, and identity that are easy to ignore when one works only locally.

"This new adventure of exploring ways of working together while socially distanced actually facilitates working with others who otherwise I might not be able to … . People are questioning everything about their universe, about all the structures we are used to, especially patriarchal structures, we are now imagining worlds where everything can be different … COVID has created this situation where everyone is welcome, we get to create a new global environment … whatever we do after COVID, we will be different, we will have a new awareness … we are going to live with what we have created during COVID even when we can go back to doing things in person."

9 The performance can be viewed at: https://www.youtube.com/watch?v=-6HqOb3ibYo&list=PLBxbddARljQ_uxn89Vefm4_nVOCxoqoRa&index=86. Part three constitutes the post-performance discussion. The new forms of interaction that telematics allow for was also stressed by Marc Jacoby, a NYC-based musician with over thiry years of experience working with children and adults with disabilities in creative contexts focused on, but not limited to, music. He observes that conducting session with youths in their home, and allowing them to see his home-setting adds a layer of intimacy and understanding to their interactions. "I learned more about them [his clients with disabilities] on Zoom then I ever did live." He goes on to add, "you see them in their house, you see pets and family members … they are letting you in to their personal environment … they feel like they are not being judged on Zoom in a way they might be in a embodied encounter." This is one way in which the seemingly impersonal nature of telematics can actually serve as a site for a deeply personal encounter.

10 If this does come to pass, the diversification of business models might be another way in which responses to COVID may well result in the culture industry being on a better financial foundation in the future.

11 See https://improvfest.ca/about/.

12 The World Wide Tuning Meditation was organized and led by Ione, Claire Chase, Raquel Klein. See: https://www.musicrebound.com/pauline-oliveros-tuning-meditation.

13 This phenomenon has been noted by organizations presenting live-streamed performances, and they are now making sure chat-functions are incorporated into their streams, and even adding question and answer periods with performers to increase a sense of belonging and participation for the virtual audience.

14 See https://www.improvisedmusic.ie/news/artists-announced-for-piece-by-piece.

15 See https://www.nicoletachatzopoulou.com/gallery.
16 See, for example, Kassam (2020), Prabhakar (2020), and Susias (2020).
17 An overview of these initiatives can be found at https://www.impalamusic-covid19.info/sector-initiatives.
18 Although this may be changing quickly as major players venture into this area, as is the case for example with the partnership between Spotify and Songkick, or Amazon's use of Twitch, and, importantly, as the technology improves. For the more mainstream sector of the music world, there have already been large-scale forays into live streaming and also collaboration with gaming platforms.
19 There is an irony here not lost on most performers. The past twenty-odd years has seen recordings radically lose their importance as a revenue stream for recording artists, as streamed and otherwise digitally mediated recording sales fell hostage to the miniscule fees platforms such as Spotify and Apple Music pay to artists. Live performance has reasserted itself as the primary revenue stream. Yet now suddenly recordings in all their forms of fixation are again important, but against a backdrop where fees paid are virtually non-existent.

REFERENCES

Compendium of Cultural Policies and Trends. 2020. "Comparative Overview: Financial Measures." *Compendium of Cultural Policies and Trends*, 23 September 2020. https://www.culturalpolicies.net/covid-19/comparative-overview-financial/.

European Commission: Culture and Creativity. 2020. "Coronavirus Response." *European Commission: Culture and Creativity*. https://ec.europa.eu/culture/resources/coronavirus-response.

European Cultural Foundation. 2020. "COVID-19 Solidarity and Emergency Response in Europe in Arts, Culture, Cultural Heritage and Creative Sectors." *European Cultural Foundation*. https://cultureactioneurope.org/files/2020/06/CAE-ECF-mapping-COVID19.pdf.

European Music Council. 2020. "Joint Letter: Effect of COVID-19 on Creative Europe and the European Cultural and Creative Sectors." *European Music Council*, March 2020. https://www.emc-imc.org/cultural-policy/statements/joint-letter-effect-of-covid-19-on-creative-europe-and-the-european-cultural-and-creative-sectors/.

European Parliament. 2020. "New Funds Must Reach Creative Sectors Immediately." Press release no. 27-03-2020, 27 March 2020. https://

cultureactioneurope.org/news/verheyen-new-funds-must-reach-creative-sectors-immediately/.

Kassam, Ashifa. 2020. "Spain Rekindles a Radical Idea: a Europe-Wide Minimum Income." *The Guardian,* 3 June 2020. https://www.theguardian.com/world/2020/jun/03/spain-rekindles-a-radical-idea-a-europe-wide-minimum-income.

Live DMA. 2020. "COVID-19 Live Music Sector – Reactions, Impact & Support." *Live DMA,* 12 March 2020. https://www.live-dma.eu/covid-19-live-music-sector-reactions-impact-support/.

Microsoft Corporation. "Apps for Office Sample Pack." Office Dev Center. Updated 20 October 2015. https://code.msdn.microsoft.com/office/Apps-for-Office-code-d04762b7.

Molitor, Claudia. 2020. "Hausmusik Kollektiv." http://www.claudiamolitor.org/#/hausmusik-kollektiv/.

Morozov, Evgeny. 2011. *The Net Delusion: The Dark Side of Internet Freedom.* New York: Public Affairs.

Nordicity. 2020. "Re:Venues, A Case and Path Forward For Toronto's Live Music Industry." *Canadian Live Music Association.* https://www.toronto.ca/wp-content/uploads/2020/10/9846-Re-Venues-FINAL-REPORT.pdf.

Pasikowska-Schnass, Magdalena. 2019. "Employment in the Cultural and Creative Sectors." European Parliamentary Research Service. October 2019. https://www.europarl.europa.eu/RegData/etudes/BRIE/2019/642264/EPRS_BRI(2019)642264_EN.pdf.

Prabhakar, Rajiv. 2020. "Universal basic income and Covid-19." *IPPR Progressive Review* 27:105–13. https://doi.org/10.1111/newe.12198

Susias, Carlos. 2020. "EAPN Covid-19 Minimum Income letter to EU Commissioner Nicolas Schmit." European Anti-Poverty Network. 24 April 2020. https://www.eapn.eu/wp-content/uploads/2020/04/EAPN-EAPN-Covid19-Minimum-Income-letter-to-Commissioner-Schmit-24-April-final-4361.pdf

Zuboff, Shoshana. 2019. *The Age of Surveillance Capitalism: The Fight for a Human Future at the New Frontier of Power.* New York: Public Affairs.

3

Can Sports Partisanship Survive in the Pandemic World?

Daniel Weinstock

INTRODUCTION

A strange thing happened during a hockey game opposing the Montreal Canadiens and the Toronto Maple Leafs held recently at Montreal's Bell Centre. During the 2021 season, games have been taking place without any fans in the stands. On this particular evening, the canned arena noises that had been used in a somewhat desultory manner until then in order to simulate the conditions of a normal game were turned up to a very high level. The colour commentator on the English network carrying the game claimed that his was due to a request from Canadiens' team captain Shea Weber. Whatever the source of the decision to increase the volume, it was clear that it was being done in order to provide the local team with a greater "hometown advantage." The sound of artificial "fans" reacting to plays in much the same way that real fans would – jeering at referee calls that went against the Canadiens, cheering goals and nice plays by the local team, and booing the opposition – might recreate, in pandemic conditions, the "sixth man" effect that contributes to making it the case that teams are statistically far more likely to win when they are at home than when they play on opposing teams' rinks (Swartz and Arce 2014).

What was striking about the decision was the fact that the piping in of canned fan noises was thought likely to yield a hometown advantage even in the absence of actual fans. The thought presumably was that in the thick of the action the members of the team might be able to leverage even obviously fake fan support into the energy boost that the real participation of fans is said to encourage. (There may have been other reasons to engage in this apparent trickery, such as improving the experience of fans watching the game at home on screens).

The broader point I want to develop on the basis of this anecdote has to do with the centrality of partisanship to team sports. Partisanship matters to sports in a number of ways. The story briefly recounted above shows that it actually matters to the athletes. They derive motivation from the palpable feeling of having tens of thousands of partisans in close proximity cheering them on. But, probably most importantly from the point of view of the business model around which professional sports are built today, it matters to the willingness of fans to disburse large sums of money to attend games, to purchase heavily marked up products while they are in attendance, to buy all manner of team-branded merchandise, and so on. Briefly stated, professional sports monetize partisanship. It is not outlandish to claim that the future of professional sports in pandemic society depends upon the ability of teams and broadcasters to "reinvent" partisanship in a radically new context, one that on the face of it does not lend itself particularly well to the development and maintenance of the requisite affective bonds between fans and teams. What follows are somewhat speculative remarks on the future of sports partisanship in pandemic society.

I will proceed as follows. First, I will address the "who cares?" objection. Why should we concern ourselves with the fate of a bloated industry paying disproportionate sums to sporting mercenaries hawking their considerable skills and athletic prowess to whoever is able to pay them most? I will argue that there are virtues to partisanship in general, and to partisanship geared toward elite professional sports teams that should at least be weighed in the balance as we come to terms with the societal transformations that may be wrought by the pandemic, and by the lasting effects that it might have even after the acute phase of the crisis is over. Second, I will focus on the physical conditions of partisanship that seem to depend upon the kinds of events that may no longer be possible in a pandemic society. The staging of professional sports tends to occur around densely crowded events bringing together tens of thousands of individuals, which may simply no longer be feasible in the years to come. Does this spell the end of partisanship? In the third and final section of this essay, I will speculate on the future of partisanship in pandemic societies, and reflect on ways in which it might be rethought in less "embodied" spaces.

THE VALUES OF PARTISANSHIP

My focus here is on sports partisanship that is focused on elite professional sports leagues. Such leagues have a number of features that distinguish them from other competitive sports contexts that I want to highlight here. First, they tend to be based in cities, or in the case of very large cities, in city neighbourhoods. Second, they bring together players who tend not to be from the cities in question. Rather, they are high-priced sporting "mercenaries" who are recruited by city-based teams on the basis of considerations that rarely have to do with the attachment of athletes to the cities in question. Third, they play in leagues that schedule games over many months over the course of the year, culminating with a playoff tournament that crowns the league's "best" team.

The kind of partisanship that I am considering here is therefore not of the kind that attaches to national sports teams, and to the tournaments in which they compete. Such teams are most often made up of athletes who devote much of their time to teams located in other countries, and they are brought together temporarily to perform in such (often highly visible) evens such as the World Cup, the Olympics, and the like. There are ethical issues that arise specifically in the case of national teams. For example, does an emphasis on national teams exacerbate the ethically questionable feelings that sometimes accompany nationalism, or on the contrary does it deflect them in morally benign ways?[1]

One of the reasons not to focus on national sports team is that, in a sense, partisanship that focuses on them piggybacks on national allegiances. Whatever one thinks of nationalism as a force in the constitution of individual identities, its presence as a potent force can hardly be denied. The COVID-19 pandemic has done nothing to undercut the potency of national allegiance. In many ways it may even have exacerbated it. Indeed, there is, and is likely for the foreseeable future that there will be, much less international travel. To the extent that such travel "enlarges" sympathies, it is possible that nationalist sentiment will be even more dominant than it already has been, given the fear that has developed everywhere of foreigners as potential carriers of illness. "Vaccine nationalism," which has clearly been present in the manner in which the early supply of vaccines has been distributed, is but one instance of this, and suggests that the conative support for national sports teams is far from being depleted any time soon.

What value is there in supporting city-based team in elite professional leagues? I would like to suggest a number of reasons why such partisanship has value.

First, partisanship might serve as an epistemic gateway to the appreciation of sporting excellence. There is a debate in the philosophy of sport between those who believe that there is value in the appreciation of sports mediated by partisan focus, and an appreciation that is grounded solely in an appreciation of excellence.[2] Regardless of where one falls on the debate, it is at least arguable that for a substantial proportion of the population, having a partisan "stake" in a game will be the way in which to develop an appreciation of the game's finer points and of the skills involved in playing it. Allegiances focused around city or neighbourhood-based teams tend to give rise to bandwagon effects: the interest placed in teams by fans tend to draw in people who may at the outset just be interested in being part of a social trend. Some of them may then come to appreciate the game "on its own terms," that is, on the basis of the skills displayed, the strategies involved, and the subtleties manifested. This benefit is moreover greatest where partisans are able to watch games performed at elite level. There are other benefits to partisanship in local sports, whether professional or amateur. But to the extent that one believes, as I do, that there is independent value in the appreciation of team sports performed at the highest level, it is at least arguable that this benefit requires as a facilitating condition that one access it by following a team in which one has a partisan interest.

Second, and relatedly, partisanship provides people with a way of experiencing commonality of purpose with others. To be a partisan is to be part of a community that extends beyond those with whom one associates on a daily basis. What is more, sports partisanship connects one with people with whom one would not normally associate or find common purpose. Sports partisanship often[3] transcends the kinds of divisions that structure everyday life, and brings one into connection with others with whom one would ordinarily share very little. As Avner de-Shalit and Daniel Bell have argued, city-based identities tend to be less politically toxic than national identities (Bell and de-Shalit 2011). City-based sports identifications thus have the potential to channel aspects of our psyches that thrive on rivalry in politically and socially benign ways.[4]

Third, the fact that elite professional sports teams are made up not of local athletes but of athletes from around the world both diffuses the risk that partisanship will come to mirror or track the kinds of politically noxious allegiances that national identity can give rise to, and opens up the possibility of the enlargement of sympathies. When players on a city-based team come from a wide range of countries (and play for these countries when taking part in international competitions), or when they are members of minority groups that are subjects of systemic discrimination in the societies of which they are a part, there is the potential that partisans will come to learn something about other places about which they may have known nothing, or about which they may have harbored negative feelings, and also potential for consciousness-raising within their own society. Arguably, the profile of Black Lives Matter within mainstream American society has been raised by the way in which it has been taken up by admired, highly visible athletes in professional sports leagues.[5]

Fourth, and finally for present purposes, I would like to point to another ethical benefit that partisanship vested in a team that participates in league matches over the course of a season that typically lasts several months. Following a team is not unlike following characters in a long-running television series. Indeed, for many of us, it is a long-running television series. Players go through crises of confidence, overcome obstacles, succeed and fail, and so on. And unlike most of us, they do much of this in plain view of partisans and of opposing fans. Just as there is moral learning involved in reflecting on the situations that characters in high-quality series go through, so there is moral work involved in following the ways in which individual players and teams deal with the often unpredictable situations that they find themselves in – injury, disappointment, aging, and so on. I do not want to overstate the degree to which the activities of millionaire athletes confront us with the full range of life's realities. Nonetheless, a season in the life of a professional sports team possesses both individual and collective narrative arcs that are comparable to the narrative arcs one finds in serial fiction. And the degree to which one is inclined to engage in the themes that are raised in these arcs depend on the degree to which we engage in sympathetic identification with their protagonists.[6]

There are likely other (broadly construed) ethical considerations involved in partisanship. Needless to say, there are also ills associated in partisanship that should also be weighed in the balance. For example, in the non-ideal world in which we live, partisanship often intersects with social rifts that betoken patterns of injustice and discrimination. In such circumstances, sports partisanship contingently connects with ethnic and class conflicts. Additionally, the development of the skills that are required in order to compete in professional sports at an elite level now require the imposition of training regimes upon children that are ethically problematic, in that they constrain the future of children by overemphasizing the development of some capacities and talents to the detriment of a balanced development that keeps a wide range of doors open.

The recognition of such potential ills should not lead us to welcome the disappearance of professional sports. As with a lot of things, the challenge is to try to secure the benefits involved in an activity while finding ways to limit or eliminate its ills. What I have wanted to make plausible in this section is that there are reasons to value partisanship in professional team sports. It provides us with the appreciation of a range of skills performed at a very high level, it connects us with others with whom one would not normally come into contact in societies rifted by class and ethnic, it has the potential to widen our sympathies and awareness, and it involves sympathetic identification with the protagonists of the "dramas" that sports seasons instantiate, and that are akin to the kinds of narrative arcs one finds in serial fiction. There are therefore reasons to hope that professional sports, and the opportunity it affords for partisanship, will survive the pandemic. What threats are there to professional sports in pandemic society? It is to this question that I now turn.

THREATS TO PARTISANSHIP IN PANDEMIC SOCIETIES

Professional sports leagues have understandably had to adopt and enforce quite draconian measures in order to resume activities in the months following the first wave of the COVID-19 pandemic. Many of these have involved isolating athletes from fans. When the National Hockey League and the National Basketball Association resumed activities, they did so inside "bubbles." A small number of facilities were selected, and insulated from the outside world so as to minimize the likelihood that the virus could make it into the playing facilities, or indeed, that it could be carried from the facilities out. Aside from those who happened to play in the facilities that had been chosen to act as "bubbles," all teams were playing away from their normal "home" arenas. In a sense this hardly mattered, as fans were excluded from facilities anyway. Seasons interrupted by the pandemic were completed in empty arenas. Fans watched games for the most part from their homes, as the restaurants and bars in which they tend to congregate in order to watch games were closed as well, or else operating at a reduced capacity and with rules inhibiting mingling among patrons in place.

As seasons resumed in the later phases of the pandemic, most sport teams were able to go back to their home arenas and fields. Social distancing requirements however made it the case that these facilities continued to operate without any fans in the stands, or a significantly reduced capacity. For some teams performing in leagues that straddle international borders that have been closed during the pandemic, this has not been possible. This has particularly affected Canadian teams playing in North American markets. While the National Hockey League was able to create a "North" division of Canadian teams who could compete against one another in their home arenas during the regular season (hoping to get into playoff rounds that will again be played in "bubbles"), basketball and soccer teams have had to remain south of the border to play in leagues in which virtually all the teams are US American. Thus, the Toronto Raptors, the only team in the NBA operating out of a Canadian city, have had to adopt Tampa, Florida, as their "home" for the 2021 season. As I write these lines, it seems all but certain that the three Canadian soccer clubs that compete in North American Major League Soccer will have to find a home in the US as well.

The question of what the future holds for mass sporting events is, at the time of writing, an open one. It seems likely that the post-pandemic world will not be a world entirely exempt of risk. We are still unclear as to the length and the level of immunity of the vaccines that are currently being administered to populations around the world, nor is there any certainty that they will adequately protect against the variants of the coronavirus that are currently multiplying around the world. There are many practices that may have to be reconsidered in a world of increased risk of infectious disease, from everyday greeting practices (will we ever shake hands with one another again?) to mass events in which tens of thousands of people are brought into close proximity with one another in order to watch cultural or sporting events. Similarly, crowded bars and restaurants in which people mingle with one another in collective areas such as dance floors and bar counters, often watching sports in close proximity to one another on large screens designed to be watched by many people, may be a thing in the past, even as restaurants and bars reopen in more controlled ways aimed at minimizing interaction among people who do not share a domestic "bubble."

While it is too early to determine whether the kinds of restrictions that have just been mooted will come into effect, or whether on the contrary we will be able to return to a world in which mass gatherings can occur relative safely, we should at least start planning for a world in which professional sports are played and watched in radically different circumstances from the ones that we have become habituated to. The question we must ask ourselves is whether partisanship can survive in conditions of moderate risk such as that which we may emerge into when the acute phase of this pandemic is behind us.

The comedian Jerry Seinfeld once made a philosophically astute observation about the prima facie absurdity of sports partisanship. A reviled player, he noted, can all of a sudden become a well-loved one if he is traded to the team of which one is a partisan. Given this fact, Seinfeld notes, "You're voting for clothes when you get right down to it."[7]

Arguably, two dimensions of team sports connect us to a particular team and to its particular members in ways that provide an answer to the serious question posed in a joking manner by Seinfeld. Both of these dimensions are connected to ethical benefits of sports partisanship that I briefly described above. First, there is the fact that following a team through the entirety of a season connects us to them sympathetically in a manner that differs from the more episodic way in which we might follow other athletes.

But this just pushes the question posed by Seinfeld back a level. What is it that make us choose to identify sympathetically with one group of athletes rather than another (remembering that, at least at the elite level, the athletes themselves are typically not from the cities in question) is a connection to place. What I have in mind here is not simply the fact that the players wear uniforms that affirm the connection to a particular place, but rather that their sporting activities are connected physically to myriad interrelated spatially embodied activities.

To begin with, teams are connected with often iconic arenas and fields that possess significant symbolic freight in constituting the identity of a city. (I remember attending a Rolling Stones concert at River Plate stadium in Buenos Aires, Argentina. When the concert ended, many spectators descended onto the field from the stands in order to claim a piece of turf from what they clearly perceived as hallowed ground). Much of the work of establishing new facilities when old ones decay or are judged inadequate to the needs of modern sports franchises is to recreate that sense of place in a new location. Thus, sports teams are not just assemblages of athletes that happen to be wearing uniforms on which the name of a city figures. They are the athletes that play in this particular space, a space that may for many inhabitants of a city bear an important affective and symbolic dimension.

What is more, the sporting events that take place in such iconic arenas, stadiums and fields are significant communal experiences. Part of the experience of attending a sporting event is not just to witness the event, but to do so with others with whom one shares an identity, with whom the fact of taking part in such an event is part of the process of collective identity formation. Watching the home team in a specific space is, to use Charles Taylor's phrase, is an "irreducibly social good." That is, part of what constitutes its good is that people take part in it together in a manner that changes the nature of the good in question (Taylor 1997).

Finally, the spatially embodied aspect of games performed in specific places in front of partisan audiences has, I would argue, an impact on partisans watching games from a distance, whether in a friendly local pub or at home. Partisans experience the irreducible social good vicariously through their awareness of the partisan activity going on within the confines of the arena or stadium. One of the odd things about watching games that were held in bubbles was that all of those embodied, spatial dimensions of events were eliminated even for those of us who were watching games on television in our homes. All of a sudden, the Seinfeldian fact that these were at some levels just an assemblage of athletes purporting to play "for" a city became apparent. Without fans cheering one side or the other, and with all of the teams playing in what was considered to be a safe "neutral" space. The realization that the many partisans watching sporting events at a distance need the sense of place and of communal activity in order to nourish their partisanship at a distance may very well have been at the origin of the decision to include artificial crowd noises to the broadcasting of events. It is possible, as I mentioned in the introduction to this essay, that the athletes themselves need these partisan crowd noises in order to trick themselves into thinking that they are actually being supported by thousands of fans (Cf. Saunders, forthcoming). But it is also likely that part of the reason for the choice has had to do with the concern that in the absence of crowd noises, fans watching games at home will feel insufficiently connected to their home team, and will over time cease to identify with them in the manner required in order to maintain partisanship.

This brief account suggests that mass partisanship, the partisanship that connects not just the minority of fans who are able to attend games in person, but also the very many fans who watch games either by themselves or with others at home or in bars and at other public venues, is constructed on the basis of spatially embodied, collective practices. Clearly, these practices are threatened in all sorts of ways by the pandemic, but also by a situation in which, post-pandemic, a reassessment of the risks involved in mass events leads either to their elimination or to a profound transformation of the way in which they are held. The need to use "bubbles" or alternate venues located across borders in cases in which international travel might still be severely restricted, the significant reduction of the numbers of people who can attend sporting events (and the concomitant lessening of the sense of these events as constituting communal "happenings" generating irreducibly social goods, and even the transformation in the rules governing the ways in which partisans can interact in bars and even in private homes (in jurisdictions where legal limitations are placed on the ability of people to visit one another's private homes), all of these phenomena risk occurring at least to some degree in "pandemic societies," and all of them risk eroding the physical, spatial grounds upon which sports partisanship is built.

WHAT IS TO BE DONE?

In the face of such foreseeable occurrences, what should be done? One answer, which might be privileged by the "purist" sports fan who watches sports not with a partisan interest, but rather in order to witness the display of athletic prowess, tactical and strategic virtuosity, and the like, would be that we should do nothing. The erosion of partisanship would on this view not put an end to sports, or to the appreciation of sports by spectators. Rather, it would dissuade the wrong kind of sports fan, namely, the fan who watches sports in order to see his or her side win, rather than in order to appreciate the sport's intrinsic virtues.

I have suggested above that there are virtues to partisanship, at least one of which should be appreciated by the purist, namely, that partisanship might for many people provide an epistemic gateway to the appreciation of the sport's "purer" properties. What this suggests is that the erosion of partisanship might alter the incentive structure in which not just spectators but also prospective athletes operate. If there are fewer partisans, then presumably, there are fewer people willing to spend money on watching sports and on purchasing the numerous ancillary products and services that accompany competitive sports. If there is less money available to athletes, then again presumably, this lessens the incentive that might exist for athletes to compete among one another to achieve the level of skill that will allow them to perform at elite levels. Now, this may, all things considered, be a good thing. The reduction in the pressure placed upon juvenile athletes to take on potentially damaging and horizon-limiting training regimens in order to achieve the requisite level of skill would certainly be a good thing, even if it leads to a reduction in the level of skill and physical prowess displayed by athletes in competitive sports. But the purist must be clear-eyed in the realization that this reduction may be one of the effects in the erosion of partisanship.

The alternative, of course, is to discover alternative ways of establishing the conative basis for partisanship in pandemic societies. If one of the ways in which pandemic society reorganizes our use of space in was that are detrimental to communal experiences in heavily symbolically freighted spaces, the challenge is substantial.

There are a number of routes that could be explored in order to achieve this goal. One would be to multiply the kinds of technological fixes that are already being used to create simulacra of "being there," such as the aforementioned use of piped in artificial crowd noises, and other devices such as the real-time projections of fans onto stadium and arena seats. Another kind of technical fix would be to alter the experience that people derive from watching broadcast sports. Platforms such as Netflix quickly came up with ways in which people could watch movies and television programs "together" through such (fairly simple) tools like "Netflix Party." Specialty websites already allow people to comment on games in real time in conversation with one another. It is likely that the search for ways in which to improve and democratize this way of watching games "together" will be one of the impacts of the move of elite professional sports into "pandemic society."

Another avenue will be to embed teams and team members more visibly into the communities that support them. Professional sports teams are already active in numbers of ways – creating sporting facilities for disadvantaged youth, making regular visits to children's hospitals, and the like. Teams will have to find other ways in which to integrate themselves into the new urban spaces, institutions and practices that pandemic society will give rise to. At the limit, one of the phenomena we may witness is a return to a time when players hailed from the cities that they played for. At present, athletes playing for professional sports teams are frequent flyers whose families often reside in one place while athletes perform in another. Athletes often return either to their countries of origin or to wherever their families live during the off season. Such peripatetic lifestyles might become more difficult in a world in which crossing borders becomes more complicated and arduous a process than it has been in the pre-pandemic world. The incentive to play close to home might start making itself felt in ways that it has not done so before. At time of writing, the coach of Montreal's professional soccer team, Thierry Henry, cited the complications brought about by the pandemic and the travel restrictions it has wrought as the reason that has led him to resign his post. Surely he is not the only athlete or coach who will find themselves facing such complexities, and choosing to work closer to home.

We can only speculate as to the manner in which pandemic society will alter the way in which elite sports are practiced, and in which partisanship is sustained. It seems clear that the way in which fans and sporting events are connected is one of the many ways in which societies will be changed as we transition toward pandemic societies.

NOTES

1 On the ethics of national sporting partisanship, see Dixon (2000).
2 For a defence of partisanship, see Dixon (2001). For a view that emphasizes the "disinterested" appreciation of partisanship, see Mumford (2012).
3 This is clearly not always the case. Especially in the case of larger cities, allegiance to a sports team is often grounded in class, religion, or ethnicity, and can sometimes exacerbate the tensions that mark cities that are rifted along such lines. Think of how importantly class figures in soccer rivalries between such teams as Boca Juniors and River Plate in Argentina, and Manchester United and Manchester City in the UK.
4 Obviously, anyone making this kind of a claim needs to reckon with the massive transnational fact of football hooliganism. I clearly cannot deal adequately with the topic within the confines of this short paper. Suffice it to say that the dominant approach to the study of hooliganism, the so-called "Leicester school," points to myriad social forces as contributing to emergence of hooliganism, rather than anything intrinsic to sports partisanship. See Shaun Best (2010).
5 For a measured voice on this matter, see Adam B. Evans et al. (2020).
6 For related arguments, see Mumford (2011).
7 See Jerry Seinfeld make this remark on the David Letterman show here: https://vimeo.com/47283296, accessed 28 February 2021.

REFERENCES

Bell, Daniel, and Avner de-Shalit. 2011. *The Spirit of Cities. Why the Identity of a City Matters in a Global Age.* Princeton: Princeton University Press.

Best, Shaun. 2010. "The Leicester School of Football Hooliganism." *Soccer and Society* 11, no. 5: 573–87.

Dixon, Nicholas. 2000. "A Justification of Moderate Patriotism in Sport." In *Values in Sport*, edited by Claudio Tamburrini and Torbjörn Tännsjö, 74–86. London: E&FN Spon.

– 2001. "The Ethics of Supporting Sports Teams." *Journal of Applied Philosophy* 18, no. 2: 149–158.

Evans, Adam B., Sine Agergaard, Paul Ian Campbell, Kevin Hylton, and Verena Lenneis. 2020. "'Black Lives Matter': Sport, Race, and Ethnicity in Challenging Times." *European Journal for Sport and Society* 17, no. 4: 289–300.

Mumford, Stephen. 2011. *Watching Sports. Aesthetics, Ethics, and Emotion*. London: Routledge.

Mumford, Stephen. 2012. "Moderate Partisanship as Oscillation." *Sport, Ethics and Philosophy* 6, no. 3: 369–375.

Saunders, Bryan. Forthcoming. "Losing the Twelfth Man: Will Empty Stadiums Eliminate Home Advantage, and Could Placebo Crowds Rectify This?" Accessed on 28 February 2021: https://doi.org/10.31236/osf.io/ujq4b.

Swartz, Tim B., and Adriano Arce. 2014. "New Insights Involving the Home Team Advantage." *International Journal of Sports Science and Coaching* 9, no. 4: 681–92.

Taylor, Charles. 1997. "Irreducibly Social Goods." In *Philosophical Arguments*. Cambridge, MA: Harvard University Press.

4

Getting Pandemic Education Outside of the Box

Andrew Potter

INTRODUCTION

It has become a commonplace bordering on the cliché to note that the COVID-19 global pandemic exposed weaknesses or fault lines in one part or another of our social infrastructure. Whether it is basic emergency preparedness, our treatment of temporary foreign workers, or the state of our long term care facilities for the elderly (to name just a few from a very long list) the pandemic has made clear the fragility and inflexibility of many of our institutions.

Perhaps nowhere have the exposed fault lines appeared so deep and so wide as in the domain of education. It is not a stretch to point out that the pandemic has revealed fundamental truths about how our society functions, and one of those truths is the absolutely central place of schools in that system.

After the World Health Organization declared a global pandemic on 11 March 2020, most Canadian schools were promptly closed. In many cases these were billed as "temporary" shutdowns, mostly intended to give public officials some breathing space while they came to grips with the scope and nature of what was coming. But those temporary closures kept getting extended, and while some jurisdictions reopened schools temporarily or on curtailed schedules, for the most part they remained shut until the scheduled end of the year and the summer break.

As the summer of 2020 wore on, back to school planning became the focal point for a number of intense and very high stakes political questions. These included the question of getting parents (but especially women) back into the workforce, the mental health of children, the social inequality that would result from the myriad ad hoc arrangements parents were making to educate their children, the basic requirements of a more general economic reopening, and workplace safety for teachers and school administrators. Making matters more complicated, schools became battlefronts in the ongoing culture war opened up by questions of whether to mandate the wearing of masks, how much social distancing was necessary, how infectious children were, and how and when students should be tested.

In short, virtually everything at stake in the pandemic managed to find its expression in the question of school reopening. Furthermore, as with most aspects of our pandemic response, one of the most significant obstacles to resolving the debate over schools has been the myopic focus on getting schools back to "normal."

Since the COVID-19 pandemic arrived in full force in March 2020, our ability to cope with the personal, professional, and public disruptions it has caused has been confounded by two related problems. The first is a collective inability or unwillingness to think creatively about the appropriate policy responses. The second is a relentless desire to get back to normal, where normal is understood entirely as "how things were on March 10." There has been little in the way of out-of-the-box thinking about how to reconfigure space or make creative use of time to manage the pandemic and its effects, to reduce harms while enabling a different form of what normal might look like.[1]

One glaring example of this blinkered thinking was the decision by many jurisdictions to allow bars and clubs (including, in some provinces, strip bars and karaoke bars) to reopen during the summer of 2020 when case counts went into a steep decline, even as epidemiologists were warning that a second wave was inevitable. Instead of, say, loosening restrictions on the consumption of alcohol in public spaces such as parks, most jurisdictions chose to let establishments open as normal, subject only to various limits on numbers and social distancing requirements.

The question of how to manage the return to schools in September 2020 and onward has been another iteration of this persistent dynamic. Almost without exception, politicians and school boards dedicated their energies to trying to reconcile all of these competing agendas within the context of the way school has always been done: twenty to thirty students in a square room with a teacher, with the occasional trip outside for a socially distanced recess or lunch or maybe gym class.

In some cases they were able to succeed, by these limited criteria. Schools in Quebec managed to open and for the most part stay open, despite a long list of outbreaks across the province that led to the temporary closures of some classes and in some cases of entire schools. But you would be hard pressed to find anyone – teachers, parents, students, administrators – who is happy. Everyone is some degree of angry about how things have gone. But given what they were trying to do, this was inevitable. If by "open schools during the pandemic" you mean some facsimile of how schools opened before the pandemic you are bound to fail, because it cannot be done.

There is an alternative approach, though, which involves flipping our entire model of education on its head. Instead of students spending most of their time indoors in a square room with occasional trips outside for some brief gulps of fresh air and exercise, the default in a pandemic should be to hold school outside with very occasional sessions indoors only when absolutely necessary.

THE VIEW FROM INSIDE THE BOX

On 11 March 2020, the World Health Organization formally confirmed that the rapidly spreading outbreak of the novel coronavirus had become a global pandemic. It did not come as much of a surprise, since Canada's first case had been confirmed in Canada in late January, with cases popping up with increasing frequency in a growing number of provinces over the next month. Even before the formal announcement of a pandemic, various public institutions had already started taking mitigation steps: testing centres had been set up in various cities, the Société de transport de Montréal had stepped up cleaning on its buses and metros, and Air Canada had cancelled flights from Italy, which was one of the early epicentres of the COVID-19 outbreak.

But with the official declaration of a pandemic things started happening very quickly, with a rolling list of closures and cancellations. The NBA cancelled its season, and was soon followed by the NHL, the World Figure Skating Championships, and other sports leagues. Via Rail stopped running its major passenger services, the airlines cancelled a growing list of scheduled flights, the St Patrick's Day parade in Montreal was postponed, and the premier of Quebec closed bars, restaurants, sugar shacks, and other public venues. And on Friday,

13 March, the schools closed in most provinces, including Quebec and Ontario. The lockdown had begun as public health officials and politicians struggled to grasp the extent of the crisis.

Yet within a few weeks, a textbook plan for how to end the lockdown, both in Canada and abroad, had started to take form. First, you close down society as much as possible in order to "flatten the curve" of transmission and get the number of cases under control. You keep pressing down until the rate of transmission drops to the point where recovery rates outpace hospitalizations, so we do not overwhelm hospitals and other health services.

Once this is done, we can slowly start to reopen society; not all at once, but in a carefully staged return. In a piece published in the early weeks of the pandemic that was typical of the thinking at the time, Andrew Coyne, writing for the *Globe and Mail*, argued that any staged reopening would have to be in the reverse order in which things were closed down, which means playgrounds and restaurants might open sooner, while the last things to return will be any sort of unnecessary mass gathering – live sporting events, movies and concerts, and so on (Coyne 2020).

For all its orthodoxy, Coyne's article is striking in that it does not once mention schools. But the school question is tricky, because, on the one hand, they are one of the most significantly social institutions in our society, and their very nature is a repudiation of the social distancing requirements that quickly became second nature during the lockdown. But on the other hand, getting some significant portion of our children back into school, particularly elementary students, was clearly a precondition for re-opening other parts of the economy. You simply cannot get parents back into the workforce in any meaningful way if they are simultaneously playing the role of full-time babysitter slash homeschooler.

That was at least part of the thinking behind the relatively early push in Quebec to reopen the elementary schools. After the initial two-week shock-treatment shuttering of schools and the overall economy in early March 2020 was extended well into April, Quebec premier François Legault started musing about getting children back in school. He asked teachers to report back to work on 4 May, with schools scheduled to reopen a few weeks later. The plan was supported by Quebec's association of pediatricians, which worried about the effects of the closures on the mental health of children as well as on their social and physical development.

But while the province made it clear that sending children to class would be totally voluntary, the reopening was met with opposition from many quarters. A parent-initiated petition to keep the schools closed until September received almost three hundred thousand signatures, while some of the province's teachers unions pushed back against what they called a "dangerous plan" (Kovac and Shields 2020). Ultimately, the ongoing rise of caseloads of COVID-19 meant that only elementary schools outside the island of Montreal reopened. Schools on the Island of Montreal remained closed until the end of the normal school year.

When the elementary schools in Quebec did finally return as scheduled in the fall of 2020, it was under very rigid social distancing rules, with cohort "bubbling" and other mitigation measures that varied by jurisdiction and grade level but generally involved a ban on the use of libraries, the cancellation of extracurricular activities, regular and thorough cleaning of desks and other classroom surfaces, and mandatory or voluntary mask wearing.

It is worth pausing to take note of a few things here.

First, it is clear that when it comes to the education system, all of society is a stakeholder. That has always been true in the broadest sense of an educated populace being a public good (that is why it is publicly funded in the first place) but the COVID-19 lockdown made it clear the manner in which that it is true in a much narrower sense as well: virtually everyone has an interest in children actually being in school. When children are not in school, the effects cascade down through our social, political, and economic infrastructure, most notably because employers suffer when parents are unable to work, or at least cannot work at their full productive capacities because they have to take care of their children.

Second, at the domestic level it has become obvious that the costs of taking care of and of homeschooling children are not borne equally. The economic shock of the pandemic led to what has been coined a "she-cession," with women suffering job loss disproportionately. But even for those women who remained employed, the costs were huge as many working mothers took on the equivalent of a second full time job in caring for their children while also continuing to work (van der Liden 2020).

Third, the costs of taking care of children who are not in school are not shared equally across social classes. Private schools were better equipped to quickly set up home schooling systems for children at home. But even for families with children in public schools, wealthier families quickly set up "pandemic pods" – essentially small learning groups with other families – to hire tutors and instructors to make up for what their children were missing. To the extent to which these pods are effective, they threaten to exacerbate pre-existing social inequalities (McMahon 2020).

And finally, taking all of this into account, it is striking just how little the debate around reopening schools has been about the pedagogical practicalities of learning. As far as the most vocal stakeholders are concerned, the back-to-school agenda has very little to do with education. Indeed, the Quebec premier explicitly argued that one of the primary reasons for re-opening the schools was not to make sure the children did not miss too much school. Rather, it was to start to build "herd immunity" in the population, a position that was denounced at the time by epidemiologists but, surprisingly, supported by Quebec's association of paediatricians (Jelowicki 2020). When all of this finally shook out and schools reopened in September 2020, it was under extremely difficult and unpleasant conditions for everyone, with learning taking a back seat to safety at every step.

This was probably inevitable, given the basic conundrum: the government wanted children back in school for reasons that had almost nothing to do with pedagogy. The teachers' unions were clearly unhappy with being asked to get back in the classroom, and as a result the schools proposed to offer something bearing only a passing resemblance to education. Yet because as a society we are stuck in a box that says if children are not at home then they must be in school, we committed to opening the schools under conditions that more closely resembled prison.

At this point, a more self-aware society would be looking around for ways to get out of the box. That is, how could we accomplish the goals we need out of schools in a way that is safer, more resilient and flexible, without the prison-like features?

One old but largely forgotten solution is to get outside.

OUTSIDE THE BOX

The COVID-19 virus is a puzzle, from the question of who it infects, how it manifests itself, and how severe it becomes. When it first appeared in late 2019, it was described as a type of influenza, and indeed a lot of the early and largely uninformed commentary about the spread of the novel coronavirus tended to downplay the significance of the infection as nothing more than a particularly nasty 'flu. But even the doctors and the epidemiologists who understood just how serious and infectious the virus was assumed that it was a respiratory illness, which is why so much of the early panic about treatment and hospitalizations was focused on the limited supply of ventilators. Eventually scientists figured out that it was not a pulmonary disease but rather primarily a cardiovascular disease where the virus targeted the endothelium, the layer of cells lining the inside of every blood vessel. This discovery helped explain many of the stranger symptoms of COVID-19 infection, including blood clots, strange rashes, myocarditis, and the spike in cases of Kawasaki disease in children.

Yet the virus demonstrates enormous heterogeneity between infected patients. Some show no symptoms at all or might just lose their sense of smell for a while, while other patients suffer severe breathing problems, strokes, and heart attacks. And whereas some patients recover quickly and completely, others, known as "long haulers," experience serious symptoms for weeks or months. More confusing is that there is no predicting who will become a longhauler, their cases are a mix of young and old, and those who had a relatively mild case and those whose infection was more severe.

This extreme heterogeneity recapitulates itself at the population level. Some countries have done very poorly fighting the pandemic, while others have done relatively well. And while in some obvious instances the poor results can be directly linked to populist political leaders who more or less denied the seriousness of the virus (such as Brazil and the United States), for the most part it remains somewhat of a mystery. Similarly, the death rates from COVID-19 vary widely between countries, but not in the way you would expect. Contrary to the usual pattern, it is the wealthier countries that have the highest death rates, with many developing countries reporting death rates ranging from one tenth to one one-hundredth of that seen in places like the United States (Mukherjee 2021).

So while there is still a lot we don't know about the virus, its modes and mechanisms of transmission, and its unpredictable morbidity, one of the earliest and most widely replicated features to emerge from the case data is that outdoors is significantly safer than indoors. An early study from China that was published in April 2020 found that out of seven thousand cases of COVID-19 transmission, only two happened outdoors (Nishiura et al. 2019). A more comprehensive review published in late November 2020 found that less than 10 per cent of all COVID-19 infections happened outdoors, with the risk of indoor transmission being almost 19 per cent higher than outdoors. And while there remain gaps in our understanding of the specific pathways and mechanisms through which the virus is transmitted, the major factor seems to be that the virus is spread through respiratory droplets that soon fall to the ground or are quickly dissolved into aerosols that simply blow away.

That stable and enduring fact about the virus should have been guiding our policy responses and reopening strategies from the earliest days of the pandemic. Whether it was opening bars or restaurants, allowing team sports or other forms of recreation, or keeping playgrounds accessible, the question, "can this be done outdoors?" should have been the primary, if not the only, consideration. Of course, not every activity is made safe simply by taking place outside. The general rule of thumb for COVID-19 transmission is that it is a function of proximity and time, and the guidance from the CDC defines "close contact with an infected person" as closer than six feet for longer than fifteen minutes. That is why outdoor rock concerts might not be much safer than one held in a club, given that it is still a lot of people packed into a tight space yelling into one another's faces for hours on end.

But when it comes to the question of how to reopen schools safely during a pandemic, the solution is obvious. We can dispense with the hard problems of whether to mandate masks in class and, if so, for what age groups. We do not have to worry about how many students should be in the classroom, whether we should spend millions on air purifiers, and whether kids should be allowed to interact outside their bubbles in the schoolyard. Teachers do not need to wear face shields or to hide behind plexiglass, and they do not need to spend recess time wiping down all of the desks and other surfaces with disinfectant. None of this would be necessary if we were to just flip the entire model of how we educate kids on its head. Instead of students spending most of their time indoors with occasional trips outside for some fresh air, the default should be to hold school outside with very occasional sessions indoors only when absolutely necessary.

In the early months of the pandemic, back in April and into May of 2020, it is understandable that officials did not rush to reopen classrooms in schoolyards, parks, and even parking lots although there was certainly a case to be made that they should have made some effort at opening summer camps as early as May (Potter 2020). But having had the better part of eight months to prepare, and given ample warnings about the inevitable second wave of the pandemic as the weather cooled in the fall, at least some of our efforts should have been dedicated to figuring out just how much schooling could have taken place outside. That this did not happen can only be seen as a failure.

To begin with, outdoor education during a public health crisis is hardly a new idea. Open air schooling was widely used as a way to control the spread of tuberculosis in the early twentieth century. The idea started in Germany in 1904, spread across Europe and over the ocean, where it was used with great success in places such as Rhode Island, in New York City, and Canada, where "forest schools" opened in Toronto in 1912. Within a decade there was a robust open-school movement in Europe and North America, with regular conferences being held on the subject until the middle of the century (Pruitt 2020).

Despite this precedent, outdoor schooling saw limited use during the 1918 influenza pandemic. Most schools in the United States closed, with the notable exception of schools in Chicago and New York City. In Canada, the outbreak hit in the fall of 1918 just as the weather was turning. In Ontario, officials tried for the most part to keep schools open with business happening as usual. But the extent of the outbreak eventually forced schools in the province to shut for as long as three months. In Quebec, most schools simply closed and many were turned into makeshift hospitals.

When the COVID-19 pandemic arrived, a handful of creative educators and public health officials looked back to the earlier lessons of the open-schools movement for guidance. One of the most widely cited is the example of the Samso Frie Skole, located on the Danish island of Samso, which fully embraced outdoor education and moved their whole operation into the forest. Pupils and teachers would walk or bike a mile every morning to their new classroom in the woods, with time indoors restricted for short lessons or in cases of very bad weather.

There were other small-scale and local attempts along these lines in both Canada and the United States. One New Hampshire private Waldorf school cut down some trees on its large wooded property and made some A-frames to serve as outdoor classrooms, while the mayor of New York City encouraged schools to find ways of using parks and streets for outdoor classes. Meanwhile, the principal of an elementary school in Gatineau, Quebec purchased tents and logs for an outdoor classroom that teachers could book for fifty-minute classes. He put up the $3,000 out of his own pocket, hoping that the school board would approve the plan – which it did (Mahoney 2020).

For the most part though, the Canadian approach to school has remained largely stuck in the deep wagon-ruts of conventional thinking. When it comes to opening schools, our central preoccupations have been over questions class sizes; of the distance between desks and how to manage social distancing in the school; over whether to allow students to have recess or lunch together; and of whether students and instructors should wear masks, at what age, and in what circumstances. That is, we have been arguing over the logistics of how to go back to doing school the way we have always done it despite the fact that we are still in the middle of a global pandemic that makes that impossible. And even on the few occasions that holding school outdoors is even mooted, it is entertained only for the sake of dismissing it as an interesting little-toy thought experiment that no one should really take seriously.

To be sure, it is not hard to come up with objections to the idea of moving education outdoors. Yet it is surprisingly easy to deal with most of them.

One obvious objection has to do with space and materials. Whatever else they are, schools are buildings, specifically designed as places where children can be taught a specific curriculum. A school is, or at least ought to be, an environment for learning, and moving schooling outside is not a simple matter, especially in urban areas where there is going to be traffic, construction, machinery, and other forms of noise and distraction.

A second is money and resources. It is one thing for a private school or academy to take initiatives on its own, using its own resources, but not every school backs onto a forest or has its own acreage from which to source logs for outdoor schoolrooms. How outdoor education can be funded and scaled across an entire public school system in towns or cities with dozens or even hundreds or schools is no minor matter.

A third question, related to the first two, has to do with fairness and equality. Even within a public system, some schools have more resources than others, some are better situated for outdoor education, and some have teachers and students who might be more amenable to the prospect. And this in turn raises the issue of the curriculum – how do you ensure a common curriculum when learning environments might be so diverse?

So let us tackle these difficulties head on.

Canada, as is widely known, is huge. There are plenty of school yards, sports fields, baseball diamonds, public parks, shopping mall parking lots, and other spaces that could easily be commandeered for outdoors classrooms. So space is not generally a problem, it is just a matter of seeing creative ways of making use of it. And while you might not be able to easily set up smart boards or wifi or any of the other trappings of modern learning, it is not hard to set up some chalk or whiteboards under a tent with students arranged in small groups around tables. If you are really having trouble getting your mind around how it might work, you might consult your local wedding planner.

Regarding money or other resources, if there is one thing that the pandemic has taught Canadians, it is that we are rich. Collectively, our governments have shown themselves totally willing, and entirely able, to spend hundreds of billions of dollars on our pandemic response. Unimaginable sums, at levels not seen outside of a wartime economy, have been thrown at various pandemic support measures. The amounts that would be required to fund outdoor education across the country, at scale, are a mere fraction of what has been spent on various income supports for individuals and businesses.

But not everything can be taught through chalk and talk, after all. What about science labs and computers and music class and art and drama and all the other things that go into what we consider an education? And what about that thing we call the curriculum, the basic elements of knowledge that we require every student in the province to acquire as a condition of moving on to the next stage of their education?

Well, what of them. Concerns with what gets taught are themselves part of the problem. The sacredness of the curriculum is part of the problem. One thing that a lot of parents of elementary students realised when faced with Zoom school or other forms of home schooling that became necessary during the pandemic is just how little actual learning of core subjects goes on in a given school day. Most of time at school, at the elementary level in particular, is spent on what really amounts to well-structured babysitting.

We would do well to acknowledge this and embrace its deeper logic. Lots of schools build field trips into their curriculum. Why not make field trips the default part of the school experience? Why not teach kids how to identify all the trees and plants in the park, how to use a compass and read a map, or how to follow the sewage system from where a toilet gets flushed to where it discharges into the nearby river or sea? What is preventing us from using this pandemic as an opportunity to rethink where and how we educate our children, and for what purposes?

Maybe this is crazy talk. And maybe the reason we are not considering any of this is not because our politicians are weak, or because our education administrators are unimaginative, or because our teachers' unions are too rigid and selfish.

Maybe it is something much more straightforward, namely, the weather. After all, much of Canada is pretty much frozen over from the end of November till early March. This is true enough, though a lot can be accomplished with heaters and blankets. Also, this is a country where millions of parents happily spend hours every weekend freezing on a bench in a hockey rink sipping their "double double" and do not think much of it.

But if it turns out that in many parts of the country it is just too cold to hold school outside in the dead of winter, then should we bite the bullet and get the kids back inside? Not necessarily. Perhaps we need to make one last, big, cognitive leap, and invert the entire school year. There is no obvious reason why the school year has to run from September to June. In a pandemic, it would make more sense to take a long holiday from the early December to late February, with the school year running from March right through the summer and into the late fall.

Is this crazy? Possibly. But it is a lot less crazy than the safety-first and education-last tunnel-vision thinking that passed for education planning in Canada during the COVID-19 pandemic.

CONCLUSION

One of the ongoing frustrations with how the COVID-19 pandemic has been handled in Canada at all levels of government is the relative absence of creative, push-the-envelope thinking. The novel coronavirus that emerged at the end of 2019 and spread across the planet has challenged all of society in ways that would have seemed unimaginable right up to the formal declaration of the pandemic in early 2020.

But nothing focuses the mind like the prospect of a hanging, as Samuel Johnson sort of said, and the prospect of illness, death, bankruptcy, or irrelevance led many individuals, enterprises, and institutions to respond with imagination and flexibility. To give just a few examples, think of how many craft breweries quickly got into the business of manufacturing hand sanitizer, or the way so many restaurants managed to keep the lights on by turning themselves into take-out or delivery businesses. Or compare Canada's venerable professional football league, the CFL, which scrubbed its entire season, with Canada's young and fragile professional soccer league, the CPL, which took advantage of the relative safety of the "Atlantic bubble" to hold a shortened but energetic season entirely on Prince Edward Island.

In comparison, politicians and policy makers frequently seemed out of their depth, daunted by the task they faced and unsure of how to respond. In the early months of the pandemic there was a great deal of talk of "testing and tracing" our way out of the pandemic, with plans floated that would see us processing millions of tests a day while using state of the art surveillance technologies to trace and isolate contacts. While that model proved highly successful in places such as Taiwan and South Korea, for whatever reason Canada was simply not up to the task. It took months to scale up testing to barely acceptable levels, by which point there was too much community spread across the country to make contact tracing viable. Meanwhile, our feeble attempt at using technology in the form of a smartphone app for alerting users to possible contacts failed in the face of federal-provincial squabbling and hyperactive concerns over privacy. With the failure of this technocratic solution, we were left with the only available alternative, namely, the "hammer and the dance" of repeated cycles of lockdown and reopening.

Given the enormous stakes, any decision over how much to lock down or over what to reopen and under what conditions became enormously political. Inevitably, schools have found themselves square in the crosshairs of this highly politicized pandemic management, and only something highly creative, such as getting schools outside, would have prevented it.

Again, there are plenty of reasons why outdoor education is difficult or risky. Outdoors is safer, but it is not completely safe. But here is the key point: this proposal does not promise to eliminate the risks to staff or students, but what it almost certainly does is reduce the risks relative to the government's plan.

But ultimately the main obstacle to something like this happening is not about risk, or money, or space, or the weather – it is about the mental models we live in. We have these built-in notions of what children are supposed to be doing at this time of year, or what getting "back to normal" is supposed to look like, and we have a very hard time thinking outside of those models. In these pandemic times, these mental models have become cognitive cages. It has made us enormously risk averse, while ignoring the fact that keeping our heads down and staying resolutely inside the box is itself a highly risky strategy, with very little in the way of apparent reward.

NOTE

1 For a good example of this sort of creative thinking, see Weinstock (2020).

REFERENCES

Coyne, Andrew. 2020. "We Can See the Way out of the Coronavirus Pandemic, but the Steps to Get There will be Slow." *The Globe and Mail*, 18 April 2020. https://www.theglobeandmail.com/opinion/article-we-can-see-the-way-out-of-the-coronavirus-pandemic-but-the-steps-to/.

Jelowicki, Amanda. 2020. "Quebec Parents Fear Sending Kids Back to School, Concept of 'Herd Immunity.'" *Global News*, 24 April 2020. https://globalnews.ca/news/6865226/coronavirus-quebec-school-herd-immunity/.

Kovac, Adam, and Billy Shields. 2020. "Teachers, Union Call Plan to Reopen Montreal Schools Dangerous." CTV *News*, 30 April 2020. https://montreal.ctvnews.ca/teachers-union-call-plans-to-reopen-montreal-schools-dangerous-1.4919823.

Linden, Clifton van der. 2020. "The Moms Are Not Alright: How Coronavirus Pandemic Policies Penalize Working Mothers." *The Conversation*, 3 September 2020. https://theconversation.com/the-moms-are-not-alright-how-coronavirus-pandemic-policies-penalize-mothers-144713.

Mahoney, Jill. 2020. "Classes Move Outdoors to Prevent COVID-19 Spread." *The Globe and Mail*, 7 September 2020. https://www.

theglobeandmail.com/canada/article-classes-move-outdoors-to-prevent-covid-19-spread/.

McMahon, Tamson. 2020. "Affluent US Parents Turn to Private 'Pandemic Pods' to Navigate New Homeschooling Reality." *The Globe and Mail*, 27 July 2020. https://www.theglobeandmail.com/world/article-affluent-us-parents-arrange-private-tutelage-from-public-school/.

Mukherjee, Siddhartha. 2021. "Why Does the Pandemic Seem to be Hitting Some Countries Harder than Others?" *The New Yorker*, 1 March 2021. https://www.newyorker.com/magazine/2021/03/01/why-does-the-pandemic-seem-to-be-hitting-some-countries-harder-than-others.

Nishiura, Hiroshi, Hitoshi Oshitani, Tetsuro Kobayashi, Tomoya Saito, Tomimasa Sunagawa, Tamano Matsui, Takaji Wakita, MHLW COVID-19 Response Team, and Motoi Suzuki. 2020. "Closed Environments Facilitate Secondary Transmission of Coronavirus Disease 2019." *medRxiv*, 16 April 2020. https://www.medrxiv.org/content/10.1101/2020.02.28.20029272v2.

Potter, Andrew. 2020. "Forget about Schools, Open the Summer Camps in the Spring." *The Globe and Mail*, 6 May 2020. https://www.theglobeandmail.com/opinion/article-forget-about-schools-open-the-summer-camps-in-spring/.

Pruitt, Sarah. 2020. "When Fears of Tuberculosis Drove an Open-Air School Movement." *History*, 30 July 2020. https://www.history.com/news/school-outside-tuberculosis.

Weinstock, Daniel. 2020. "Harm Reduction in Pandemic Times." *Max Bell School of Public Policy*, 21 April 2020. https://www.mcgill.ca/maxbell-school/article/articles,-policy-challenges-during-pandemic/briefing-harm-reduction-pandemic-times.

5

The COVID-19 Pandemic and the Loss of the Urban

Quill R Kukla

There is a long history of associating dense cities with contagion and lack of sanitation during public health crises, and so we might assume that cities are especially risky places during the COVID-19 pandemic. In contrast, it turns out that at a population level, cities are the safest places to be to be during the pandemic. Cities are healthier places than non-cities in general, with an overall 2.4-year bump in lifespan for city dwellers (Litman 2020). Moreover, most infection risks are associated with activities that are not specific to cities, such as long-distance travel, at-home gatherings, and worksites for essential workers. While contagion rates in cities are somewhat higher, cities also have better public health infrastructure and lower infectious disease mortality rates overall (Litman 2020). Indeed, according to Todd Litman, "although city residents are more exposed to infectious diseases, rural residents are more likely to die if infected, and urban living provides large health and safety benefits making cities significantly safer and healthier overall" (Litman 2020, 2). In fact, Litman concludes that "For most households, the safest, healthiest and most resilient home is located in a walkable urban neighborhood where commonly-used services and activities are easy to access on foot and by bicycle" (Litman 2020, 22). The real contagion risk comes not from density, but from crowding, which is often confused with density. Density is the number of people per unit of land, whereas crowding is the number of people per room. Litman writes, "Density is not actually correlated with higher transmission, and in fact, higher density counties have significantly lower virus-related mortality rates, possibly due to better health care" (Litman 2020, 12). Crowding is associated with poverty, which is a real predictor of COVID risk, unlike city living per se.

But even though the risks of COVID-19 are not higher in cities, the pandemic may give us other reasons to leave the city, based on our changing needs and preferences. Many of the immediate effects of the pandemic seem to push towards an abandonment of cities: a huge increase in teleworking means that many people do not need to live near their workplace, and they also may want more space for a home office, both of which push people away from expensive city centres with smaller residential spaces. A fear of sharing crowded spaces with others may drive city dwellers to want to privatize formerly public activities, stimulating a desire for private lawns, home gyms, and the like, which pushes people out of cities and into more suburbanized spaces. Moreover, many of the former benefits of living in the city – bustling streets, amenities such as restaurants and retail, events involving large crowds such as concerts – no longer exist, or are not usable by those of us who are cautious. Meanwhile, for the many people who work at home now, there are no longer motives to stay in the city to cut down on commuting time. And until the market restabilizes, it still costs more to live in the city. For all these reasons, people may choose to leave the city because of the pandemic. In other words, while abandoning the city for health reasons alone may be misguided, abandoning it for quality-of-life reasons may make sense, as the form that quality-of-life takes has changed for many of us during the pandemic.

In the first part of this paper, I explore what may happen to cities in the wake of the pandemic if we just let the market take its course, and then I look at what planning and policy steps we can take to prevent cities from emptying out and dying. In the second part, I argue that even excellent planning, while potentially saving cities, may leave what we know as city life fundamentally altered; the basic experience of living in cities, and of being a city dweller, and the human value of cities, may be changed in substantial ways.[1]

Indeed, I will claim, the very steps that planners need to take in order to keep people in cities are the same steps that will change those cities in their essence. What emerges instead may have its own charms and values, but for those of us who love city life as we know it, the pandemic may be a cause for permanent grief.

Many cities feel different in the midst of the pandemic, with businesses shuttered, rush hours thinned, and streets emptied. But how will cities be affected permanently by these changes, assuming that we do not intervene at the level of policy or design? There are two types of changes we can expect: changes that are a direct response to the pressures of the pandemic, and secondary changes from shifts in the market caused by new patterns of living and working in the wake of COVID.

It is hard to guess how much and for how long individuals will be concerned about contagion, in ways that affect their daily behaviour. Will people continue to wear masks and avoid physical contact and proximity with one another of their own accord, once the pandemic abates? Regardless of such ongoing daily choices, we can predict some substantial shifts in the urban landscape, based the current pressures of the pandemic. We are already seeing increasing demand, among those who can afford it, for single family housing, as opposed to apartments with shared common spaces. We can also expect an increased market for housing with better ventilation, and for housing near parks and other outdoor amenities. We may see a devaluation of residential high-rises with small shared foyers and elevators; incidentally, this shift would have other health benefits, as such high rises are associated with lower mental health among residents (Evans 2003). As housing that is safer from contagion is built to accommodate a new market, this housing, without policy interventions, is likely to be more expensive than existing unsafe housing, thereby enhancing inequality in cities. Moreover, if we start to destroy and replace unsafe housing, we will displace poorer residents from cities. Thus the pandemic has the potential to redistribute people in a way that partially empties out the city core, with poor people left behind in city centres with fewer services and opportunities.

How will the secondary effects of the pandemic shift urban geography? Many firms have successfully shifted their operations online, thereby saving enormous operating costs, opening up their potential labour pool, and giving their employees more flexibility as to where to live. It is highly unlikely that all or even most of these firms will shift back to brick and mortar, in-person operations. Many professional, office, service, and retail jobs will become permanently virtual (Bereitschaft and Scheller 2020, 9). In pre-COVID times, geography dictated function, with different parts of cities supporting different sorts of businesses and services, but these principles do not apply as many businesses move to online operations, especially given that very few cities are still organized around manufacturing. This changes the fundamental economic dynamics of cities; there is no longer a reason for firms to agglomerate in expensive downtown areas, or in any one area at all. This will lead not only to massive decentralization, but also to the hollowing out of downtowns. The hollowing out comes not just from the primary loss of employment centres that formerly needed to be located downtown, but from secondary loss of businesses such as restaurants and newsstands that used to support commuters. Moreover, in the midst of this shift, large chains, which are less dependent on geography for survival and can better weather a long suspension or dip in their operations, are more likely to survive in some form or another than are independent businesses. For all these reasons, we are likely looking at a more homogenous, less centralized urban landscape, post-COVID.

The economic and geographic effects of people's newfound mobility are just starting to emerge. For instance, COVID is likely to redistribute people into cheaper cities, not just to move them out of cities. Some companies, like Redfin, are already scaling income to residential location in ways that shape and incentivize where people live (Buyahar 2020). We do not know how this sort of trend will affect cities, but its impact on how people are distributed might be profound. Through all of this, crucially, many people cannot work remotely, because their jobs are manual, and they do not and will not have increased mobility. Such folks are disproportionately working class. For this reason as well, we may see a situation in which poorer urban residents are stranded in dying cities. This may have the advantage of providing them with lower costs of living, but it will make our urban geography even more inequitable than it already is, reversing the revitalization and revaluation of city cores that has characterized the last few decades.

To what extent can cities be saved by good planning, and what would that look like? In the wake of the pandemic, we will likely need to reorient the last several decades of planning trends. The focus of cutting-edge planning has been so-called "smart growth" and "new urbanism," which emphasize dense neighbourhoods, more compact living spaces, multi-use streets, small set-backs, and other design features meant to encourage crowding and mixing (Bereitschaft and Scheller 2020, 11). point out that much of the focus of the new urbanism has been on finding ways of building the proximity, interaction, and crowding typical of cities into planned communities and suburbs, whereas now we seem to be entering an era where instead we build the distancing, separation, private space, and controlled character of the suburbs into cities, if we are to keep them safe and convince people to stay in them. We need design features that allow people to enjoy cities while moving through space in orderly ways that build in physical distance and keep people interacting with intimates rather than strangers.

Decentralization seems to be a nearly inevitable outcome of the pandemic, at least to some extent, unless we were to introduce draconian policies to force people and businesses to stay in place. The traditional city form with a dense core surrounded by sprawl may be made obsolete by the pandemic. The question is whether the decentralized city can be made both safe and appealing with proper planning, or whether it will turn into unmitigated sprawl made up mostly of privatized household spaces, with dead zones where dense cores used to be. Urban designer Michael Mehaffey suggests that we need to replace areas that used to involve the crowded, uncontrolled mixing of people with more complex spaces that allow both sociality and distancing. These might include parks and trails, walking and biking infrastructure, and streets devoted to outdoor dining and retail with design features to keep people apart, such as pocket parks between tables. To save cities, we will need to fundamentally reconceive many streets as being for pedestrians rather than for cars. During the pandemic, many streets have already been closed to traffic and given over to outdoor dining, or tuned into "slow streets" open only to residents and emergency vehicles, with lower speed limits, so as to allow pedestrian use. This is more plausible than it used to be, as commuting traffic has gone down, perhaps permanently.

In addition to simple health interventions such as widespread handwashing stations and the normalization of mask and hand sanitizer availability, post-pandemic architecture might emphasize porches and balconies, which allow connection to public space and the possibility of socializing with those on the street from a safe distance (Mehaffey 2020; Bereitschaft and Scheller 2020). Such spaces are neither public nor private. They serve as home territories for those who own them, but open up towards sociality rather than closing in towards privacy. This architectural shift may be positive, quite apart from its health benefits, providing what Jane Jacobs called "eyes on the street" as well as a zone that bridges private and public space. Michael Mehaffy writes: "'Social distancing' requires just the kind of physical separation that is afforded by structures like porches. We can continue to interact with others, maintaining an important degree of 'social solidarity,' but we can also continue to maintain separation to the degree considered safe and appropriate – 'sociable distancing,' perhaps. This degree of user control provides a paradoxical benefit, as the research suggests. It tends to *encourage* social interaction, by giving users more confidence to interact with others at the level desired, instead of offering only the binary choice of full exposure or full retreat into seclusion." (Mehaffy 2020)

It is a major question whether planners will be able to save the city's role in providing "third places" (Oldenburg 1999), that is, places that are neither home nor work, neither private nor public, but rather "ours" in a communal sense. Third places are places for socializing, playing, and just co-existing in a fluid and unstructured but patterned way. Such places have insiders for whom they are home territory, and they form the basis for fluid communities that need not be based on formal affiliations. They can include barbershops, coffee shops, and bars, for instance. Ray Oldenburg and others after him have claimed that flourishing life requires such third places for most of us. Third places are much more common in cities, where sharing space is the norm and activities happen outside home or work in communal places.

COVID has shut down most third places, or made those of us who are cautious afraid to use them. Can we retain the communal, social nature of third places, and their functioning as comfortable territories, without the ability to crowd one another and enjoy spontaneous close encounters? We are already seeing a great deal of innovation in the attempt to save the establishments that typically function as third places. For instance, one Paris café has put teddy bears in alternating seats in order to keep people distant, and other cafes have followed suit. We have all seen restaurants that have divided their outdoor seating using pods or bubbles to enclose diners, and some restaurants even seat customers under individual Plexiglas shields. What is not yet clear is whether establishments can retain their phenomenological and social character as third places with these sorts of design features in place. Will we be able to build community across them, or are they specifically designed so as to prevent the very embodied forms of interaction that build community? It is unclear to what extent we can use design solutions to save third places, but doing so would be a major step in retaining the point of living in cities and using city spaces.

It seems that we may at least potentially be able to make cities relatively attractive and safe in the wake of the economic and health impacts of the pandemic, through the judicious planning of a less centralized, more structured city with built-in possibilities for distanced interaction. But my discussion of third places raises a more general concern, which will be at the centre for the rest of this paper. I worry that planning that is designed to reduce our uncontrolled contact with one another is inherently anti-urban. Part of what is essential to the phenomenology and form of life of the city, I argue, is precisely its uncontrolled character, the way we bang up against one another in spontaneous and unpredictable ways. Living in a city generally involves living in close proximity to many other people, including strangers and neighbours with whom we do not have an intimate relationship, and it typically involves complex spontaneous contact with these strangers. Even wealthy city dwellers typically live close up to others, often in the same building, and have to move through crowds of other bodies in order to get through their day. Negotiating this uncontrolled mixing is, I claim, at the core of city living, and any sort of new city that plans it away will lose this core essence.

Bereitschaft and Scheller point out that part of the point of going out in the city and using shared space is taken away if there are design features and norms in place that prevent spontaneous mingling; thus it is not clear how much things like socially distanced eating pods outside restaurants will keep street life and businesses alive (2020, 5). But I want to make a slightly different point, which is that even if we do manage to keep such places alive, we might do so by losing the core of what makes a city feel urban. All these creative forms of social control through design cannot escape the fact that it is specifically the uncontrolled character of city streets, the spontaneity of their encounters, and the lack of fear of otherness and strangers, that is at the centre of their urban feel. Thus the pandemic may cost us a rich, historied, inherently valuable form of life, which is the only form of life known to many of us.

Jane Jacobs's 1961 classic *The Death and Life of Great American Cities* celebrated the buzz and diversity of urban neighbourhoods with flourishing ecologies. Jacobs argued that proximity and diversity, and complex and fluid movements through space, gave neighbourhoods life. She recommended a variety of techniques, from short city blocks to porches and windows facing the street, that would encourage the mixing of strangers and pump life into an urban neighbourhood. Earlier conservative theorists such as Louis Wirth (1929) saw cities as inherently alienating, in virtue of being made up of passing encounters between strangers. But in Jacobs and in leftist theorists after her, there is an appreciation of openness to diversity and complexity as a lived phenomenological value nurtured by city life. Later twentieth-century leftist theorists such as Iris Young (1990), Mary Louise Pratt (1991), and Richard Sennett (1992) argued compellingly that part of the essential pleasure and power of a city is the way it opens us to difference, unassimilated otherness, disorder, and a multitude of passing transactions.

It is also essential to urban life that many of the activities that are privatized in the suburbs and in rural areas are shared and public in the city. Whereas in general, suburban public spaces (like roads, supermarkets, and community centres) are designed to support private family spaces, in the city the dependence tends to be reversed; private spaces are much smaller and less separated off from other places, and built around the expectation that their inhabitants will be out in public and communal spaces. In cities, more of our activities are designed to be communal activities, compared to suburbs and rural areas; activities such as working out, swimming, or eating outdoors, for instance, can be privatized and domesticated in suburban homes with rec rooms, pools, and lawns, but city homes are not designed with the space or layout to privatize such activities, which happen in communal gyms, city pools, and parks instead.

City life is unpredictable in a way that suburban, small town, and rural life tends not to be; just the sheer number and diversity of folks up next to one another make it much more likely that things will not go as expected, and that we need to be ready at each moment to adjust our expectations and responses and our perceptual framing. Both Iris Young (1990) and Richard Sennett (1970) influentially discussed how cities are distinctively spaces in which we are called upon to negotiate unexpected circumstances, with people who are unfamiliar to us (and perhaps even unlikeable to us). Not sharing in or fully understanding what we encounter is part of the distinctive experience and even the pleasure of city living, Young convincingly claims (1990, 258–9).

In "City Life and Difference," Young defines the "normative ideal" of city life as "the being together of strangers ... different groups dwell alongside one another, of necessity interacting in city spaces ... City life [is] an openness to unassimilated otherness." (1990, 251) She argues that the pleasures and distinctive character of city life revolve around this constant confrontation with and negotiation of difference and disorder. Cities are riddled and veined through with what Mary Louise Pratt calls "contact zones," which are places where expectations and norms bump messily up against one another; contact zones are "social spaces where cultures meet, clash, and grapple with each other" (1991, 34).

Because living quarters in cities tend to be much smaller and closer together, and because spaces are shared and overlapping, city dwellers are constantly, as a matter of course, accommodating themselves to others. These others are often strangers in two senses: they are people we do not know except in passing (literally), and they are often people who are very different from the sorts of people we are or know intimately. The latter is so even if our intimate circle is quite diverse; still, city living bumps us up against people from countries we know little about, people with life circumstances dramatically different from our own, and so forth. Urban sidewalks, plazas, and alleys often serve as socially complex points of contact in which public and private life spill over into one another. City dwellers must control how much they impede on others and also accept a certain level of intrusion from them, and such impositions are constantly being negotiated. The mere fact of having to accommodate other bodies, at home and in public space, has profound effects upon the lived, embodied experiences of city dwellers.

Is any of this this possible after the pandemic? If the only way in which we can save cities is by orchestrating our movements in controlled ways that avoid direct or spontaneous contact with those who are not already our intimates, will they be recognizable as supporting city life at all? If we are made inherently wary of interacting with anyone other than our intimates, and if our shared spaces are set up to minimize these interactions, to separate and control the flow of people through space, will distinctively urban forms of life survive, or will we in effect canalize and suburbanize urban space in order to keep it occupied?

It is possible that one might accept that cities have been characterized by proximity, spontaneous encounters with strangers, and shared space, and that COVID will change this in permanent ways, but to find this change neutral. Perhaps this is just a shift to a different set of embodied patterns. Why should we consider it a loss? I think the loss here is substantial for at least two kinds of reasons. The first is that it is a disruptive and disorienting change for those of us who live in cities; the subjective loss of a way of life that is inculcated into our embodied agency and existence is real and not small. The second is that, without ranking ways of life, there are distinctive virtues to city life in its pre-pandemic form that will be objective losses if they vanish.

Consider first the subjective losses to city dwellers. We all learn to be at home in spaces by mastering what architectural theorist David Seamon has called "place ballets." In a place ballet, movements flow together in ways essentially supported by and integrated with a place (Seamon 2002). For instance, consider someone whose job it is to stack produce in a grocery store, while helping customers. We cannot understand their embodied practice except in relationship to how the space is divided into aisles and sections, and contains objects with specific sizes, shapes, and maintenance needs; it is not like they could practice this stacking or customer assistance at home. Conversely, we cannot interpret the space of the store as meaningful unless we see it as having been organized by people who use it and move through it. In such cases, the space and its users form a tightly interwoven system that essentially involves embodied users interacting with each other and with a material space. Markets, train stations, and school yards are all examples of places characterized by distinctive place ballets: kids on a school playground divide themselves up and move in certain ways, with different children claiming different pieces of space and using them in different, coordinated ways, for example. These ways of moving make no sense except as oriented to and embedded within a particular material place. The shape of the schoolyard equipment, the location of a shady tree, and the placement of benches are all intimately integrated into the place ballet of the schoolyard.

The point is that city dwellers have been inculcated into specific place ballets, which make us at home in our bodies and spaces. Part of what it is to move around as ourselves and to be at home in the space around us is to engage in these place ballets. We hop on the subway, line up to buy an espresso, navigate cars and pedestrians at busy intersections. These place ballets give us a sense of place and a sense of self and agency. But COVID has disrupted these place ballets, which were characterized in essence by proximity and the flow of contact with strangers. Right now, our movements through city spaces are halting, self-conscious, and artificial, as we measure out distances and work to avoid others, without our naturally inculcated senses of appropriate personal space and movement to help us. We are exceptionally reflective as we move through space right now, and the distances between us are uniform and rigidly calculated. All other people on our streets show up as immediate threats. Our sense of risk and safety has been thrown into chaos; everything seems risky and we have little to no settled or expert ability to determine how risky a situation is, not least because threats are mostly invisible. Our sense of self and place is disrupted by the unavailability of comfortable place ballets. If we redesign cities so as to build in different patterns of movement, new place ballets will develop. But this will still constitute a loss of home and embodied identity for those who lived in cities pre-pandemic. We should take this seriously as an existential loss, however successful redesigned cities are from the standpoints of economics and health.

Moreover, from an impersonal point of view, and without giving an overall ranking of different forms of geographic life, we might well think that there are virtues built into the ways of living of pre-pandemic city dwellers, that are at risk of being lost. Richard Sennett influentially argued that urban community should not be centered on intimate relationships. Sennett claims that purified, homogenous spaces that emulate the private domestic home lessen our contact points with unpredictable complexity, not only limiting the skills we develop, but also reducing our openness and flexibility when it comes to developing new skills. Cultural norms and material and economic structures in the suburbs close off family life from the rest of life, unlike the plazas, streets, foyers, and thin walls of the city. For Sennett, the fact that we have multiple contact points and shared spaces with random diverse strangers in the city has direct normative value for human flourishing. He argues that purified spaces that neatly divide up public and private terrains and lessen contact points between non-intimates, such as are built into the traditional design of suburbs, reduce our ability to cope with the unexpected and our acceptance of contingency, complex social interactions, and difference. Meanwhile, Richard Sampson (1992) points out that the seclusion and privatization of suburban White middle-class life means activities such as drinking, arguing, and hanging out, which are street activities in shared space for urbanites, are activities done at home with family for this group. Sampson argues that people for whom these activities are privatized do not have an opportunity to develop skills at perceiving the distinction between normal, friendly public versions of these activities and threatening ones. They quickly read any public drunkenness, argument, or such like, as the threat of unmanageable disorder rather than being able to tell when it is part of the place ballet of the space. In fact, city dwellers are consistently more tolerant of difference and less authoritarian than their suburban and rural counterparts (Thompson 2012). We can hypothesize that these systematic differences in attitude can be partially traced to our embodied practices.

There are special skills that city dwellers develop in virtue of living in an unpredictable space of proximity to others. Becoming at home in a city involves developing the skill of coping with new and unexpected situations, and with people and things we do not completely understand. We need to learn how to judge and adjust on the fly, and how to tolerate uncertainty. City living requires that we be fast and competent at moving between different skillsets and adjusting our expectations, responding smoothly and quickly to new sounds, interactions, obstructions, and so forth. In order to navigate a city successfully, we need a large background store of place knowledge. We need to be able to tell quickly when someone needs help or is just playing us; we need to be alert to people in our way, or in need of our seat. As we move around the city, we do things like join and wait in queues; dodge slow walkers and oblivious umbrellas; recognize the needs of strangers who move and take up space differently; catch the attention of a cab driver or a barista; pet some dogs and avoid others. Along our path, people talk to us and move around us; maybe they even yell at us or ask us for things. We need to know how to distinguish between the harmless and the dangerous drunk. We have to negotiate a large and subtle set of codes for personal space and eye contact; these vary by neighbourhood and by demographics but also by specific location (a queue versus a park) and even by time of day (a subway car in rush hour versus late at night). Walking city streets often requires negotiating various risks and exigencies, although this may be in addition to and intertwined with experiencing distinctive pleasures in urban movement. While city interactions require attention and mindfulness, a competent dweller who has mastered these skills will be able to bring perceptual frameworks and problem-solving strategies on board fluidly, expertly, and unreflectively. Many of our skills and perceptual practices are sedimented into our bodies and embody implicit and perhaps uncodifiable norms – our shifting sense of how to balance eye contact, personal body space, and privacy is a good example.

Our bodies and perceptual capacities are deeply shaped by this sort of city-specific skill mastery. The way we hold our body and perceive our surroundings in urban spaces varies from city to city, and demographic to demographic, and neighbourhood to neighbourhood. The skills we develop and the norms our bodies internalize shape our embodied perceptions and sense of self and place. One can vividly see tourists who have not internalized these local skills and stances and perceptual capacities flounder through a city, their motions clunky and ineffective.

Will we lose these skills if city spaces are intensively redesigned so as to be orderly and organized, with people flowing neatly past one another without contact? This is a risk of pandemic planning. All the public health messaging during the pandemic has encouraged us to restrict our interactions to our immediate family. The abandonment of busy downtowns, and post-pandemic planning that focuses on distance and separation, may well continue this privatization of socializing and our use of space. If we rebuilt city space so as to emulate the suburban focus on the home and the domain of intimate relationships, we risk losing valuable skills and flexibility that have traditionally attached to city life.

Michael Kimmelman (2020) argues that the pandemic not only harms city dwellers, but undercuts our resilience in the face of harm. He points out that when we face a crisis, it is our ability to come together and act cooperatively that is most likely to let us repair. Empirically, he is right: communities survive disasters better when they have resilient social support networks, and isolation is one of the most important risk factors during a shared crisis; social connection literally saves lives during an ecological disaster (Klienberg 1999; Cutter et al 2008). But the pandemic has forced us to take the opposite approach – to stay more isolated the worse things become. Kimmelman claims that the pandemic is distinctively anti-urban.

City spaces, he writes, were built to be used together, so those of us in cities are now occupying spaces maximally ill-suited to this crisis: "social distancing ... not only runs up against our fundamental desires to interact, but also against the way we have built our cities and plazas, subways and skyscrapers. They are all designed to be occupied and animated collectively." (Kimmelman 2020)

But this is only part of the story. In response to Kimmelman, Kevin Rogan points out in "The City and the City and Coronavirus" (2020) that as many of us mourn the loss of our urban lives, millions of urban dwellers are still forced to go to work under unsafe conditions. For many of us, who can work from home or who have the means to take a break from work, suffering from isolation is itself a privilege. Rogan points out that the romantic idea that we are all suffering from loss of togetherness depends on the myth that we were together rather than separated by structural inequality to begin with. Building on Rogan's point, not only are millions of poorer city dwellers forced to move through crowded space even as the rest are forced to isolate at home, but when we do move through the city, our bodies are not treated equally. Unsurprisingly, Black and Brown bodies are being differentially targeted for policing and harassment for breaking curfews or violating masking and distancing rules during the pandemic (Noor 2020). Our losses are not the same as one another's; there is no easy "we" in the city, despite our sharing space.

I think that both Kimmelman and Rogan are right. Agency in cities is deeply unequal and cities are fractured in all sorts of ways, and the pandemic has made these divisions even more vivid. But at the same time, cities are materially built on principles of proximity, shared space, and close-up interaction, and so the current moment is fundamentally anti-urban, insofar as we are minimizing and stigmatizing such uses of space. We can avoid romanticizing cities while acknowledging that many city dwellers are facing an embodied existential crisis on top of the economic and health crises the pandemic has wrought.

We may need to redesign city space in order to keep it safe and populated, by building in design features that keep the flow of people distanced and orderly, and which encourage home-based activities and privilege intimate encounters over mixing with strangers. But these redesigns risk compromising both our embodied sense of home, and the distinctive virtues of urban life. Of course, humans are creative and resilient, and new forms of life with their own distinctive value will likely emerge. It is also possible that as the pandemic fades into a memory, urban life in its traditional form will resurface, at least to an extent. Despite such hope, those of us who love and feel at home in cities have real reasons to grieve.

NOTE

1 This second half of the paper will draw heavily upon the preface and chapter two of my book, *City Living: How Urban Dwellers and Urban Spaces Make One Another* (2021), although my argument there is different and for the most part does not concern the pandemic. Some paragraphs are reused here.

REFERENCES

Bereitschaft, Bradley, and Daniel Scheller. 2020. "How Might the COVID-19 Pandemic Affect 21st Century Urban Design, Planning, and Development?" *Urban Science* 4, no. 4: 56–78.

Buyahar, Noah. 2020. "The Work-from-Home Boom is Here to Stay. Get Ready for Pay Cuts." *Bloomberg News*, 17 December 2020.

Cutter, Susan L., Lindsey Barnes, Melissa Berry, Christopher Burton, Elijah Evans, Eric Tate, and Jennifer Webb. 2008. "A Place-Based Model for Understanding Community Resilience to Natural Disasters." *Global Environmental Change* 18, no. 4: 598–606.

Evans, Gary W. 2003. "The Built Environment and Mental Health." *Journal of Urban Health* 80, no. 4: 536–55.

Jacobs, Jane. 1961. *The Death and Life of Great American Cities*. New York: Vintage.

Kimmelman, Michael. 2020. "Can City Life Survive Coronavirus?" *New York Times*, 17 March 2020.

Klinenberg, Eric. 1999. "Denaturalizing Disaster: A Social Autopsy of the 1995 Chicago Heat Wave." *Theory and Society* 28, no. 2 (April): 239–95.

Kukla, Quill R. 2021. *City Living: How Urban Dwellers and Urban Spaces Make One Another*. Oxford: Oxford University Press.

Litman, Todd. 2020. "Pandemic-Resilient Community Planning." *Victoria Transport Policy Institute*.

Mehaffy, Michael. 2020. "Why We Need 'Sociable Distancing.'" *Congress for the New Urbanism*, 30 March 2020.

Noor, Poppy. 2020. "A Tale of Two Cities: How New York Police Enforce Social Distancing by the Color of Your Skin." *The Guardian*, 4 May 2020.

Oldenburg, Ray. 1999. *The Great Good Place: Cafes, Coffee Shops, Bookstores, Bars, Hair Salons, and Other Hangouts at the Heart of a Community*. Boston: Da Capo Press.

Rogan, Kevin. 2020. "The City and the City and Coronavirus." *Failed Architecture*, 6 April 2020.

Sennett, Richard. 1992. *The Uses of Disorder: Personal Identity and City Life*. New York: WW Norton & Company.

Thompson, Michael J. 2012. "Suburban Origins of the Tea Party: Spatial Dimensions of the New Conservative Personality." *Critical Sociology* 38, no. 4: 511–28.

Wirth, Louis. 1938. "Urbanism as a Way of Life." *American Journal of Sociology* 44, no.1: 1–24.

Young, Iris Marion. 1990. "City Life and Difference." In *Justice and the Politics of Difference*, 226–256. Princeton: Princeton University Press.

2

Transforming Work and Restarting the Economy in a Post-Pandemic Era

6

Technology and Globalization in the Post-COVID Economy

Etienne Lalé and Sophie Osotimehin

INTRODUCTION

On 25 January 2020, the first international day of protest against 5G technology took place in hundreds of cities in both industrialized and developing countries. Protesters argued that 5G technology poses a serious threat to health and the environment, to privacy and cybersecurity, and to energy consumption, and called for a moratorium on the adoption and wide-scale implementation of this technology. This event was soon eclipsed by the coronavirus crisis. In the United States, the first few cases were diagnosed at the end of January. The epidemic unfolded in Europe in February and March, and on 11 March the World Health Organization (WHO) declared the COVID-19 outbreak a global pandemic. If anything, tensions around 5G technologies only escalated during the COVID crisis. With half of humanity on lockdown in April 2020, the surge of telework, e-learning, and online socializing amplified the need for high-speed broadband internet services. In the meantime, amid growing geopolitical tensions between the United States and China, the Trump administration urged European leaders to ban Chinese companies from Europe's 5G infrastructure on national-security grounds. While the race to roll out 5G seems unstoppable, concerns have emerged that the post-COVID era could witness a technological fragmentation of the world economy between two "Internet systems," a Chinese one and a Western one.

The example of 5G technologies illustrates well the intricate relationships between technology, globalization, and the pandemic.

It brings to light the existence of trends that predate the crisis – dissensions about the adoption of a new technology, in a context of increasing fragmentation of the world economy. And it begs the question of whether the COVID-19 crisis is a *krisis* in the Ancient Greek meaning of the word, that is to say a turning point. Will the pandemic bring prior trends in technological change and globalization to a halt? Or, instead, will it amplify the developments that started before the pandemic? These are the questions that we address in this chapter. To answer them, our approach is to systematically provide context and perspective we see relevant to understand the long-lasting impact of the crisis on technology and globalization. There is much to say about the interaction between the crisis and technology on the one hand, and that between the crisis and globalization on the other hand. Therefore, we first examine these two topics in isolation from each other. We then discuss what we see as the unifying, underlying theme: how economic disparities will be addressed after the pandemic. We argue that this issue will deeply shape the evolutions of the post-COVID economy.

PART I: TECHNOLOGY

The way we work, spend our leisure time, or shop have all been profoundly altered during the pandemic. Information and communication technologies (ICT) and digital services have been a lifeline during the crisis as many of these activities moved online in an effort to limit in-person contacts. In the US, it is estimated that half of all employed persons worked entirely or partly from home in May 2020 (Bick et al. 2020). The videoconferencing company Zoom reported a fivefold increase in its number of clients in the third quarter of 2020, relative to the same quarter last fiscal year. In a period during which many companies were struggling financially, the online retailer Amazon reported year-on-year increases in its total sales of 37% in the third quarter of 2020. Without the support of ICT and digital services, the lockdowns that were put in place during the pandemic could never have lasted long enough to "flatten the curve."

Although exceptional in its magnitude, the surge in the use of ICT and digital services during the pandemic is only the acceleration of a long-run trend towards the digitization of our economies for most sectors. The crisis is transformative only for a few sectors.

To put current developments in perspective, let us remind ourselves that our economies have been operating more and more in the digital space since the invention of the computer. A few numbers showing the pre-COVID growth of the use of digital services and online shopping illustrate this fact. The digital economy, which includes online trade, computers, software, and online services, grew in the US at a remarkable 6.8% annual rate from 2005 to 2018.[1]

Before the crisis, the tech companies, Google, Amazon, Facebook, Apple, and Microsoft were already among the largest firms by market capitalization. Online retail sales went from less than 1% of total retail sales in 2000 to 11% at the end of 2019 (US Department of Commerce 2020). The pandemic pushed the share of online retail to 14% in the third quarter of 2020. Like in online retail, in many areas, the acceleration of digital services is noteworthy but maybe not as transformative as one could have thought.

Pandemic-related change has been more radical for sectors like health or education, in which the movement towards digitization had been much slower and online services were scant before the crisis. For example, a recent study of 16 million American patients shows that virtual medical consultation accounted for less than 1% of total visits before the pandemic. By June 2020, virtual consultations had reached about 20% of total visits (Patel et al. 2020). Doctolib, a French digital health firm, reported that its video consultations in Europe increased during the pandemic from one thousand to a hundred thousand a day. Higher education is also profoundly affected. Online learning became the norm in many universities across the world, and Massive Online Open Courses (MOOCs) grew exponentially during the pandemic. For instance, the online provider of MOOCs Coursera reports that enrollment went from 1.6 million to 10.3 million between mid-March and mid-April – a 543% increase.

Which of these Changes Will Persist in the Post-COVID Economy?

This is an open question as of this writing, but several elements strongly point to permanent shifts towards digitization and online services. First, after being forced to experiment these technologies and new services, many firms and consumers would discover they have a taste for them. As an example, early surveys suggest that working-from-home arrangements would stay in high-demand when the pandemic is over (Barrero et al. 2020). Another important force suggesting that changes will persist post-pandemic is the digital investments that firms have made in order to continue operating during the pandemic. Economists call them "sunk costs," in the sense that these costs cannot be easily recouped once they have been incurred. Firms will continue using these new digital processes now that these up-front costs have been paid. Finally, in some sectors the pandemic has forced regulators to lift barriers that had hampered the development of online services. In France, regulators relaxed the rule that allowed video medical consultations only after a first in-person visit. In the US, Medicare expanded its coverage of remote consultations beyond rural areas. It is unlikely that these regulations will revert to what they were before the pandemic.

More importantly, to understand whether and how these changes will matter for the post-COVID economy, we must ask ourselves how they will affect productivity. In turn, this will inform us about future implications for labour markets.

The key point is that the acceleration of digitization opens the way to more computerization and automation. Indeed, with the shift to paperless information and the development of digital services, more data becomes available to feed machine-learning algorithms and more tasks become amenable to automation. In the retail industry, for example, the development of e-commerce will increase automation since robots can more easily operate in warehouses than in brick-and-mortar stores. Beyond the forced adoption of these new technologies during the pandemic, the increase in digitization and automation may also be driven by firms' willingness to reduce their exposure to future epidemic risks. As digital information facilitates the optimization of production and automation lowers production costs and improves quality, these changes will bolster productivity. In the medium to long run, this improvement in productivity will be accentuated by the reallocation of activities and workers towards firms that were quicker to adopt new technologies.[2]

As Computerization and Automation Expand, What Will Happen to Workers Whose Jobs Will Disappear in This Process?

This is not the first time society is anxious about technological progress displacing workers and creating unemployment. This question has surged many times in the past, particularly in periods of accelerating technological change. In his 1930 writing about the "Economic Possibilities for our Grandchildren," John Maynard Keynes warned his readers about the pressing issue of technological unemployment. So did Wassily Leontief who grimly predicted that "the role of humans as the most important factor of production is bound to diminish in the same way that the role of horses in agricultural production was first diminished and then eliminated by the introduction of tractors" (Leontief 1983). History has proved both of them wrong. The three technological revolutions that we have witnessed since the nineteenth century have not made human labour redundant. In fact, the employment rate, calculated as share of employed workers out of the working-age population, has been roughly constant throughout this period.

While there is no debate that technological progress causes some workers to lose their jobs, the question of how long those workers will remain unemployed and how important this issue is in the long run is much more complex. By reducing the number of workers needed to produce the same quantity of goods, automation reduces labour demand. At the same time, however, automation drastically cuts production costs and therefore lowers prices and increases demand for goods. If demand and output increase sufficiently, then labour demand and employment will actually increase after automation. Given the lack of downward trend in the employment rate, the consensus among economists is that the increase in demand is sufficiently strong that technological unemployment is not an issue.

In a recent work, Acemoglu and Restropo (2018) propose a complementary explanation. They argue that viewing technological change has a force that only substitutes machines for humans is restrictive. Technological change also leads to the creation of new tasks – tasks in which humans have a comparative advantage. As they explained using Leontief's analogy "the difference between human labor and horses is that humans have a comparative advantage in new and more complex tasks. Horses did not." This comparative advantage is what allows employment and the labour share to remain stable even if the number of tasks that is automated grows over time. Key to their analysis is also the fact that technological change is endogenous: a wave of automation lowers the effective cost of producing with labour, discouraging further efforts to automate additional tasks and encouraging the creation of new tasks.[3] While higher unemployment remains a possibility, taken together, these elements do suggest that, like previous episodes of technological adoption, digitization will not create mass unemployment in the near future.

Digitization will, however, exacerbate the polarization of the labour market. Polarization refers to the rapid employment growth in jobs at the bottom and top of the skill distribution relative to middle-skill jobs.[4] Several works by David Autor and co-authors (see, for example, Autor et al. 2006) help understand the relationships between the development of computers and increasing automation of tasks on the one hand, and polarization on the other hand. The main idea is that not all tasks are affected by computerization and automation in the same way; computers can replace workers in some tasks while they can contribute to the workers' inputs and raise their productivity in other tasks. In the words of economists, the key distinction is whether computers are substitute or complement to workers for the various tasks performed on the job. As emphasized by Autor et al (2006), routine tasks (either cognitive or manual) are more susceptible to computerization. The demand for workers who perform routine tasks, such as bookkeeping or repetitive assembly work, and who are typically middle-skill workers, declines with automation. By contrast, non-routine manual tasks, such as janitorial or home-care work, are harder to automate. Computers, hence, do not substitute for the least-skilled workers, who are typically employed in these occupations. Finally, Autor et al. (2006) show that if computers are complementary to non-routine cognitive tasks, the demand for workers performing these types of tasks, such as physicians or financial analysts, increases. Hence, by accelerating digitization, the pandemic crisis will contribute to increasing computerization and automation, which in turn leads to more labour market polarization.[5]

With recent advances in machine learning and mobile robotics and the surge in data brought about by the increasing digitization of our economies, the range of tasks that can be automated is constantly broadening. In fact, since Autor and co-authors wrote their paper in 2006, technological advances have permitted the automation of many tasks considered non-routine. Improvement in pattern recognition has made possible the automation of non-routine cognitive tasks, such as translation, which until recently were deemed too complex to be automated.[6] At the same time, progress in mobile robotics has widened the scope of computerization towards non-routine manual tasks. In a much-discussed work, Frey and Osborne (2013) find that with these recent technological advances, 47% of jobs in the US are at high risk of computerization. These are jobs that do not involve tasks that remain challenging to computerize (perception and manipulation, creative intelligence, and social intelligence tasks). In short, assembly line or clerical jobs are far from the only jobs at risk of being displaced by computers.

To sum up, technology developments in the aftermath for the pandemic crisis will likely amplify inequality across workers. We will discuss policy responses in the last section of this chapter. Before doing so, to fully understand the post-COVID challenges that increased inequality will pose, we must place them in a global context.

PART II: GLOBALIZATION

Globalization, broadly defined, refers to the acceleration of the flow of goods and services, people, capital, and technologies all over the planet. Most indicators used to measure these flows exhibit the same profile in 2020: they fall precipitously with the outbreak of the COVID crisis. For example, the world trade monitor of the Netherlands' Bureau of Economic Analysis indicates that world merchandise trade fell by 15% between the beginning of 2020 and mid-March;[7] foreign direct investment flows, for which 2020 data are not yet available, are expected to fall by 40% relative to 2019;[8] the number of international commercial flights dropped by 80% between the end of February and mid-April.[9] By these metrics, it seems that globalization suffered a sudden regress during the COVID-19 crisis. This being said, the picture is not entirely bleak. The crisis has also coincided with an increased flow of ideas exchanged all over the planet, as well as a burst in scientific collaboration well illustrated by the development of a vaccine against the new virus.

Besides the collapse of international trade and investment, several developments related to policy making and international relations cast a larger shadow over the process of globalization. Indeed, multilateral cooperation has been seriously challenged during the crisis. Perhaps the most emblematic example was the announcement made on 14 April 2020 that the US were to halt funding to the World Health Organization. Another telling example were the series of uncoordinated border closures in Europe, openly violating the Schengen regulations. In parallel, the COVID crisis also witnessed a resurgence of protectionist policies and isolationism in both industrialized and developing countries.[10] The crisis laid ground for a my-country-first rhetoric that seems to appeal to a large part of the public opinion.

More generally, the crisis has been perceived by many as an indication that economies were excessively interconnected, and that the appropriate policy response would be to sever some of these connections to prevent future health and economic crises from spreading over the world so rapidly.

The backlash against globalization is, however, not new. The pandemic crisis took place in a context where globalization had already started to slow down.

To put current developments in perspective, it is worth starting by noting that globalization is a process that evolves through waves – that is to say bursts of progress, often followed by periods of regress. During the forty-year period that begun around 1870, the world economy experienced what has become known as "the first globalization." Largely propelled by the invention of the steamship, which reduced shipping time and costs, international trade developed rapidly during that period, so much so that export as a share of world GDP went from 6% at the beginning of the period to 14% on the eve of WWI.[11] Not only were the flows of goods, capital, and people high across borders during that period, but there were also fierce political debates on trade openness and the desirability of implementing trade barriers to protect the domestic economy. This era of globalization came to an end with WWI and the Great Depression. After a few decades, the globalization process resumed, and the world economy experienced another wave of globalization. A distinctive feature of this wave, which started in the early 1980s, is the emergence of so-called global value chains. To quote Antràs (2020)'s definition, "a global value chain, or GVC, consists of a series of stages involved in producing a product or service that is sold to consumers, with each stage adding value, and with at least two stages being produced in different countries. A firm participates in a GVC if it produces at least one stage in a GVC." Much of our discussion of the future of globalization will revolve around the role of GVCs.

The latest wave of globalization had started to lose strength prior to the pandemic. As shown recently by Pol Antràs (2020), a battery of indicators, such as world trade as a share of world GDP, portfolio investment inflows, and foreign direct investment from multinational companies, have grown at a slower rate since the 2007–09 recession compared to the 1986–2008 period.[12] Antràs calls the years 1986 to 2008 the era of "hyper-globalization," which he argues had been fuelled by mainly three factors. First: automation and the ICT revolution that helped the development of global production networks. Second: trade liberalization, through the lowering of tariffs and making of binding trade commitments via the GATT/WTO and regional agreements. Third: the fall of the "iron curtain" and China's transition to a market economy, which created an enormous increase in the number of workers who participate in the world free-market economy. At least two of these factors – trade liberalization and the spread of the free-market economy – are one-off events, suggesting that hyper-globalization could not have continued at the same pace.[13] As a result, when COVID-19 struck the world economy, it had already entered a new era that can be described as "slowbalisation" – a term coined by the bank Morgan Stanley a year before the COVID crisis.

An important dimension of the slowbalisation era is that it witnesses sporadic but fierce protests against globalization throughout the world. These protests are largely rooted in resentment related to what economists call the "distributional effects" of international trade, that is to say the consequences in terms of income inequality. Pressing concerns about these consequences began to mount well before the 2007–09 recession. For instance, in the US, income inequality had been on the rise at least since the early 1980s. Although not the only factor explaining this trend, international trade (and in particular trade integration with China) is widely perceived as a key driver of rising inequality.[14] Since the 2000s, these protests have led to the emergence of populist parties and leaders with a de-globalisation policy agenda.[15] Well before the COVID crisis, populist movements had been gaining ground in multiple countries, with Orbán becoming the Prime Minister of Hungary in 2010, the United Kingdom voting to leave the European Union in 2016, and the Trump administration launching a tariff war against China in 2018. Add to these observations the fact that the WTO has been in an impasse for years with the current round of Doha negotiations; it is clear that the policy challenges faced by globalization started long before the pandemic.

Will the Pandemic Change These Pre-Existing Trends? And How?

The COVID crisis certainly demonstrates the vulnerability of economies to disruptions or "shocks" originating abroad. The key point we wish to make is that there is no reason to believe that the world economy in general, and firms involved in GVCs in particular, had been myopic about the possibility of being hit by some of these shocks. The reason is twofold. First, these shocks are not as rare as one would think. Add together force majeure events (e.g., an acute climate event, a pandemic); geopolitical events (e.g., a financial crisis in a given region of the world, a military conflict); interferences from malicious actors (e.g., a cyber attack); or idiosyncratic events (e.g., an industrial accident), then a firm engaged in international trade should expect some disruption of its economic activity over a not-too-long period of time. Second, the disruptions entailed by these events are very costly, and therefore firms likely keep a close eye on the occurrence of these shocks. In a 2020 report, the McKinsey Global Institute evaluates that these disruptions cause top international firms to suffer, on average, a loss worth 42% of one year's revenue every decade.[16] In the report, the Institute surveys 605 leading business executives about their strategy to increase the resilience of their firms. Forty-four per cent of them report that they would sacrifice short-term efficiency to build resilience through, for example, dual sourcing, making inventories of critical products, and so on.

If anything, the COVID crisis helped reveal that GVSs were perhaps too vulnerable to the disruptions caused by these shocks. If firms that participate in GVCs find it worth making investments to avoid these disruptions, what will be their strategy to increase resilience? And how will this shape the future of globalization?

Reducing exposure to international shocks by re-shoring parts of the production process (essentially, a reversal of the process that has been fueling the current wave of globalization) seems unlikely. Indeed, at least two factors run counter to this scenario. One: the presence of large sunk costs when firms engage in offshoring and outsourcing. For instance, an important component of the firms' participation in GVCs is related to search costs, meaning the costs involved in finding the "right" business partner. Besides, the value of trade links involves significant relational capital – economists call it match-specific capital – that would be destroyed with a re-shoring of production. Two: the continued search for lower production costs which, among other costs, include the effects of the disruption of production chains. This force has driven much of the offshoring of manufacturing during the era of "hyper-globalization." Concentrating production in the domestic economy reduces exposure to international shocks but at the cost of increasing vulnerability to domestic shocks. To lower disruption costs, a more effective strategy is to build resilience by relying on a more diversified pool of suppliers. In sum, for firms that already participate in GVCs and for those that will join this process, it seems likely that the post-COVID era will be characterized by a re-bound towards more diversification – a re-boost of globalization.

There is one element that might nuance this statement, however. As already mentioned, automation and the ICT revolution have been instrumental in the development of hyper-globalization. The development of digital platforms should continue to foster firm participation in GVCs, and thereby to boost globalization. But recent technological advances might also act in the reverse direction, if new automation becomes a substitute to offshoring; 3D printing might be one such example. This technology has now reached a stage of development where it can be easily adapted and incorporated into firms' production process. In particular, a key feature of 3D printing is that it is highly versatile and portable, which makes it possible to take production to local markets. By being closer to customers, local manufacturing allows to save on transportation costs and becomes cost-competitive compared to mass production in foreign countries. This suggest that manufacturing 3D printing could induce firms to re-shore parts of their production process to the domestic economy and sever their links with some of their foreign suppliers. At the time of writing this chapter, empirical evidence on the substitutability between new technologies and offshoring is still too scarce to reach definite conclusions on this matter. As an aside, note that if firms were to relocate part of their production in the domestic country by using these technological improvements, the number of jobs brought back on the homeland would be close to zero.

Whereas changes in GVC firms' strategies are unlikely to reverse globalization, more serious threats to globalisation exist. The main threat comes from trade policy. Recall that trade liberalization, which is one of the factors that propelled the era of hyper-globalization, is the result of policy choices. Were more protectionist policies adopted across the world, the international flow of goods and people could be drastically altered. As discussed above, the pandemic occurred in a context of mounting discontent about globalization. The crisis has most likely exacerbated this resentment, notably by widening inequality between workers. It has disproportionately hurt low-income workers, reflecting the toll the crisis took on hotels, restaurants, and other businesses in the hospitality sectors (Kurmann et al. 2020).

If working-from-home arrangements remain prevalent in the post-COVID economy, many jobs in these sectors will be permanently destroyed, leading this rise in inequality to persist well beyond the COVID crisis. In fact, inequality may widen even further in the coming decades since, as explained earlier, the acceleration in digital trends will amplify the polarization of the labour market. The rise in inequality and the hollowing out of the middle class will continue to tip the political agenda towards anti-globalization policies.

CONCLUSION

As we have seen, the trends in technology and globalization are interrelated in many dimensions – the most important of which being the rise in inequality, a consequence of technological change (and to a lesser extent of globalization), and at the same time a key factor behind the backlash against globalization. To conclude this chapter, we wish to highlight that the rise in inequality and the resulting push towards deglobalization are not set in stone; these evolutions hinge on the path taken by future policies. Income gaps between low-, middle-, and high-wage workers are shaped by tax and other redistributive policies as much as by underlying technological shifts. Take North America and European countries, for instance. These groups of countries have substantially different levels of inequality even though the same technology and globalization factors are at play for both groups. The wealthiest 1% of Americans hold 37% of total wealth whereas the same group holds 23% of wealth in France. What is striking is that transatlantic differences in inequality are observed also on pre-tax income, indicating that the progressivity of the tax code is not the only element shaping the distribution of income.[17] Beyond tax policy, we see two areas where policies can play a critical role in curbing the trend analyzed in this chapter. First: competition and anti-trust policies. Giant tech companies and digital platforms will leave the crisis even stronger than they entered it. The enormous market power of these firms can only tilt the income distribution in favour of the richer section. This is an area where better and more effective anti-trust laws can make a difference. Second: education and training policies. The acceleration of automation will make universal access to higher education and adequate training policies even more important than before in reducing income gaps. More emphasis should be put on developing skills that complement computers, such as creativity and social intelligence.

The pandemic will leave the world economy more digitized and more productive. Without the appropriate policy responses, it will leave it less equal and less global than before.

NOTES

1. Growth rate of the value added of the digital economy (Bureau of Economic Analysis 2020).
2. This reallocation of resources towards high-productivity firms, which is central for aggregate productivity growth, typically accelerate during downturns (e.g., Foster et al., 2016). This productivity-enhancing feature will be present in the current recession as well, although the large COVID-19 relief packages implemented in many countries may reduce the strength of this channel.
3. However, Acemoglu and Restropo (2018) also show that technological change can reduce employment (increase unemployment) if automating tasks becomes increasingly easier relative to creating new tasks.
4. There is a vast literature on the polarization of labour markets, showing that this phenomenon has been observed since the late 1980s in many industrialized economies; see, among many others, Goos and Maning (2003) for evidence for the United Kingdom and Autor et al (2006) for US evidence.
5. This aspect is not specific to the pandemic, in the sense that recessions in general are times of increased labour market polarization. Recent work by Jaimovich and Siu (2020) shows that the reduction in the proportion of middle-skill jobs is concentrated in periods of recession: 88% of the job loss in middle-skill, routine occupations since the mid-1980s has occurred during economic downturns.
6. Brynjolfsson and McAfee (2014) provide a vivid description of recent progress in artificial intelligence, robotics, and digital technologies.
7. See CPB Netherlands Bureau for Economic Policy Analysis. 2021.
8. Calculations from the Organization for Economic Co-operation and Development (2021).
9. According to the trade barometers monitored by the World Trade Organization (WTO).
10. We should note that these protectionist policies were of a somewhat unusual nature. While standard protectionist measures aim at slowing down imports of foreign goods to protect the domestic economy, the goal of policies that were in place during the crisis was instead to prevent the export of certain goods, such as face masks and artificial respirators.

11 Figures from the World Economic Forum 2021.
12 The trend change in the international flow of people is, however, is not so clear. The share of international migrants in the world population, which was on the rise during the 2000s, continues to grow after the 2007–09 recession at about the same rate.
13 Whether the other factor – automation and the ICT revolution – is also contributing to the slowdown of globalization after the 2007–09 recession is unclear, as will be discussed in the last paragraphs of this section.
14 As has been discussed in Part I: Technology, labour market polarization induced by computerization and automation is another key contributor to the increase of income inequality across workers.
15 The 2007–09 economic crisis, which started as a financial crisis in the US but then spread globally and triggered a sovereign debt crisis in Europe, probably played a role, by showing the dangers of an unregulated, hyper-globalized finance industry.
16 This number is computed on average across sectors. There is a lot of variation across sectors: for firms in the pharmaceutical industry, the expected revenue loss is worth 24% of one year of their revenues, while for firms of the aerospace industry the expected loss is at 67%.
17 The top 1% earn 20% of national income in the US vs 10% in Europe (Chancel 2019).

REFERENCES

Acemoglu, Daron, and Pascual Restrepo. 2018. "The Race Between Man and Machine:
Implications of Technology for Growth, Factor Shares, and Employment." *American Economic Review* 108, no. 6 (June): 1488–1542.

Antràs, Pol. 2020. "Conceptual Aspects of Global Value Chains." *World Bank Policy Research* Working Paper no. 9114 (February).

Antràs, Pol. 2020. "De-Globalisation? Global Value Chains in the Post-COVID-19 Age." *National Bureau of Economic Research* Working Paper no. 28115 (November).

Autor, David H., Lawrence F. Katz, and Melissa S. Kearney. 2006. "The Polarization of the US Labor Market." *American Economic Review* 96, no. 2 (May):189–94.

Barrero, Jose Maria, Nicholas Bloom, and Steven J. Davis. 2020. "Why Working from Home Will Stick." *University of Chicago Becker Friedman Institute for Economics* Working Paper no. 2020-174 (December).

Bick, Alexander, Adam Blandin, and Karel Mertens. 2020. "Work from Home After the COVID-19 Outbreak." *Federal Reserve Bank of Dallas* Working Paper no. 2017 (June).

Brynjolfsson, Erik, and Andrew McAfee. 2014. *The Second Machine Age: Work, Progress, and Prosperity in a Time of Brilliant Technologies.* New York: W. W. Norton & Company.

Chancel, Lucas. 2019. "Ten Facts about Inequality in Advanced Economies." *World Inequality Database* Working Paper 2019–15 (October).

CPB Netherlands Bureau for Economic Policy Analysis. 2021. "World Trade Monitor." CPB Economic Analysis. https://www.cpb.nl/en/worldtrademonitor.

Frey, Carl Benedikt, and Michael A. Osborne. 2017. "The Future of Employment: How Susceptible are Jobs to Computerisation?" *Technological Forecasting and Social Change* 114 (January): 254–280.

Maarten Goos and Alan Manning. 2003. "McJobs and MacJobs: The Growing Polarisation of Jobs in the UK." In *The Labour Market Under New Labour: The State of Working Britain*, edited by Richard Dickens, Paul Gregg, and Jonathan Wadsworth, 70–85. London: Palgrave Macmillan.

Foster, Lucia, Cheryl Grim, and John Haltiwanger. 2016. "Reallocation in the Great Recession: Cleansing or Not?" *Journal of Labor Economics* 34, no. S1 (January): S293-S331.

Jaimovich, Nir, and Henry E. Siu. 2020. "Job Polarization and Jobless Recoveries." *Review of Economics and Statistics* 102, no. 1 (March): 129–147.

Kurmann, André, Etienne Lalé, and Lien Ta. 2020. "The Impact of COVID-19 on Small Business Employment and Hours: Real-time Estimates with Homebase Data." *ESG-UQAM Chaire en macroéconomie et prévisions* Working Paper 2020–02 (April).

Leontief, Wassily. 1983. "National Perspective: The Definition of Problems and Opportunities." In *The Long-Term impact of Technology on Employment and Unemployment*, edited by The National Academy of Engineering, 3–7. Washington: The National Academies Press.

McKinsey Global Institute. 2020. "Risk, Resilience and Rebalancing in Global Value Chains." McKinsey & Company. 6 August 2020. https://www.mckinsey.com/business-functions/operations/our-insights/risk-resilience-and-rebalancing-in-global-value-chains#.

Nicholson, Jessica R. 2020. "New Digital Economy Estimates." *US Bureau of Economic Analysis* (August).

Organization for Economic Co-operation and Development (OECD). 2020. "Foreign Direct Investment Flows in the Time of COVID-19." http://www.oecd.org/coronavirus/policy-responses/foreign-direct-investment-flows-in-the-time-of-covid-19-a2fa20c4/.

Patel Sadiq Y., Ateev Mehrotra, Haiden A. Huskamp, Lori Uscher-Pines, Ishani Ganguli, and Michael L. Barnett. 2020. "Trends in Outpatient Care Delivery and Telemedicine During the COVID-19 Pandemic in the US." *JAMA Internal Medicine*, 16 November 2020.

US Department of Commerce. 2020. "Quarterly Retail E-Commerce Sales." *US Census Bureau News* 4th Quarter (February).

World Economic Forum. 2021. https://www.weforum.org/.

7

Is Teleworking Here to Stay? Learning from the COVID-19 Experimentation

Tania Saba, Gaëlle Cachat-Rosset, Kevin Daniel André Carillo,
Alain Klarsfeld, Josianne Marsan

INTRODUCTION

For about a decade beginning in the late 1990s, telework received increasing attention from researchers and practitioners in a range of disciplines, including management, psychology, information systems (IS) and transportation engineering (Gajendran and Harrison 2007). Surprisingly, this attention gradually declined in the ensuing decade (Raghuram et al. 2001). Moreover, despite the rapid development of technology since the late 1970s, the use of telework has remained low in Canadian workplaces. Prior to the pandemic, in 78% of companies, less than 10% of staff worked remotely. Only 13% of employees teleworked regularly in 2018, and generally for just a few hours per week (Deng et al. 2020). This is only slightly higher than the rate of 11% who were teleworking in 2008 (Turcotte 2010). It is common knowledge that not all jobs are suited to telework, and that the situation varies greatly from sector to sector. Nevertheless, in 2020 the "telework capability" of the Canadian economy was estimated to be about four out of every ten workers (or 38.9% of jobs). The proportion of jobs that would be suited to telework is even higher for government jobs, where it is estimated to be close to 60% (Deng et al. 2020).

Past experience shows that telework is an effective way to ensure business continuity in the context of major disruptions, particularly in natural or health emergencies (Donnelly and Proctor-Thomson 2015; Mello et al. 2011). With the onset of the COVID-19 pandemic in early spring 2020, many employers and businesses in Canada very quickly shifted to teleworking. Indeed, by the end of March 2020, 39% of Canadian workers were already teleworking (Deng et al. 2020). And while this rate initially declined as lockdowns were lifted, to a low of 26% in September, it started to rise again in the autumn with the increase in COVID-19 cases. As of December 2020, 29% of workers in Canada were teleworking, with the highest rates in Ontario, Quebec, and British Columbia (Statistics Canada 2021). In August 2020, the share of businesses in which at least half of the workforce worked remotely in these provinces stood at 57%, 52%, and 51%, respectively (Statistics Canada 2020).

This intense use of telework during the COVID-19 pandemic has prompted many organizations to express their readiness to adopt telework in a more sustained way once the pandemic ends (OECD 2020). In light of this shift, our chapter explores the potential of telework as a central and strategic way of organizing work in Canada. Specifically, we aim to identify the conditions in which employees would telework, both voluntarily and effectively. This will help guide the actions of organizations to promote telework as a new "normal" work organization.

In this chapter, we present an integrated framework that attempts to explain how, based on the telework experience in the specific context of COVID-19, employees shape their intentions to continue teleworking once the constraints of the pandemic are no longer felt. First, the main factors of adjustment to pandemic-induced telework are analyzed. We then determine the influence of these factors on employees' intention to continue teleworking after the pandemic ends. We conclude this chapter by examining the theoretical and practical implications to be considered should telework become a new mode of work organization.

WILL ADJUSTMENT TO PANDEMIC-INDUCED TELEWORK HELP PREDICT ITS POST-PANDEMIC DEPLOYMENT?

In line with Raghuram et al. (2001), we define pandemic-induced telework adjustment as employees' level of adjustment to the environmental demands of a new telework context triggered by a global health crisis. The theories of reasoned action (Ajzen and Fishbein 1977, 2000; Fishbein and Ajzen, 1975) and planned behaviour

(Ajzen 1985, 1991) provide us with a relevant overall framework to support the assumption that the intention to continue teleworking will predict future behaviour after the pandemic ends (Fekadu and Kraft 2001). We also mobilize the Conservation of Resources Theory (COR; Hobfoll 1989) to explain why employees would want to continue teleworking. It is reasonable to assume that over time, teleworkers would have acquired more innovative information and communication technologies (ICTs) and technological applications, improved the design of their home working environment, adapted work processes and means of communication, or achieved a better work-life balance (Carillo et al. 2020; Rubino et al. 2012). Based on COR and the principle of the "primacy of resource loss" (Hobfoll 2001), it could be argued that teleworkers would be motivated to maintain the gains resulting from the new telework-related resources developed to adjust to the COVID-19 pandemic. The loss of such resources would therefore be psychologically damaging to individuals and likely to generate tensions (Hobfoll 2001; Halbesleben et al. 2014).

THE EFFECT OF TELEWORK ADJUSTMENT VARIABLES ON INTENTION TO CONTINUE TELEWORKING

Our conceptual framework was derived from the crisis-induced telework adjustment framework introduced in the Theory of Work Adjustment (Dawis and Lofquist 1984) and the Interactional Model of Individual Adjustment (Nelson 1990). The framework comprises five groups of variables (see Figure 7.1).

Central to our framework are the components of adjustment to telework, including the intention to continue teleworking after the pandemic ends. Adjustment to telework depends on five factors. The first refers to the environment in which teleworkers carried out their work during the pandemic, that is, the conditions of their remote location, workload, and the overlap of work hours with personal life. The second factor refers to organizational efforts to support teleworkers and to prevent professional isolation. Job characteristics, which make up the third factor, play an important role in determining teleworkers' level of autonomy, the interdependence of tasks, and thus the extent to which the employment system is compatible with telework. The fourth factor takes into account the level of stress resulting from the constraints of the environment or the risks

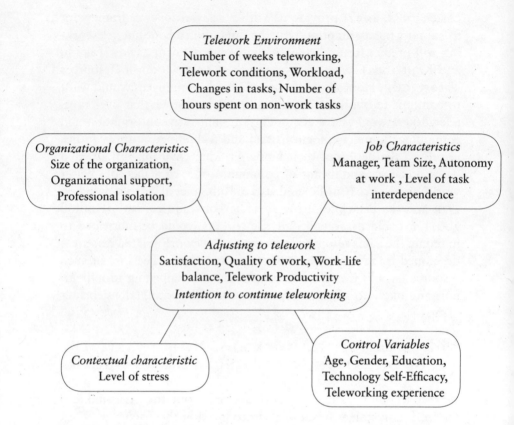

Figure 7.1 | Conceptual framework to analyze telework adjustment and intention to continue teleworking.

caused by the pandemic. Finally, the fifth factor comprises individual characteristics, such as age, gender, education, and comfort level with technology. These were used to examine the variation in telework adjustment according to the individual profiles of teleworkers.

Many of the variables in our framework derive from studies on teleworking, with special attention paid to variables that are specific to the COVID-19 pandemic. The latter include stress levels, the teleworking environment, professional isolation, and organizational support.

To test our framework, we conducted a cross-sectional study over several months. We surveyed 3,239 teleworkers in Quebec during the period of 4 April–30 July 2020. We analyzed the data at monthly intervals to verify changes in teleworkers' perceptions of their adjustment. The survey was promoted on digital platforms and social media. A screening question ensured that data was collected only for individuals who were teleworking when the survey was being administered. We were able to gather data from a diverse sample of teleworkers from a wide variety of industries and backgrounds, and to capture the different aspects and specificities of teleworking during the pandemic. The average age of the sample was 42.08 years (range 19–73 years), and 74% were female. The average tenure was 8.17 years; 28% of respondents held a management position; 68% worked for companies with over five hundred employees (8% between two hundred and five hundred employees; 10% between fifty and two hundred; 14% fewer than fifty employees); 46% of respondents had a graduate degree and 37% an undergraduate one.

PREDISPOSITION TO CONTINUE TELEWORKING

Just over half of the respondents (51%) would like to continue to telework if given the choice to do so after the pandemic ends. Approximately 26% strongly intended to continue to telework, while 25% somewhat intended to do so. Among the respondents, 40% said that since they began teleworking, they were more productive and 36% said that they were better at doing their job.

Over time, teleworkers felt that they had become more efficient and more responsive to their new work environment. After an average of almost six weeks of teleworking, respondents reported a very high level of satisfaction (82%). The proportion of respondents who reported being "very" satisfied increased from 36% to 47% from mid-April to late July. Moreover, teleworkers' perception of their productivity while teleworking increased from 11% to 24% in the same time period. Far from growing tired of teleworking, the proportion of respondents who said that they "strongly" wished to continue to telework if given the choice increased from approximately 16% in mid-April, to 35% in mid-May, and to 47% in July.

Enabling Factors

As expected, organizational characteristics played an important role in adjusting to telework (Wang et al. 2020). It should be noted that

72% of respondents felt that they had received support from the organization since the implementation of telework. Organizational support was considered a significant determinant for each of the five adjustment criteria, which form the central cell of our framework: greater satisfaction, increased productivity, improved quality of work, better work-family balance, and the intention to continue teleworking. Indeed, the intention to continue teleworking tends to be stronger in larger organizations, which are better equipped to support their teleworkers.

In addition, telework has historically been presented as a mode of work-family flexibility (Clark 2000; Hill et al. 1998; Kossek et al. 2006; Piszczek and Berg 2014). During the COVID-19 pandemic, one-third of the respondents reported that they had to spend at least one hour of their work time on family responsibilities. Despite the difficult context, including school and day care closures, summer vacations, and limited access to summer camps, two out of three respondents felt that they had been able to balance work and family while teleworking. Once again, the ability to balance work and personal life improved over time. The percentage of respondents who strongly agreed that telework provided them with a better work-family balance increased from 25% in mid-April to 39% in July.

Risk Factors

A very large majority of respondents (85%) said that they had experienced good working conditions and were able to function well while working remotely. Respondents reported taking on a greater workload while teleworking. Unexpectedly, this increased workload resulted in a better adjustment to teleworking. Employees seemed to appreciate being: less rushed by traffic during business hours; able to devote more time to their work; more productive and able to improve the quality of their work. Conversely, when telework altered their tasks, employees showed less adjustment to teleworking and a lower intention to continue teleworking.

Job characteristics played an important role in the adjustment of teleworkers (Ashforth et al. 2000). Greater autonomy at work resulted in greater satisfaction with telework and a better work-life balance. Conversely, respondents who said that they were dependent on their colleagues' work to carry out their own tasks were less likely to intend to continue teleworking.

Initially, managerial functions were particularly disrupted by teleworking due to the dispersion of team members (Ruiller et al. 2019). Early study results showed that managers had the lowest levels of adjustment to telework across all five adjustment criteria in our framework. They reported lower levels of satisfaction, productivity, work quality, work-life balance, and intention to continue teleworking. Perhaps this is not surprising given that managers not only had to deal with the sudden and forced introduction of telework, just like all employees, but also had to support their teams throughout this major change.

However, while the preliminary study results of April and May 2020 showed that managers had the lowest levels of adjustment and a lower intention to continue teleworking, by July the managers reported the highest levels of adjustment. Indeed, their intention to continue to telework increased from 35% in mid-April, to 52% in mid-June, and to 70% in July – a marked change in managers' attitudes towards telework.

Our results confirmed that the feeling of isolation is one of the major factors that negatively influence adjustment to telework (Kurland and Cooper 2002; Orhan et al. 2016). We analyzed two forms of professional isolation – social and organizational. Regarding the former, 56% of respondents reported feeling isolated from co-workers quite often or very often. In terms of organizational isolation, 24% of respondents felt that they were isolated from organizational decisions or important meetings, or that career coaching was being neglected. While social isolation emerged as a significant negative influence on all adjustment parameters, the effect of organizational isolation requires a more nuanced interpretation. Strangely, the lower frequency of interactions related to formal organizational information (such as advising teleworkers of organizational changes, consulting on operational decisions, or conveying strategic information) seems to have been beneficial to teleworkers. It is safe to assume that this is because fewer such interactions allowed teleworkers more time to focus on their work. Thus, teleworking has revealed certain shortcomings in the organization of work, and this is probably one of them. These results underline the importance of revisiting the frequency, relevance, and channels for the efficient transmission of strategic and operational information (Baruch 2000).

Finally, given that the survey was conducted in the context of a global health crisis, it is not surprising that stress was found to have a significant negative impact on the adjustment to teleworking (Mann and Holdsworth 2003; Perry et al. 2018). Despite the fact that 81% of respondents said that they had never or almost never felt stressed, in this difficult situation, the general level of stress experienced by individuals negatively influenced their appreciation of telework. Although the direct influence of stress is negative, it was found to be strongly associated with professional isolation, telework environment, and organizational support. Thus, stress seems to be losing its explanatory capacity to more proximal factors that have a direct influence on adjustment to telework. Stress appears to be less related to adjustment to telework, and much more likely to be caused by the increased demands of telework that are not compensated by adequate resources (Karasek 1979).

Teleworkers' Sociodemographic Profiles

Individual characteristics, such as gender, age, level of education, and comfort with technology, seem to influence telework adjustment less than other factors, such as telework environment, job characteristics, or organizational support.

Our results indicate that younger workers are more reluctant to continue to telework. This counters earlier literature that assumes that telework posed more issues for older workers (Sharit and Czaja 2009). But in the context of the pandemic, where telework is imposed and full-time, this result is consistent with our other finding of higher perceived isolation among younger respondents.

The lower intention to pursue telework expressed by workers with a higher education level leaves room for questions. The intention to continue teleworking may depend on occupational level and its associated responsibilities, which may require greater dependence on other workers. Another explanation is that more highly educated teleworkers, seeking career advancement, may favour avoiding professional isolation even if that means less access to flexible work schedules. Women react in the same way as men when it comes to intention to continue teleworking. This suggests that the pandemic may result in more gender equality, in spite of doubts raised by some (Cannito and Scavarda 2020; Carli 2020) and suggestions that motivations to pursue telework may differ between women and men (Sullivan and Lewis 2001).

Finally, the intention to continue teleworking remains highly dependent on the ability of teleworkers to master technological complexity.

Facilitating learning, and increasing familiarity and ease with technology are essential to telework, which is set to increase in the midst of the digital shifts and technological disruptions in the workplace.

PANDEMIC-INDUCED TELEWORKING TO PLANNED TELEWORK ORGANIZATION: THE ESSENTIAL ELEMENTS

While pandemic-induced telework has inherited some of its characteristics from conventional telework, it appears to have particular aspects that make it a unique context with specific conceptual boundaries. More particularly, the sudden, mandatory, and unprepared nature of pandemic-induced telework alters the person-environment relationship (i.e., the employee to work-home environment), thus triggering adjustment behaviours to adjust to the new work situation (Golden and Gajendran 2019).

Building on a conceptual framework that incorporated the Theory of Planned Behavior as well as other theories that are conducive to explaining telework adjustment, we were able to determine predictors of the intention to continue teleworking after the pandemic ends. Through the COVID-19 pandemic, telework emerged as a real transition between two perspectives: on the one hand, the view of telework as an organizational practice that leaves it up to employees to decide on the organization of working time under flexibility policies; and on the other hand, a vision of telework as a work system that sustains flexible arrangements, but in an organized manner and within a coherent and efficient organizational design. Given the way telework has been carried out during the pandemic and the anticipation of its post-pandemic development, we need to further develop a theoretical framework to incorporate this new complexity.

Our study highlights both the key anticipated elements and the risks involved in setting up a teleworking system in an organization. It suggests that the following practical issues must be considered.

Analyzing Jobs and Evaluating the Impact of Telework on Work Performance

According to the theory of contingency, the development of any organizational design, such as the one required by telework, must be coherent with environmental constraints both external and internal to the organization (Mintzberg 1977; Ouchi 1979). The technical system that defines the work organization and power relations also influences the success of the design's implementation. Structural elements, such as the degree of centralization or decentralization of relations, the level of control, and the formalization of the behaviours of various stakeholders must be reconsidered to ensure feasibility (Mayo et al. 2009). The experience of teleworking during the pandemic increased the workload and changed in the tasks to be performed by respondents. While the increased workload had a positive impact on the adjustment to telework, the change in tasks had a negative impact instead. Analyzing the flow and organization of work to identify adjustments to be made in teleworking and developing technologies to maximize teleworkers' productivity are required.

Adapting the Scope of Work and Responsibilities to Reflect the Interdependence of Work and Increase Autonomy

Consistent with the results of studies conducted during the pandemic, telework makes it more complex to divide tasks among employees who are members of the same work team and between employees and managers (Chong et al, 2020). It involves adapting management practices so that they become more goal- and results-oriented (Felstead et al. 2003; Liden et al. 2006; Van der Vegt et al. 2001). It is essential to define objectives, tasks, and intermediate follow-up steps (Lautsch et al. 2009). Regular exchanges on work progress would be beneficial. Practices aimed at developing the capacity to manage workloads and work time should be planned. In accordance with previous research, adjusting to telework requires changing control mechanisms so that they focus more on outcomes than on behaviours (Beauregard et al. 2019; Cooper and Kurland 2002). The replacement of traditional controls with trust should ultimately maximize the benefits of telework (Handy 1995).

POSITIONING TELEWORK IN THE DIGITAL SHIFT: ADAPTING TECHNOLOGIES AND WORKSPACES

Re-skilling Teleworkers and Managers

Teleworking must accompany the evolution of work in more interdependent environments that call for more transversal skills. Revisiting practices aimed at strengthening trust, a sense of belonging and communication, as well as determining new evaluation and performance criteria are becoming essential. Training and developing comfort with technology and digital literacy are key (Galluch et al. 2015; Kim and Kankanhalli 2009; Pyöriä 2003). Respondents indicated the positive effect of being comfortable with technology on both telework productivity and their intention to continue teleworking. Creating or strengthening communities of practice in the use of ICTs allows for continuous learning and the use of expert resources when required (Kazekami 2020; Saba et al. 2021).

Reconfiguring Workspaces as an Integral Part of Teleworking

ICTs are at the heart of telework, and can both cause social distancing and help reduce feelings of isolation. ICTs are evolving and have the potential to enrich the teleworking experience by deploying remote collaborative tools as well as virtual meeting and augmented reality tools.

Despite strong intentions to continue teleworking after the pandemic ends, respondents clearly indicated the importance of maintaining contact between colleagues and avoiding situations of professional and social isolation. Thus, irrespective of the technological tools and beyond the pandemic, the reconfiguration and rearrangement of workspaces must be an integral part of telework development plans. In order to encourage interaction between employees, to strengthen team dynamics and the sense of belonging to the organization, employees must maintain meetings for discussion and exchange, training days, regular social events, outdoor activities, and so on. This will require redesigned workspaces to meet these objectives and enhance the positive impact of these activities.

Thinking About and Planning How to Use Collaborative Platforms to Establish Communities of Practice for Sharing between Organizations, Especially between Small and Mid-Size Enterprises

Our findings show that small and mid-size enterprises found it more difficult to provide support for teleworking and take the digital shift.

EXAMINING THE CONSISTENCY OF WORKING CONDITIONS AND THE LEGAL FRAMEWORK

Identifying the Needs of Employees to Have an Appropriate Teleworking Environment

Telework policies benefit from addressing the need for home-based work equipment, access to professional computer tools, and data security. A sound occupational health and safety framework can help organizations establish safe working conditions at home and make the necessary accommodations.

Assessing Telework, Foreseeing its Effects on Working Conditions and Adjusting the Telework Organization

Like any other organizational model, a telework system should be assessed periodically and adjusted as needed. This will help to ensure that it continues to meet the expectations of teleworkers and their managers, as well as those of the organization. Teleworkers must be surveyed regularly to evaluate their adjustment to telework, the difficulties they encounter, and the effectiveness of the actions put in place to support them at home. A teleworker community of practice could also be fostered for sharing information and experience, or providing peer support.

CONCLUSION

Due to the pandemic, at the time of writing, organizations had been forced to experiment with telework for almost a year. Our findings point to the importance of telework in contemplating the reorganization of work in the future. Compatible with considerations of well-being, work-life balance, and respect for the environment by limiting travel, telework offers a new way of reconfiguring work in the digital era (Belzunegui-Eraso and Erro-Garcés 2020). Our study has identified conditions that organizations can put in place to promote telework's influence on productivity and well-being and limit its potential risks. In a knowledge-based economy where more autonomous jobs predominate, telework is positioned as a promising alternative way of organizing work. Our findings highlight both the key anticipated elements and the risks involved in setting up a teleworking system in an organization.

Our study has obvious limitations. Our conclusions are drawn from data collected from a sample of teleworkers in Quebec between April and July 2020. The survey design has provided cross-cutting and in-depth understanding of the factors affecting how a population of workers can, through experience in times of crisis, learn and shape their attitudes towards continuing to telework. Longitudinal research designs would provide additional insights into how employees' adaptation evolves over time and influences the transformation of telework into an organizational design that is sought beyond such crises.

The authors would like to acknowledge the financial support of the Quebec Research Funds and the International Observatory on Societal Impacts of AI and Digital Technology.

REFERENCES

Ajzen, Icek. 1985. "From Intentions to Actions: A Theory of Planned Behavior." In *Action Control*, 11–39. Berlin: Springer.
– 1991. "The Theory of Planned Behavior." *Organizational Behavior and Human Decision Processes* 50: 179–211.
Ajzen, Icek, and Martin Fishbein. 1977. "Attitude-Behavior Relations: A Theoretical Analysis and Review of Empirical Research." *Psychological Bulletin* 84, no. 5: 888–918.
– 2000. "Attitudes and the Attitude-Behavior Relation: Reasoned and Automatic Processes." *European Review of Social Psychology* 11, no.1: 1–33.
Ashforth, Blake E., Glen E. Kreiner, and Mel Fugate. 2000. "All in a Day's Work: Boundaries and Micro Role Transitions." *Academy of Management Review* 15, no. 3: 472–91.
Baruch, Yehuda. 2000. "Teleworking: Benefits and Pitfalls as Perceived by Professionals and Managers." *New Technology, Work and Employment* 15, no. 1: 34–49.
Beauregard, Alexandra, Kelly Basile, and Esther Canónico. 2019. "Telework: Outcomes and Facilitators for Employees." In *The*

Cambridge Handbook of Technology and Employee Behavior, edited by Richard N. Landers, 511–43. Cambridge: Cambridge University Press.

Belzunegui-Eraso, Angel, and Amaya Erro-Garcés. 2020. "Teleworking in the Context of the Covid-19 Crisis." *Sustainability* 12, no. 9: 1–18.

Cannito, Maddalena, and Alice Scavarda. 2020. "Childcare and Remote Work during the COVID-19 Pandemic. Ideal Worker Model, Parenthood and Gender Inequalities in Italy." *Italian Sociological Review* 10, no. 3S: 801–20.

Carillo, Kevin, Gäelle Cachat-Rosset, Josianne Marsan, Tania Saba, and Alain Klarsfeld. 2020. "Adjusting to Epidemic-Induced Telework: Empirical Insights from Teleworkers in France." *European Journal of Information Systems*: 1–20. https://doi.org/10.1080/0960085X.2020.1829512.

Carli, Linda L. 2020. "Women, Gender Equality and COVID-19." *Gender in Management: An International Journal* 35, no. 7/8: 647–55.

Chong, SinHui, Yi Huang., and Chu-Hsiang Chang. 2020. "Supporting Interdependent Telework Employees: A Moderated-Mediation Model Linking Daily COVID-19 Task Setbacks to Next-Day Work Withdrawal." *Journal of Applied Psychology* 105, no. 12: 1408–22. https://doi.org/10.1037/apl0000843.

Clark, Sue Campbell. 2000. "Work/Family Border Theory: A New Theory of Work/Family Balance." *Human Relations* 53: 747–70.

Cooper, Cecily, and Nancy Kurland. 2002. "Telecommuting, Professional Isolation, and Employee Development in Public and Private Organizations." *Journal of Organizational Behavior* 23: 511–32. https://doi.org/10.1002/job.145.

Deng, Zechuan, René Morissette, and Derek Messacar. 2020. "Faire tourner l'économie à distance: le potentiel du travail à domicile pendant et après la COVID-19." Catalogue de Statistique Canada, no. 45280001. Ottawa: Statistique Canada. https://www150.statcan.gc.ca/n1/pub/45-28-0001/2020001/article/00026-eng.pdf.

Donnelly, Noelle, and Sarah Belle Proctor-Thomson. 2015. "Disrupted Work: Home-Based Teleworking (HBTW) in the Aftermath of a Natural Disaster." *New Technology, Work and Employment* 30, no.1: 47–61.

Fekadu, Zelalem, and Pål Kraft. 2001. "Self-identity in Planned Behavior Perspective: Past Behavior and its Moderating Effects on Self-Identity-Intention Relations." *Social Behavior and Personality: An International Journal* 29, no. 7: 671–85.

Felstead, Alan, Nick Jewson, and Sally Walters. (2003). "Managerial Control of Employees Working at Home." *British Journal of Industrial Relations* 41, no. 2: 241–64.

Fishbein, Martin, and Icek Ajzen. 1975. *Intention and Behavior: An Introduction to Theory and Research*. Boston: Addison-Wesley.

Gajendran, Ravi S., and David A. Harrison. 2007. "The Good, the Bad, and the Unknown about Telecommuting: Meta-Analysis of Psychological Mediators and Individual Consequences." *Journal of Applied Psychology* 92, no. 6: 1524–41. https://doi.org/10.1037/0021-9010.92.6.1524.

Galluch, Pamela S., Varun Grover, and Jason B. Thatcher. 2015. "Interrupting the Workplace: Examining Stressors in an Information Technology Context." *Journal of the Association for Information Systems* 16, no.1: 1–47.

Golden, Timothy D., and Ravi S. Gajendran. 2019. "Unpacking the Role of a Telecommuter's Job in their Performance: Examining Job Complexity, Problem Solving, Interdependence, and Social Support." *Journal of Business and Psychology* 34: 55–69.

Halbesleben, Jonathon R.B., Jean-Pierre Neveu, Samantha C. Paustian-Underdahl, and Mina Westman. 2014. "Getting to the 'COR': Understanding the Role of Resources in Conservation of Resources Theory." *Journal of Management* 40, no. 5: 1334–64.

Handy, Charles. 1995. "Trust and the Virtual Organization." *Harvard Business Review* 73, no. 3: 40.

Hill, Edward J., Brent C. Miller, Sarah P. Weiner, and Joe Colihan. 1998. "Influences of the Virtual Office on Aspects of Work and Work/Life Balance." *Personnel Psychology* 51, no. 3: 667–83.

Hobfoll, Stevan E. 1989. "Conservation of Resources: A New Attempt at Conceptualizing Stress." *American Psychologist* 44, no. 3: 513–24. https://doi.org/10.1109/NETWKS.2008.4763690.

Hobfoll, Stevan E. 2001. "The Influence of Culture, Community, and the Nested-Self in the Stress Process: Advancing Conservation of Resources Theory." *Applied Psychology*. https://doi.org/10.1111/1464-0597.00062.

Karasek, Robert A. 1979. "Job Demands, Job Decision Latitude, and Mental Strain: Implications for Job Redesign." *Administrative Science Quarterly* 24: 285–308.

Kazekami, Sachiko. 2020. "Mechanisms to Improve Labor Productivity by Performing Telework." *Telecommunications Policy* 44, no. 2: 1–15.

Kim, Hee-Woong., and Atreyi Kankanhalli. 2009. "Investigating User Resistance to Information Systems Implementation: A Status Quo Bias Perspective." *MIS Quarterly* 33, no. 3: 567–82.

Kossek, Ellen Ernst., Brenda A Lautsch, and Susan C. Eaton. 2006. "Telecommuting, Control, and Boundary Management: Correlates of Policy Use and Practice, Job Control, and Work-Family Effectiveness." *Journal of Vocational Behavior* 68, no. 2: 347–67. https://doi.org/10.1016/j.jvb.2005.07.002.

Kurland, Nancy B. and Cecily D. Cooper. 2002. "Manager Control and Employee Isolation in Telecommuting Environments." *Journal of High Technology Management Research* 13: 107–26.

Lautsch, Brenda A., Ellen Ernst Kossek, and Susan C. Eaton. 2009. "Supervisory Approaches and Paradoxes in Managing Telecommuting Implementation." *Human Relations* 62, no. 6: 795–827. https://doi.org/10.1177/0018726709104543.

Liden, Robert C., Berrin Erdogan, Sandy J. Wayne, and Raymond T. Sparrowe. 2006. "Leader-Member Exchange, Differentiation, and Task Interdependence: Implications for Individual and Group Performance." *Journal of Organizational Behavior* 27, no. 2: 723–46. https://doi.org/10.1002/job.409.

Mann, Sandi, and Lynn Holdsworth. 2003. "The Psychological Impact of Teleworking: Stress, Emotions and Health." *New Technology, Work and Employment* 18, no. 3: 196–211.

Mayo, Margarita, Juan-Carlos Pastor, Luis Gomez-Mejia, and Cristina Cruz. 2009. "Why Some Firms Adopt Telecommuting while Others Do Not: A Contingency Perspective." *Human Resource Management* 48, no. 6: 917–39. https://doi.org/10.1002/hrm.

Mello, Alvaro, Francisco de Assis Goncalves, and Fernando Lima. 2011. "Lessons Learned from September 11th: Telework as an Organizational Resource to the Business Continuity Planning (BCP)." *Journal of Japan Telework Society* 9, no. 1: 46–51.

Mintzberg, Henry. 1977. "Policy as a Field of Management Theory." *Academy of Management Review* 2, no. 1: 88–103.

Nelson, Deborah L., James Campbell Quick, and Mark E. Eakin. 1988. "A Longitudinal Study of Newcomer Role Adjustment in US Organizations." *Work and Stress* 2, no. 3: 239–53.

Organisation for Economic Co-operation and Development (OECD). 2020. "Productivity Gains from Teleworking in the Post COVID-19 Era: How Can Public Policies Make it Happen?" OECD. https://www.oecd.

org/coronavirus/policy-responses/productivity-gains-from-teleworking-in-the-post-covid-19-era-a5d52e99/.

Orhan, Mehmet A., John B. Rijsman, and Gerta M. van Dijk. 2016. "Invisible, Therefore Isolated: Comparative Effects of Team Virtuality with Task Virtuality on Workplace Isolation and Work Outcomes." *Journal of Work and Organizational Psychology*, 32, no. 2: 109–22. https://doi.org/10.1016/j.rpto.2016.02.002.

Ouchi, William G. 1977. "The Relationship Between Organizational Structure and Organizational Control." *Administrative Science Quarterly* 22, no. 1: 95–113.

Perry, Sarah Jansen, Cristina Rubino, and Emily M. Hunter. 2018. "Stress in Remote Work: Two Studies Testing the Demand-Control-Person Model." *European Journal of Work and Organizational Psychology* 27, no. 5: 577–93. https://doi.org/10.1080/1359432X.2018.1487402.

Piszczek, Matthew M. and Peter Berg. 2014. "Expanding the Boundaries of Boundary Theory: Regulative Institutions and Work-Family Role Management." *Human Relations* 67, no. 12: 1491–1512.

Pyöriä, Pasi. 2003. "Knowledge Work in Distributed Environments: Issues and Illusions." *New Technology, Work and Employment* 18, no. 3: 166–180.

Raghuram, Sumita, Rahgu Garud, Batia Wiesenfeld, Vipin Gupta. 2001. "Factors Contributing to Virtual Work Adjustment." *Journal of Management* 27: 383–405.

Rubino, Cristina, Sara Perry, Alex Milam, Christiane Spitzmueller, and Dieter Zapf. 2012. "Demand-Control-Person: Integrating the Demand-Control and Conservation of Resources Models to Test an Expanded Stressor-Strain Model." *Journal of Occupational Health Psychology* 17, no. 4: 456–72.

Ruiller, Caroline, Beatrice Van Der Heijden, Frédérique Chédotel, and Marc Dumas. 2019. "You Have Got a Friend": The Value of Perceived Proximity for Teleworking Success in Dispersed Teams." *Team Performance Management* 25, no. 1-2: 2–29. https://doi.org/10.1108/TPM-11-2017-0069.

Saba, Tania, Sosina Bezu, and Murtaza Haider. 2021. *New Working Arrangements Skills for the Post-Pandemic World.* Future Skills Center and Public Policy Forum. March 2020.

Statistics Canada. 2021. *Série d'enquêtes sur les perspectives canadiennes 1: La COVID-19 et travailler de la maison, 2020.* https://www150.statcan.gc.ca/n1/fr/daily-quotidien/200417/dq200417a-fra.pdf?st=Fr172HBr

– 2020. Table: 33-10-0228-01. "Percentage of Workforce Teleworking or Working Remotely, and Percentage of Workforce Able to Carry Out a Majority of Duties During the COVID-19 Pandemic, by Business Characteristics." https://www150.statcan.gc.ca/t1/tbl1/en/tv.action?pid=3310022801.

Sullivan, Cath, and Susanne Lewis. 2001. "Home-Based Telework, Gender, and the Synchronization of Work and Family: Perspectives of Teleworkers and their Co-Residents." *Gender, Work and Organization* 8, no. 2: 123–45.

Turcotte, Martin. 2010. "Le travail à domicile: une mise à jour, 2008." Publication no11-008-X. Statistique Canada. 7 December 2010. https://www150.statcan.gc.ca/n1/pub/11-008-x/2011001/article/11366-fra.pdf.

Van der Vegt, Gerben S., Ben J.M. Emans, and Evert van de Vliert. 2001. "Patterns of interdependence in work teams: A two-level investigation of the relations with job and team satisfaction." *Personnel Psychology* 54, no. 1: 51–69.

Wang, Bin, Yukun Liu, Jing Qian, and Sharon K. Parker. 2020. "Achieving Effective Remote Working During the COVID-19 Pandemic: A Work Design Perspective." *Applied Psychology*. https://doi.org/10.1111/apps.12290.

8

Occupational Health and Safety Lessons Learned: Moving Forward after the Pandemic

Katherine Lippel, Barbara Neis, Phil James

INTRODUCTION

The COVID-19 pandemic has served to both confirm and accentuate trends in the regulation of occupational health and safety (OHS) that have long been argued to be damaging. In doing so, it has illustrated mechanisms by which governments can sacrifice workers in the interests of other social and economic objectives. In this chapter we examine gaps in effective regulatory protection which have become evident during the course of the pandemic, drawing examples from Canada and the United Kingdom. We first present three occupational contexts in which organizational factors contributed to the disproportionate exposure of workers to the hazards of COVID-19. Some preventive measures created new health hazards for workers, unintentional consequences that led nonetheless to adverse working conditions. We then address regulatory challenges associated with management of the pandemic looking both at protections for workers' health and public health. Overlapping jurisdictions contribute to diffuse protections for workers.

COVID-19 AND WORKERS' HEALTH AND SAFETY: REGULATORY BLIND SPOTS

We focus here on three issues related to the organization of work that contribute to regulatory failure in the protection of workers' health: the precarious nature of employment, including precarious migration and precarious employment status; organizational and employment factors at play in the mobile workforce, and organizational issues related to the health care sector.

Precarious Employment in a Pandemic

Sargeant and Tucker (2009) described the layers of vulnerability that undermine regulatory effectiveness of OHS legislation for migrant workers. In the Canadian context, the most vulnerable are undocumented migrants, then documented migrant workers, but precariously employed Canadian workers also experience many of these vulnerabilities. During the pandemic, all three categories work in sectors deemed essential by the government.

Many of these workers are precarious labour migrants (including temporary foreign workers and undocumented workers). They are less likely to seek testing or health care as many are, or believe they are, ineligible for free public healthcare; many fear deportation. Some documented and undocumented labour migrants live in employer-provided housing where it is impossible to socially distance from the other residents. By November 2020, nearly two thousand migrant workers on farms in Canada had contracted the virus and three had died. In Ontario, migrant agricultural workers were ten times more likely to contract COVID-19 than the general population (Kelley, Wirsig, and Smart 2020).

Temporary employment agencies provided workers to care homes, abattoirs, and farms, workers who were often untrained and unprotected, working in multiple facilities. Some contracted COVID-19 in their workplaces and spread it to their other workplaces and their families. Unsurprisingly, the poorest neighbourhoods in Montreal and Toronto were those with high levels of community spread as many of these precarious workers reside in densely inhabited low-cost housing (Chung et al. 2020; Lippel 2020; Lippel and Visotzky-Charlebois, 2021; Wallace and Moon 2020). As indicated by the results from a spatial analysis of testing and COVID-19 cases in metropolitan Toronto, their work, living, and travel conditions place these workers and their families at higher risk of COVID-19 infection and they often live in areas with lower levels of testing (Wallace and Moon 2020).

Outbreaks in abattoirs sometimes involved temporary employment agency workers bussed in daily from cities to facilities where the client companies had no contact information for them, undermining the possibility of contact tracing (Lippel 2020).

As both the Quebec National Institute for Public Health (INSPQ) and the Ombudsman of Quebec reported, about 10 per cent of health care workers worked in multiple facilities (De Serres et al. 2020; Protecteur du Citoyen 2020, 8–9), some via temporary employment agencies, others having part time contracts in several facilities.

Mobile Work in a Pandemic

The pandemic impacts not only employment, but also mobility to and within work. Most "essential workers" continually engage in mobility to and, in some cases, within work throughout the pandemic. Their work-related mobility is often extended and complex: it can entail commutes ranging from two hours or more daily, to less frequent long-distance commuting, as with fly-in and fly-out and drive-in and drive-out workers. It can entail mobility within work as with long-haul trucking and seafaring. Based on the 2016 census, Canada's mobile labour force, including international labour migrants, comprised approximately 16 per cent of the overall labour force (Neis and Lippel 2019).

These various types of long-distance labour commuting and mobility within work can be associated with complex travel itineraries involving multiple modes of transportation to reach the worksite or port of departure, crossing jurisdictional boundaries as between Canadian provinces and between countries, and can require overnight stays including living at or near work in camps, hotels, or mobile workplaces. Extended and complex mobility for work entails potential exposures and dealing with pandemic-related infection prevention programs at home, during the commute, at the worksite, and while living at work. Since travel time is generally not considered working time (Gesualdi-Fecteau, Nakache, and Matte Guilmain 2019), exposures and related illness on the road would normally not be covered by workers' compensation (Lippel and Walters 2019) but it is not easy to distinguish between these and exposures at work. Here, drawing on a broader Working Paper (Neis, Neil, and Lippel 2020), we explore OHS-related dilemmas experienced by truckers, seafarers, and interjurisdictional fly-in and fly-out and drive-in and drive-out workers during the pandemic.

From the outset trucking has been deemed an essential service in Canada. Some is short-haul and takes place close to home and within a particular region. Some shorter-haul and most long-haul trucking requires traversing jurisdictional borders between provinces in Canada, and between Canada and the US. As with all essential workers, truckers have to deal with the risk of infecting or being infected by family members and friends at home. They are at risk of infection at pick-up and delivery sites and in restaurants, stores, and garages along the road where they seek to access services such as meals, washrooms, showers, and repairs. Canadian truckers have been exempted from pandemic-related international travel limits and quarantine requirements between Canada and the US and from interprovincial limits on travel. They are often trucking between locations with high and low infection rates and across jurisdictions with variable infection-prevention mechanisms in place. There has been a lack of surveillance of trucking-related cases of COVID-19 on the part of the Public Health Agency of Canada (Malone 2020). While reduced commuting and other travel due to travel controls and lockdowns has in some ways made trucking easier, provincial government-initiated and industry mechanisms for controlling infection, such as the closure of restaurant dining rooms, have affected truckers by limiting their access to food and washrooms while on the road ("Le camionnage" 2021). Prolonged periods without access to washrooms were an issue early in the pandemic and continued to challenge some truckers as recently as January 2021. These constraints can affect the mental and physical health of truckers and contribute to the risk of humiliation and social isolation, particularly for women; they also force drivers to drive longer than they would like (CBC News 2021). Difficulties accessing washrooms have also been reported for delivery workers in Toronto (Brar, Arora, and Sra 2020).

Internationally and interprovincially mobile truckers encounter a patchwork of COVID-19 prevention requirements over which they have no control as they transit between jurisdictions (Mills 2020). Truckers interact – when they cross borders – with other workers and members of the public with variable requirements for masking and infection control although steps have been taken to minimize contact at drop-off and pick-up sites by having local staff handle off- and on-loading (Yarr 2020). Trucks are the main point of interface between warehouses and manufacturing outlets and customers. Manufacturing and warehouses in the Greater Toronto Area have been among the worksites with the highest number of COVID-19 cases after health care (Mojtehedzadeh 2021). Some truckers with health conditions are reported to have stopped trucking during the pandemic; some temporary foreign workers employed in trucking in Prince Edward Island have been living in their trucks (Yarr 2020). To reduce risk of infection to family, truckers limit trips home and extend driving time – contributing in turn to the risk of fatigue and social isolation (Mills 2020). Overall, trucking is a high-risk occupation associated with stress, fatigue, motor vehicle crashes, and other hazards. COVID-19 threats and infection control measures are likely exacerbating those hazards.

Seafaring is also a high-risk occupation. Globally, there are an estimated 1.65 million seafarers (Hebbar and Mukesh 2020; ILO 2020). More than 90 per cent of goods are moved by sea and shipping thus plays a critical role in global supply chains (Doumbia-Henry 2020). Most seafarers are deemed to be essential workers and are expected to go to work in Canada and globally. Seafarers may commute long distances between their residence and ports of departure and disembarkation and are employed in mobile workplaces (Shan and Neis 2020). They may work regionally, but many are interjurisdictionally mobile, and live on their worksite for months at a time. Outbreaks were common on cruise ships during the first wave of the pandemic and had devastating impacts on both customers and crews leading to a shutdown of the cruise industry in Canada and major contractions elsewhere (Marchant 2020). There have been outbreaks and cases on board other types of ships, including ferries, but there is no known summary of cases (Stannard 2020). Controlling the spread of COVID-19 on board vessels once an infection occurs is challenging. Vessels with cases on board are likely to experience difficulty finding a port of refuge and accessing appropriate medical care (Stannard 2020).

OHS and human rights consequences result from COVID-19 related policies: cancellation of shore leave, constraints on access to medical care, delays in crew changes, problems with crew repatriation including difficulties accessing flights and the refusal of some countries to allow entry of their own seafarers (Pauksztat 2020). These measures have reduced the risk of outbreaks onboard ships allowing the industry to continue to operate but have resulted in excessively prolonged periods at work and confinement on vessels for hundreds of thousands of seafarers with negative consequences for seafarer fatigue and mental health (Pauksztat 2020; Zarocostas 2020). As argued by Shan (2020a, 2020b), in the absence of core governance measures, problems will be ongoing – although differentially spread across groups of seafarers.

Thousands of Canadian and some international workers are fly-in and fly-out and drive-in and drive-out workers who engage in extended and complex intra- and inter-jurisdictional mobility to work in mines, oil and gas construction and extraction, remote hunting and fishing camps, tree-planting, and other operations. These workers are employed on rotations ranging from several days a week to months and seasons, with varying opportunities to return to their home communities (Cresswell, Dorow, and Roseman 2016). Their work often takes place on remote and transient (as in the case of road and pipeline construction) worksites. Many are housed in work camps and other facilities in nearby communities. These types of work are associated with a range of OHS issues on the road, at work, and living at work (Lippel and Walters 2019; Ryser, Halseth, and Markey 2020). In Canada, work in most of the sectors associated with fly-in and fly-out and drive-in and drive-out has been considered essential during COVID-19 and so rotational workers have had to choose between risk of infection and other challenges associated with mobility in the pandemic context, and the loss of current and possible future employment (Neis, Lippel, and Neil 2020, submitted). The negative impacts of COVID-19 on employment options contributes to these pressures (Dorow 2020; Ryser, Halseth, and Markey 2020). Despite COVID-19 infection protocols on site, during travel, and in home jurisdictions, work camps and sites in Alberta and British Columbia have seen multiple COVID-19 outbreaks. The Kearl Lake camp in the northern Alberta oilsands was associated with more than one hundred cases in April and May 2020, and there were multiple smaller outbreaks at oilsands sites in November 2020 (Graney 2020; Malbeuf 2020). Outbreaks have occurred at construction sites in northern British Columbia and in mines in northern Canada, including in Nunavut (Alex 2020; Leahy 2020; McKay 2020). Some workers infected at these sites tested positive onsite and were required to stay and self-isolate until recovered. Others developed symptoms after their return to their home communities fueling local outbreaks, social media criticisms, and associated opposition to work camps and related projects in host communities (CBC News 2020; Simmons 2020) and to rotational workers and their families in source communities in regions like Atlantic Canada (Cooke 2020; Mullin 2020).

Care Work in a Pandemic

As of January 2021, 32,905 health care workers in Quebec had contracted COVID-19, representing 15.8 per cent of all cases in that province (Statistique Canada 2021, tableau 13-26-0003). In the first wave, 13,581 had contracted COVID-19 (De Serres et al. 2020), a rate ten times higher than that of the general population, while in Australia the infection rate of health care workers was only 2.69 times higher than the general population (Quigley et al. 2021). A study of 5,074 of the Quebec health care workers who contracted COVID-19 confirmed that over 40 per cent had insufficient access to adequate training and personal protective equipment, either because it was unavailable or because it was deemed by governmental decree to be unnecessary (De Serres et al. 2020). A subsequent study of health care workers who had contracted COVID-19 during the second wave, and a control group of workers in the same sector who were not infected showed very high levels of psychological distress in both groups, related to workplace psychosocial hazards (Pelletier et al. 2021).

Understaffing meant that workers continued to report to work despite a positive test result. Mandatory overtime was imposed in many facilities and in May 2020 the average weekly overtime hours of the 26 per cent of nursing personnel who worked overtime was seventeen hours (Carrière et al. 2020). Failure to implement basic prevention techniques including separating residents and patients with COVID-19 from those who were not ill was pervasive both in health care facilities and in care homes, often because of staff shortages (Protecteur du Citoyen 2020, 8).

Restructuring of the public health care sector in Quebec as part of major austerity measures adopted in recent years led to centralized decisions, a key factor in catastrophic outcomes in long-term care facilities according to the Quebec Ombudsman (Protecteur du Citoyen 2020, 11–12).

Care homes during the first wave were, in Canada as in the UK and other countries, the locus of many of the deadliest outbreaks. While this has received significant attention, (Jackman 2020; Lagacé, Garcia, and Bélanger-Hardy 2020) fewer studies (Armstrong, Armstrong, and Bourgeault 2020) consider working conditions of the staff prior to the onset of the pandemic.

COVID-19 and UK Workers

Experiences in the UK have echoed Canadian experiences in revealing that workers, often those in low paying occupational contexts, have been proportionately more likely to contract COVID-19 and to die from it. Yet from the outset it was clear that such workers were likely to be particularly vulnerable to infection.

For male workers, analysis by the UK Office for National Statistics (ONS 2020b) revealed a disproportionate vulnerability to death among seventeen occupational groups, including taxi drivers, security guards, bus and coach drivers, and so-called elementary workers. For women, statistically higher rates have been found amongst care or home care workers and sales and retail assistants. Of seventeen occupations with increased death rates following lockdown, eleven had higher proportions of Black, Asian, and minority ethnic workers, indicating again how, in conjunction with work-related factors, COVID-19 has reinforced social inequalities.

More widely, clusters have emerged from one end of the country to another in a range of industries and employment settings, including the health sector, distribution centres, transport operations, and food processing plants (Middleton, Reintjes, and Lopes 2020). Reinforcing evidence of the role of the workplace in the spread of COVID-19, Public Health England data have pointed to a strong association between prior "workplace or education" activity and the onset of symptoms among people testing positive for the disease (O'Neill 2020b).

Developments regarding care staff reinforce parallels between Canadian and UK experiences. Care homes, from the outset, were major centres of COVID-19 outbreaks and death. In the first wave 18,562 residents of care homes in England died, representing almost 40 per cent of all deaths involving COVID-19 in England during this period (ONS 2020a). Indeed, such was the scale of the failure to protect residents, that Amnesty International (2020) was moved to produce a report detailing its causes. Those identified encompass the transfer to homes of untested hospital patients, insufficient personal protective equipment and poor guidance surrounding its use, gaps in staffing, misuse of "Do Not Attempt to Resuscitate" forms, denial of access to hospitals, and poor regulatory oversight. Infections had in part spread through the sector because of its reliance on temporary employment agency personnel who worked in more than one home.

Perhaps even more disturbingly, the government's claim to have "thrown a protective shield" around care homes continues to be an example of rhetoric running ahead of reality. For example, ONS surveillance data for the week of 21 January 2021 revealed that of the 1,878 outbreaks across the country, 875 were in care homes, with another 120 and 245 being in education and workplace settings, respectively (Public Health England 2020; "Workforce Nationality Figures" n.d.). Furthermore, given that around one in six of the adult social care workforce is non-British, many of the workers affected will be migrants, sometimes employed on temporary or zero-hours forms of employment.

In short, UK experiences, like those in Canada and elsewhere (Quinlan 2021), have confirmed that workplace settings have provided an important platform for the spread of COVID-19, highlighted the vulnerability to infection among public-facing occupational groups, including health care staff and mobile workers such as taxi and coach drivers, and home care workers employed in multiple locations who are often migrants employed on non-standard employment arrangements. They have also pointed to how these vulnerabilities have compounded existing inequalities, including ethnic and health-related ones, and drawn attention to government failures to protect staff through the provision of adequate personal protective equipment, testing, and oversight regimes.

REGULATION OF OCCUPATIONAL HEALTH AND SAFETY: SUCCESSES AND GAPS

Competing roles to regulate OHS and more broadly public health in the context of a pandemic have led to contrasting results, depending, in part, on whether the public health regulator already had a mandate to protect workers' health prior to the pandemic. Challenges are particularly great in the context of regulatory fuzziness as with interjurisdictionally mobile workers and the precariously employed. In Quebec, both the public health network and the OHS regulator are legally mandated to govern workplace health, which is not the case in either Ontario or the UK. Workers who live in one jurisdiction and work in another are governed by different regulatory bodies for work, home, and sometimes travel between work and home as with rotational workers, temporary foreign workers, and seafarers. In this section we explore the interactions between different regulators.

Who is the Regulator of Occupational Health and Safety in a Pandemic?

Canada is a federation with fourteen sovereign regulators having overlapping jurisdiction on public health, food safety, health care, OHS, labour standards, and workers' compensation, including the federal government and that of provinces and territories (Attaran and Houston 2020; Lippel 2016; Robitaille 2020). All have undergone major cutbacks to the public health care system, and particularly to the public health branches of those systems as a result of several waves of austerity measures, including measures driven by federal cutbacks to transfer payments to the provinces.

Each province has their particular bias: some, like Ontario and Alberta, are led by governments with a strong neo-liberal agenda that sometimes reflects anti-worker animus (Brophy et al. 2021). In Ontario, the current premier repealed (the two) paid sick days recently guaranteed to all workers by the previous government within days of taking power in 2018 (The Canadian Press 2018). He has since denied that paid sick days are necessary in the fight against COVID-19 (Fox 2021), turning a deaf ear to claims by critics that workers are going to work ill because of fears that they will lose their jobs and income if they call in sick (Syed and McLaren 2021).

Others are driven by political agendas directing hostility to other governments, as is the case in Quebec, where blaming the federal government bolsters the popularity of the provincial regulator. Quebec blames Ottawa for failing to purchase sufficient vaccines, and fundamentally for providing insufficient funding to allow the province to respond adequately to the pandemic. Despite horrific loss of life, the Quebec premier and the public health director, Dr. Horacio Arruda are both hugely popular (Castonguay 2020). Authors in English Canada support a strong federal hand, including the implementation of the federal *Emergencies Act*, so that the federal regulator can take control of prevention measures (Flood and Thomas 2020). However, it is unlikely that Quebec residents would have shown as much compliance with confinement measures if ordered by the federal government. As Premier Legault noted, "I am a nationalist, I like helping Québécois. It's a privilege to be able to help them, to try to save a maximum number of lives" (Castonguay 2020, our translation).

In the same interview, the premier says his greatest regret is to not have raised salaries of personal support workers prior to the pandemic; he is most proud of having ordered, in May 2020 (Labbé 2020), that ten thousand new personal support workers be paid during training over the summer to allow them to work in care homes, with access to better salaries and better working conditions, a discourse different from that of his Ontario counterpart, whose government in October 2020 provided a temporary increase in salaries to personal support workers (Davidson 2020).

Throughout Canada, during the first wave, personal protective equipment was in insufficient supply, a failure of both the federal government and those of Ontario (Brophy et al. 2021) and Quebec (Lippel and Visotzky-Charlebois 2021), that had allowed supplies to dwindle in a context of austerity, despite damning reports produced after the SARS epidemic in 2005 that pointed to failures in guaranteeing access to personal protective equipment that led to dozens of health workers' deaths (Brophy et al. 2021).

The lack of personal protective equipment, including gowns and masks (medical and N95), motivated public health officials in Quebec to misinform the public as to their usefulness and to severely ration supplies. Nurses, doctors, and paramedics were told that ordinary medical masks sufficed when treating COVID-19 patients. The Quebec Ombudsman noted that, "The directives for using personal protective equipment seemed to be based more on the quantities available than on safety standards" (Protecteur du Citoyen 2020, 8).

From the outset in Quebec the OHS regulator, the Commission des normes, de l'équité, de la santé et de la sécurité du travail (CNESST) integrated guidance from the Quebec public health authorities (INSPQ) in its operations, so that workers who exercised their right to refuse dangerous work under the *Act Respecting Occupational Health and Safety*, were told by CNESST inspectors that the guidance of INSPQ determined whether or not they could require specific personal protective equipment, such as N95 masks. This has been an issue before the courts since the adoption of a decree in June 2020 (Direction générale de la santé publique 2020; Lippel and Visotzky-Charlebois 2021) and in March 2021 the Tribunal administratif du travail (TAT) ordered that fit-tested N95 masks be provided to health care workers working with patients who are suspected carriers of COVID-19 on the basis of the precautionary principle. The CNESST has since adapted its guidance material accordingly, and the TAT decision is under review in Quebec Superior Court (PGQué 2021). The issue of aerosol transmission of the virus is the underpinning of this debate, as the need for N95 masks is based on the premise of aerosol transmission, an issue controversial in many jurisdictions (Alyazidi et al. 2021).

Collaboration between the OHS and public health authorities is not unusual in Quebec; the network of public health doctors is an integral part of the OHS regulatory regime. This is not the case in other Canadian provinces, where public health authorities appear less focused on the working conditions of essential workers (Stall et al. 2021). The INSPQ epidemiologists specialized in occupational hazards were quick to track the cases among health care workers and survey those who had become ill in order to ensure better prevention for the second wave (De Serres et al. 2020). We know that as of January 2021, 3,900 workplaces in Quebec have had outbreaks of the virus, excluding schools, day cares, and health care establishments (Meloche-Holubowski 2021). Similarly, information on workers' rights is an integral part of multi-lingual guidance produced by public health authorities relating to COVID-19 (Montreal Health 2020), and the OHS authority (CNESST) successfully prosecuted an employer for failure to comply with public health guidance targeting construction work.[1]

In Ontario several legal decisions were rendered during the first wave (Lippel 2020), and its policy allows nurses to ask for N95 masks but the masks are not explicitly required by legislation nor are they always available (Weeks 2020). Yet, despite uneven access to equipment (Brophy et al. 2021) the workers' compensation board (WSIB) refused paramedics' claims for compensation for COVID-19 stating that "paramedics would not have gotten sick on the job if they were wearing proper [personal protective equipment]," (Shetty 2021) a questionable argument, even were it to be true, in the context of a no-fault system.

In Quebec, as of 6 January 2021 the workers' compensation board (the CNESST) had accepted 13,312 claims for COVID-19 from health care workers alone, and denied 350, or 3 per cent of decided cases, while Ontario, a larger province, accepted 7,962 and denied 887 or 10 per cent of decided cases as of 22 January (WSIB Ontario 2021). It is of note that the CNESST has created a policy presumption that front-line health care workers who contract COVID-19 are presumed to have contracted it at work (CNESST 2020). British Columbia also adapted its presumptive policies in relation to COVID-19 (Proctor 2021), but other Canadian jurisdictions have yet to do so.

Beyond the political drivers of practices in these various, often competing, jurisdictions, overlap in jurisdiction within a given territory further undermines regulatory effectiveness. A case in point is illustrated by an outbreak of COVID-19 in two poultry processing plants in British Columbia. Within the food processing industry, federal authorities have jurisdiction on food inspection while provincial authorities have jurisdiction on OHS within the plant. The *Globe and Mail* reported that BC and Ottawa share responsibility for food and worker safety in those poultry plants. The BC public health officer noted, "We would expect that they go hand in hand. But sometimes, people who are responsible for the food safety part may not recognize some of the key things that happened on the worker safety side of things" (Hunter 2020).

In summary, in the jurisdictions studied, the OHS regulator took a back seat to public health officials in Quebec, and to the provincial government in Ontario. Previously integrated processes between the OHS inspectorate and public health occupational health services led to a smoother collaboration in Quebec, whereas in Ontario OHS inspectors complained that they were unable to do their jobs (Mojtehedzadeh 2020), seemingly by reason of political pressures from the government. Furthermore, aside from the issues related to overlapping authority within the same territorial jurisdiction, some of the issues we have identified are attributable to multiple provincial, national, and international jurisdictions that regulate in silos. The situation of temporary foreign workers illustrates this point.

Precariously employed international migrants entering Canada are ostensibly protected from inadequate housing by federal immigration regulations, rules that are under revision in light of the egregious failures in protecting these workers from COVID-19 during the first wave of the pandemic (CLC 2020). While the federal government has jurisdiction on work permits for immigration purposes, research has shown that the implementation of the conditions set out in draft contracts provided to federal immigration authorities by Canadian employers are not enforced either by immigration authorities or authorities in charge of labour legislation, at the best of times (Cedillo, Lippel, and Nakache 2019).

During the pandemic, abuses were documented in several provinces. In Ontario, at least seven farm workers have died and it became clear that the housing provided prevented them from socially distancing and those conditions contributed to the spread of the virus, multiple clusters affecting temporary foreign workers in agriculture (Baum and Grant 2020; Grant and Bailey 2021). In Quebec, despite federal subsidies to farmers to allow them to provide workers with appropriate housing, housing provided was often inadequate; sometimes workers were charged extra for the improved housing (Meza 2020). The federal government appears to have abdicated its responsibility to workers in an effort to facilitate the economic needs of farmers (Baum and Grant 2020), while OHS authorities hesitate to intervene on housing issues.

Similarly, fly-in and fly-out workers in Canada were afterthoughts in the planning of each province, and confinement measures had serious social and economic consequences for the workers and their families. Those communities that failed to integrate a prevention plan that included essential mobile workers found themselves with outbreaks attributable to their movement between work and home. Alberta concluded that work in the oilsands was "essential" while failure to prevent outbreaks in camps led to consequences for home provinces and territories, including Indigenous communities, far less likely to have health facilities and emergency care required to manage the outbreaks.

Is Canada unique in its jurisdictional challenges? Let us turn now to the UK.

Regulation in the UK

The Health and Safety Executive (HSE) is the UK's regulatory authority for OHS. Accountable to the Secretary of State for Work and Pensions, its day-to-day activities are overseen by a tripartite board. HSE inspectors have oversight of workplaces in higher risk sectors, with the remainder falling under the jurisdiction of Environmental Health Officers employed by local authorities.

For most of the period since its establishment under the *Health and Safety at Work Act 1974* the HSE has operated in unsupportive political contexts marked by deregulatory pressures and budget cuts (Tombs and Whyte 2010, 2013). The period of Conservative-Coalition government rule from 2010 has been particularly tough in this regard. Over the course of it, HSE funding has fallen from £239 to £121 million in 2019–20. When inflation-adjusted, this amounts to a reduction of 58 per cent in central government funding. These funding cuts have inevitably affected staffing. Between 2009–10 and

2019–20, total HSE full time equivalent posts declined by 36 per cent (from 3,702 to 2,371) and frontline staff, including all inspectors, by 35 per cent (1,617 to 1,059). In turn, these declines have resulted in considerable reductions in inspections and enforcement action. HSE was therefore poorly placed to address the regulatory challenges arising from the pandemic. Its capacity to monitor the adequacy of what employers were doing to protect workers from infection was further reduced when, in late March, it decided to largely withdraw inspectors from undertaking workplace inspections, rather ironically, on safety grounds. Given that the Care Quality Commission, the body responsible for regulating the health and safety of care home residents in England and Wales took similar action, this meant that as COVID-19 infections spread rapidly through care homes, they did so in the absence of virtually any regulatory oversight: *Hazards Magazine* reported that between March and mid-June, HSE had not made a single visit to a care home and, by the end of September, it had conducted just eight such visits (O'Neill 2020a).[2]

Eventually, in the face of pressure to address the lack of workplace oversight, the government announced that HSE would receive additional funding, but just £14 million, to undertake "spot checks" and make workplaces "COVID-secure." Given that HSE is responsible for regulating 5.5 million duty holders, it has been estimated that, at the time of writing, these spot checks had reached less than 0.5 per cent of these duty holders (James 2021). Yet this picture of regulatory failure gets worse since the HSE has been complicit not only in the production of government guidance on the management of COVID-19 which makes virtually no reference to the legal duties of employers and the penalties associated with a failure to comply with them, but has also produced guidance of its own that suffers from the same deficiency (HSE n.d.). So there has been the extraordinary sight of a regulator effectively disowning the law for which it is responsible: law that includes highly relevant regulations dealing with personal protective equipment, workplace hygiene, and the control of substances hazardous to health. On top of this, HSE has apparently been happy to support guidance that arguably misrepresents and understates the legal obligations of employers to protect workers from the risk of infection via the provision of masks and face protection (James 2021) and to produce guidance on involving workers that similarly says almost nothing about the legal rights and protections that workers possess or the actions employers should take to enhance and support collective processes of workforce consultation and representation.

The story of regulatory failure does not end here. At least publicly, HSE has also been strikingly absent from debates surrounding the opening of workplaces during the pandemic. This has been particularly apparent with regard to union-government disagreements regarding the safety of staff in schools and universities, where HSE has been largely invisible and content to stand on the sidelines even though the focus of these disagreements is a matter of OHS. In other words, the focus is precisely what HSE exists to regulate.

These various failings of HSE have seemingly stemmed from processes of marginalisation and regulatory capture (James 2021). In the case of the former, Public Health England, not the HSE, has taken the lead in producing UK government guidance on the workplace management of COVID-19: a dominance of public health considerations that provide a further echo of Canadian experiences it would seem. Meanwhile, there seems little doubt that the actions of HSE have very much reflected its subservience to the wishes and ideological preferences of the UK's Conservative government: an interpretation lent weight by the more pro-worker guidance produced by the Scottish and Welsh governments, as well as press criticisms of HSE's role in the reapproval of outdated supplies of personal protective equipment and the suggestion that it had come under political pressure in this regard.

HOW COULD WE HAVE DONE BETTER?

In Ontario, SARS in the early 2000s led to multiple fatalities among health care workers, followed by commissions and reports that provided roadmaps to prevent similar tragedies. Those lessons were not learned, but what can we now learn from the current pandemic?

A first issue is that of the independence of OHS regulators from government. Experiences during the pandemic have reinforced the vulnerability of regulators of OHS to financial and policy pressures from government that are detrimental to worker interests. How can such bodies be put on a footing that better provides and protects their independence? One option is the application, by analogy, of the United Nations' Paris Principles relating to the status and functions of National Human Rights Institutions. These principles require such bodies to embody "the pluralist representation of the social forces (of civilian society)," and make clear that, where government departments are represented, this should only be in an advisory capacity. They also require that "adequate funding" be provided to enable them to be "independent of government and not be subject to financial control which might affect its independence" (James 2021, 37).

Secondly, the integration of workers' health as an explicit mandate of the public health authorities, a model that exists in Quebec but not in other jurisdictions studied, is worth scrutiny. From a worker perspective, this might be a mixed blessing. Increased oversight by the INSPQ on the OHS regulator's practices meant that there was less emphasis on the interest of the workers' health as the INSPQ also takes into consideration the health of others, like that of children whose wellbeing is predicated on being in school. Decisions about opening schools went beyond the OHS considerations, promoting risk-taking for workers in the interest of the children, whose mental health and development may be more at risk than their risk of being exposed to COVID-19, and in the interest of the economy, open schools optimizing productivity of teleworkers. Yet at least in Quebec, the public health authorities were explicitly concerned with workers' health, as shown by their epidemiological work in the health care sector (DeSerres et al. 2020; Pelletier et al. 2021) and their active contact tracing in workplaces. A long history of collaboration between the OHS and the public health authorities mandated by the OHS legislation allowed for rapid deployment of workplace specific guidance (CNESST n.d.). In other provinces the health and safety authorities and the public health authorities seemed to work in silos (Watters 2021), giving the impression that they believe workers bring COVID-19 to work from their communities (Stall et al. 2021), while it is highly likely that the transmission goes from workplaces to communities in many cases.

Finally, work organization is often an invisible variable in the regulation of OHS, and risk assessments that take this into consideration by both the OHS regulator and the public health authorities would have reduced the spread of COVID-19 and the burden born by workers. Shining light on invisible workforces including mobile workers, precarious migrants, and the precariously employed would have done a great deal in preventing transmission to workers and from workers to communities. Ensuring precarious workers, including migrants, have access to health care and social benefits is an essential step in protecting not only those workers, but their colleagues and the communities in which they live, a conclusion applicable in all jurisdictions (Clibborn and Wright 2020; Reid, Ronda-Perez, and Schenker 2021; Quinlan 2021).

The authors would like to acknowledge Lesley Butler's help with identifying potential sources for the article and with formatting. This support was funded by the Social Sciences and Humanities Research Council.

NOTES

1   CNESST c. *8653631 Canada Inc.*, 2020 QCCQ 6684. Communication from informant from the CNESST, 25 January 2021.
2   In Scotland, HSE is also responsible for the health and safety of residents.

REFERENCES

[Government of Quebec] *Act Respecting Occupational Health and Safety.* 2020. CQLR c. S-2.1, 20 October. http://legisquebec.gouv.qc.ca/en/pdf/cs/S-2.1.pdf

Alex, Cathy. 2020. "'Terrible Sadness': Company Confirms 25 COVID-19 Cases, Including 1 Death, Connected to Lac Des Iles Mine." CBC, 28 April 2020. https://www.cbc.ca/news/canada/thunder-bay/lac-des-iles-25-cases-one-1.5546898.

Alyazidi, Raidan, Joel Anderson, David Fisman, Ted Haines, Anne A. Huang, Amir Khadir, Victor Leung, et al. 2021. "Time for Government to Take Aerosol Transmission of COVID-19 Seriously," *Labour & Industry: A Journal of the Social and Economic Relations of Work.* 4 January 2021. https://ricochet.media/en/3423.

Amnesty International. 2020. "As If Expendable: The UK Government's Failure to Protect Older People in Care Homes during the COVID-19 Pandemic." *The Amnesty International report.* London: Amnesty International Publications. https://www.amnesty.org.uk/files/2020-10/Care%20Homes%20Report.pdf?kd5Z8eWzj8Q6ryzHkcaUnxfCtqe5Ddg6=.

Armstrong, Pat, Hugh Armstrong, and Ivy Bourgeault. 2020. "Privatization and COVID-19: A Deadly Combination for Nursing

Homes." In *Vulnerable: The Law, Policy and Ethics of COVID-19*, edited by Colleen Flood, Vanessa MacDonnell, Jane Philpott, Sophie Thériault, and Sridhar Venkatapuram, 447–62. Ottawa: University of Ottawa Press. http://ruor.uottawa.ca/handle/10393/40726.

Attaran, Amir, and Adam R. Houston. 2020. "Pandemic Data Sharing: How the Canadian Constitution Has Turned into a Suicide Pact." In *Vulnerable: The Law, Policy and Ethics of COVID-19*, edited by Colleen Flood, Vanessa MacDonnell, Jane Philpott, Sophie Thériault, and Sridhar Venkatapuram, 91–104. Ottawa: University of Ottawa Press. http://ruor.uottawa.ca/handle/10393/40726.

Baum, Kathryn Blaze, and Tavia Grant. 2020. "Ottawa Didn't Enforce Rules for Employers of Migrant Farm Workers during Pandemic." *The Globe and Mail*, 13 July 2020. https://www.theglobeandmail.com/canada/article-how-ottawas-enforcement-regime-failed-migrant-workers-during-the/.

Brar, Amanpreet, Abhimanyu Arora, and Gurbaaz Sra. 2020. "Opinion | While We 'Shop Local,' Don't Forget about Ontario's Delivery Drivers. Their Stories of Working Way below Minimum Wage, COVID Scares, and No Washroom Breaks." *Toronto Star*, 21 December 2020. https://www.thestar.com/opinion/contributors/2020/12/21/while-we-shop-local-dont-forget-about-ontarios-delivery-drivers-their-stories-of-working-way-below-minimum-wage-covid-scares-and-no-washroom-breaks.html.

Brophy, James T., Margaret M. Keith, Michael Hurley, and Jane E. McArthur. 2021. "Sacrificed: Ontario Healthcare Workers in the Time of COVID-19." *New Solutions: A Journal of Environmental and Occupational Health Policy* 30 (4): 267–81. https://doi.org/10.1177/1048291120974358.

CLC (Canadian Labour Congress). 2020. "Comments on the Government of Canada's Proposal to Establish Minimum Requirements for Employer-provided Accommodations for the Temporary Foreign Worker Program (TFWP) Across Canada." December 2020.

Carrière, Gisèle, Jungwee Park, Zechuan Deng, and Dafna Kohen. 2020. "Overtime Work among Professional Nurses during the COVID-19 Pandemic." *StatCan COVID-19: Data to Insights for a Better Canada*. Statistics Canada. https://www150.statcan.gc.ca/n1/pub/45-28-0001/2020001/article/00074-eng.htm.

Castonguay, Alec. 2020. "François Legault: Passer à l'histoire." *L'actualité*, December 2, 2020. https://lactualite.com/politique/francois-legault-passer-a-lhistoire/.

CBC News. 2020. "COVID-19 Outbreak Declared at Coastal GasLink Accommodation Sites in Northern B.C." *CBC*, 21 December 2020. https://www.cbc.ca/news/canada/british-columbia/covid-19-outbreak-coastal-gaslink-1.5849605.

– 2021. "Truckers Face 'Dehumanizing' Challenges Finding Washrooms on the Road." *CBC*, 17 January 2021. https://www.cbc.ca/news/canada/toronto/truck-drivers-denied-washrooms-1.5876587.

Cedillo, Leonor, Katherine Lippel, and Delphine Nakache. 2019. "Factors Influencing the Health and Safety of Temporary Foreign Workers in Skilled and Low-Skilled Occupations in Canada." *New Solutions: A Journal of Environmental and Occupational Health Policy* 29 (3): 422–58. https://doi.org/10.1177/1048291119867757.

Chung, Hannah, Kinwah Fung, Laura E. Ferreira-Legere, Branson Chen, Lisa Ishiguro, Gangamma Kalappa, Peter Gozdyra, et al. 2020. "COVID-19 Laboratory Testing in Ontario: Patterns of Testing and Characteristics of Individuals Tested, as of 30 April 2020." Toronto, ON: ICES. https://www.ices.on.ca/Publications/Atlases-and-Reports/2020/COVID-19-Laboratory-Testing-in-Ontario.

Clibborn, Stephen, and Chris F. Wright. 2020. "COVID-19 and the Policy-Induced Vulnerabilities of Temporary Migrant Workers in Australia." *Journal of Australian Political Economy*, no. 85: 62–70.

CNESST. 2020. "Questions et réponses – COVID-19." 14 January 2020. https://www.cnesst.gouv.qc.ca/fr/prevention-securite/coronavirus-covid-19/questions-reponses-covid-19#indemnisation.

– n.d. "COVID-19 Toolkit." https://www.cnesst.gouv.qc.ca/en/prevention-and-safety/covid-19/covid-19-toolkit.

Cooke, Ryan. 2020. "Rotational Workers Feel All Eyes on Them after N.L.'s Influx of Cases from Alberta." *CBC*, 24 November 2020. https://www.cbc.ca/news/canada/newfoundland-labrador/rotational-workers-newfoundland-labrador-covid-19-1.5812552.

Cresswell, Tim, Sara Dorow, and Sharon Roseman. 2016. "Putting Mobility Theory to Work: Conceptualizing Employment-Related Geographical Mobility." *Environment and Planning A: Economy and Space* 48 (9): 1787–1803. https://doi.org/10.1177/0308518X16649184.

Davidson, Sean. 2020. "Ontario Announces Pay Raise for Nearly 147,000 Personal Support Workers." *CTV News Toronto*, 1 October 2020. https://toronto.ctvnews.ca/ontario-announces-pay-raise-for-nearly-147-000-personal-support-workers-1.5127904.

De Serres, Gaston, Sara Carazo, Armelle Lorcy, Jasmin Villeneuve, Denis Laliberté, Richard Martin, Pierre Deshaies, et al. 2020. "Enquête épidémiologique sur les travailleurs de la santé atteints par la COVID-19 au printemps 2020." *Institut national de santé publique du Québec.* https://www.inspq.qc.ca/publications/3061-enquete-epidemiologique-travailleurs-sante-covid19.

Direction générale de la santé publique. 2020. "Ordonnance Du Directeur National de Santé Publique Concernant Le Port Des Équipements de Protection Respiratoires et Oculaires." Ministère de la Santé et des Services sociaux. https://publications.msss.gouv.qc.ca/msss/fichiers/directives-covid/archives/20-MS-05553-02_PJ_Ordonnance_DNSP_port_protection_respiratoire_oculaire.pdf.

Dorow, Sara. 2020. "COVID-19 and (Im)Mobile Workers in Alberta's 'Essential' Oil Industry." *On the Move Partnership.* 20 May 2020. https://www.onthemovepartnership.ca/covid-19-and-immobile-workers-in-albertas-essential-oil-industry/.

Doumbia-Henry, Cleopatra. 2020. "Shipping and COVID-19: Protecting Seafarers as Frontline Workers." *WMU Journal of Maritime Affairs* 19 (3): 279–93. https://doi.org/10.1007/s13437-020-00217-9.

Flood, Colleen M., and Bryan Thomas. 2020. "The Federal Emergencies Act: A Hollow Promise in the Face of COVID-19?" In *Vulnerable: The Law, Policy and Ethics of COVID-19*, edited by Colleen Flood, Vanessa MacDonnell, Jane Philpott, Sophie Thériault, and Sridhar Venkatapuram, 105–14. Ottawa: University of Ottawa Press. http://ruor.uottawa.ca/handle/10393/40726.

Fox, Chris. 2021. "Doug Ford Says There Is 'No Reason' for Ontario to Offer Paid Sick Leave Program Despite Criticism." *CTV News Toronto*, 18 January 2021. https://toronto.ctvnews.ca/doug-ford-says-there-is-no-reason-for-ontario-to-offer-paid-sick-leave-program-despite-criticism-1.5271656.

Gesualdi-Fecteau, Dalia, Delphine Nakache, and Laurence Matte Guilmain. 2019. "Travel Time as Work Time? Nature and Scope of Canadian Labor Law's Protections for Mobile Workers." *NEW SOLUTIONS: A Journal of Environmental and Occupational Health Policy* 29 (3): 349–70. https://doi.org/10.1177/1048291119867750.

Graney, Emma. 2020. "Kearl Lake Coronavirus Outbreak Now Linked to over 100 Cases in Four Provinces." *The Globe and Mail*, 10 May 2020. https://www.theglobeandmail.com/business/article-kearl-lake-coronavirus-outbreak-now-linked-to-over-100-cases-in-four/.

Grant, Tavia, and Ian Bailey. 2021 "Five Migrant Farm Workers Have Died since Mid-March, Four While in COVID-19 Quarantine, Advocacy Group Says." *The Globe and Mail*, 5 May 2021.

https://www.theglobeandmail.com/canada/article-five-migrant-farm-workers-have-died-since-mid-march-four-while-in/.

Hebbar, Anish Arvind, and Nitin Mukesh. 2020. "COVID-19 and Seafarers' Rights to Shore Leave, Repatriation and Medical Assistance: A Pilot Study." *International Maritime Health* 71 (4): 217–28. https://doi.org/10.5603/IMH.2020.0040.

HSE (Health and Safety Executive). n.d. "HSE: Information about Health and Safety at Work." Accessed 30 January 2021. https://www.hse.gov.uk/.

Hunter, Justine. 2020. "B.C. to Set Its Own COVID-19 Workplace Safety Rules after Outbreaks." The *Globe and Mail*, 30 April 2020. https://www.theglobeandmail.com/canada/british-columbia/article-bc-to-set-its-own-covid-19-workplace-safety-rules-after-outbreaks/.

International Labour Organization (ILO). 2020. "General Observation on Matters Arising from the Application of the Maritime Labour Convention, 2006, as Amended (MLC, 2006) during the COVID-19 Pandemic." https://www.ilo.org/wcmsp5/groups/public/---ed_norm/---normes/documents/publication/wcms_764384.pdf.

Jackman, Martha. 2020. "Fault Lines: COVID-19, the Charter and Long Term Care." In *Vulnerable: The Law, Policy and Ethics of COVID-19*, edited by Colleen Flood, Vanessa MacDonnell, Jane Philpott, Sophie Thériault, and Sridhar Venkatapuram, 338–54. Ottawa: University of Ottawa Press. http://ruor.uottawa.ca/handle/10393/40726.

James, Phil, ed. 2021. *HSE and COVID at Work: A Case of Regulatory Failure*. Liverpool: Institute of Employment Rights.

Kelley, Mark, Karen Wirsig, and Virginia Smart. 2020. "Bitter Harvest." CBC, 29 November 2020. https://newsinteractives.cbc.ca/longform/bitter-harvest-migrant-workers-pandemic.

Labbé, Jérôme. 2020. "Québec veut recruter 10 000 préposés aux bénéficiaires en offrant des formations payées." *Radio-Canada*, 27 May 2020. https://ici.radio-canada.ca/nouvelle/1706748/coronavirus-bilan-quebec-francois-legault.

Lagacé, Martine, Linda Garcia, and Louise Bélanger-Hardy. 2020. "COVID-19 et Âgisme: Crise Annoncée Dans Les Centres de Soins de Longue Durée et Réponse Improvisée?" In *Vulnerable: The Law, Policy and Ethics of COVID-19*, edited by Colleen Flood, Vanessa MacDonnell, Jane Philpott, Sophie Thériault, and Sridhar Venkatapuram, 329–38. Ottawa: University of Ottawa Press. http://ruor.uottawa.ca/handle/10393/40726.

Leahy, Stephen. 2020. "Mines Are Hotspots for Spread of Covid-19, Study

Finds." *The Guardian*, 5 June 2020 (sec. Environment). http://www.theguardian.com/environment/2020/jun/05/mines-coronavirus-hotspots-report-us-canada.

Lippel, Katherine. 2016. "L'avenir Du Droit de La Santé et de La Sécurité Du Travail Dans Le Contexte de La Mondialisation. *Ottawa Law Revue/Revue de Droit d'Ottawa* 47 (2): 535–56. https://doi.org/10.2139/ssrn.2749634.

– 2020. "Occupational Health and Safety and COVID-19: Whose Rights Come First in a Pandemic?" In *Vulnerable: The Law, Policy and Ethics of Covid-19*, edited by Colleen M. Flood, Vanessa MacDonnell, Jane Philpott, Sophie Thériault, and Sridhar Venkatapurum, 473–86. Ottawa: University of Ottawa Press. https://ruor.uottawa.ca/handle/10393/40726.

Lippel, Katherine, and Maxine Visotzky-Charlebois. 2021. "Survol Des Enjeux Juridiques Portant Sur Le Droit de La Santé et La Sécurité Du Travail En Contexte de La COVID-19." In Barreau du Québec, *Développements récents en droit de la santé et de la sécurité du travail 2021*, 71–96. Montréal: Éditions Yvon Blais.

Lippel, Katherine, and David Walters. 2019. "Regulating Health and Safety and Workers' Compensation in Canada for the Mobile Workforce: Now You See Them, Now You Don't." *New Solutions: A Journal of Environmental and Occupational Health Policy* 29 (3): 317–48. https://doi.org/10.1177/1048291119868805.

Malbeuf, Jamie. 2020. "COVID-19 Outbreaks Declared at 6 Oilsands Sites." CBC, 19 November 2020. https://www.cbc.ca/news/canada/edmonton/fort-mcmurray-oilsands-outbreaks-1.5807705.

Malone, Kelly Geraldine. 2020. "'Alarmed': Health Critic Calls for More Data on COVID-19 in Trucking Industry." CBC, 7 June 2020. https://www.cbc.ca/news/canada/manitoba/trucking-industry-covid-19-data-1.5602109.

Marchant, Natalie. 2020. "These Startling Pictures Show the Impact of COVID-19 on the Cruise Industry." *World Economic Forum*. 6 November 2020. https://www.weforum.org/agenda/2020/11/impact-coronavirus-pandemic-cruise-ships/.

McKay, Jackie. 2020. "Workers Trapped at Nunavut Mine in Midst of COVID-19 Outbreak Growing Anxious, Says Employee." CBC, 6 October 2020. https://www.cbc.ca/news/canada/north/hope-bay-nunavut-mine-covid-1.5752889.

Meloche-Holubowski, Mélanie. 2021. "Les éclosions en milieu de travail demeurent nombreuses au Québec | Coronavirus." *Radio-Canada*,

30 January 2021. https://ici.radio-canada.ca/nouvelle/1766606/
eclosions-milieu-travail-emploi-covid-coronavirus.

Meza, Karla. 2020. "Des travailleurs étrangers forcés de payer pour leur quarantaine." *Le Devoir*, 27 July 2020. https://www.ledevoir.com/societe/583090/les-travailleurs-etrangers-temporaires-tenus-de-payer-des-frais-pour-leur-quarantaine.

Middleton, John, Ralf Reintjes, and Henrique Lopes. 2020. "Meat Plants – a New Front Line in the Covid-19 Pandemic." *BMJ* 370: m2716. https://doi.org/10.1136/bmj.m2716.

Mills, Stu. 2020. "The Long Haul: Ottawa Trucker Riding out Pandemic on Increasingly Inhospitable Highways." *CBC*, 20 April 2020. https://www.cbc.ca/news/canada/ottawa/the-long-haul-ottawa-trucker-riding-out-pandemic-on-increasingly-inhospitable-highways-1.5535980.

Mojtehedzadeh, Sara. 2020. "Many Ontario Workers Are Trying to Refuse Work Due to COVID-19 Fears – but the Government Isn't Letting Them." *Toronto Star*, 27 April 2020. https://www.thestar.com/business/2020/04/27/many-ontario-workers-are-trying-to-refuse-work-due-to-covid-19-fears-but-the-government-isnt-letting-them.html.

– 2021. "What's an Essential Workplace and Who's an Essential Worker? Ontario's New Lockdown Rules under Scrutiny." *Toronto Star*, 12 January 2021. https://www.thestar.com/news/gta/2021/01/12/whats-an-essential-workplace-and-whos-an-essential-worker-ontarios-new-lockdown-rules-under-scrutiny.html.

Montreal Health. 2020. "Informations Multilingues." *Government of Québec*. https://santemontreal.qc.ca/population/coronavirus-covid-19/informations-multilingues/.

Mullin, Malone. 2020. "The Price of Shame: N.L.'s Rotational Workers Reveal Hidden Consequences of Social Media Trolling." *CBC*, 7 December 2020. https://www.cbc.ca/news/canada/newfoundland-labrador/price-of-shame-1.5827087.

Neis, Barbara, and Katherine Lippel. 2019. "Occupational Health and Safety and the Mobile Workforce: Insights from a Canadian Research Program." *New Solutions: A Journal of Environmental and Occupational Health Policy* 29 (3): 297–316. https://doi.org/10.1177/1048291119876681.

Neis, Barbara, Kerri Neil, and Katherine Lippel. 2020. "Mobility in a Pandemic: COVID-19 and the Mobile Labour Force: Working Paper." *On the Move Partnership*. https://www.onthemovepartnership.ca/wp-content/uploads/2020/08/COVID-and-Mobile-Labour-Force-Working-Paper-August-2020.pdf.

– Submitted. "On the Move in the Midst of a Pandemic: Canada's Essential Mobile Workers and Their Families." In *Families, Mobility, and Work*, edited by Barbara Neis, Christina Murray, and Nora Spinks. St John's, NL: Memorial University Press.

O'Neill, Rory. 2020a. "ABDICATION: HSE Has Been Missing in Action throughout the Covid-19 Crisis." *Hazards*. https://www.hazards.org/coronavirus/abdication.htm.

– 2020b. "Laid Bare: The Scandal of Expendable Workers before, during and after Covid." *Hazards*. https://www.hazards.org/coronavirus/laid-bare.htm.

ONS (Office for National Statistics). 2020a. "All Data Related to Deaths Involving COVID-19 in the Care Sector, England and Wales: Deaths Occurring up to 12 June 2020 and Registered up to 20 June 2020 (Provisional)." London: *Office for National Statistics*. https://www.ons.gov.uk/peoplepopulationandcommunity/birthsdeathsandmarriages/deaths/articles/deathsinvolvingCOVID19inthecaresectorenglandandwales/deathsoccurringupto12june2020andregisteredupto20june2020provisional/relateddata.

– 2020b. "Coronavirus (COVID-19) Related Deaths by Occupation, before and during Lockdown, England and Wales: Deaths Registered between 9 March and 30 June 2020." London: *Office for National Statistics*. https://www.ons.gov.uk/peoplepopulationandcommunity/healthandsocialcare/causesofdeath/bulletins/coronaviruscovid19relateddeathsbyoccupationbeforeandduringlockdownenglandandwales/deathsregisteredbetween9marchand30jun2020.

Pauksztat, B., M. Grech, M. Kitada, and R. B. Jensen. 2020. "Seafarers' Experiences during the COVID-19 Pandemic: Report." Malmö: World Maritime University. http://dx.doi.org/10.21677/wmu20201213.

Pelletier, Mariève, Sara Carazo, Nathalie Jauvin, Denis Talbot, Gaston De Serres, and Michel Vézina. 2021. "Étude sur la détresse psychologique des travailleurs de la santé atteints de la COVID-19 au Québec durant la deuxième vague pandémique" Institut national de la santé publique du Québec. https://www.inspq.qc.ca/publications/3135-detresse-psychologique-travailleurs-sante-atteints-covid19.

Procureur général du Québec c. 2021. Tribunal administratif du travail, 500-17-116442-214, 22 April 2021(C.S.Québec).

Les professionnel(le)s en Soins de Santé Unis (PSSU-FIQP), CHSLD Vigi Dollard-des-Ormeaux and CNESST, INSPQ, and Procureur général du Québec et Centrale des syndicats nationaux (CSN). 2020. QCTAT 3362, [2021] AZ-51709629 (TAT).

Protecteur du Citoyen. 2020. "The Québec Ombudsman's Status Report: COVID-19 in CHSLDs during the First Wave of the Pandemic." Quebec City. https://protecteurducitoyen.qc.ca/sites/default/files/pdf/rapports_speciaux/progress-report-chslds-covid-19.pdf.

Proctor, Jason. 2021. "Air Canada Flight Attendant Wins Fight over COVID-19 Workers' Compensation." CBC, 30 January 2021. https://www.cbc.ca/news/canada/british-columbia/flight-attendant-workers-compensation-covid-1.5894340.

Public Health England. 2020. "National Flu and COVID-19 Surveillance Reports." *GOV.UK*. 8 October 2020. https://www.gov.uk/government/statistics/national-flu-and-covid-19-surveillance-reports.

Quigley, Ashley L., Haley Stone, Phi Yen Nguyen, Abrar Ahmad Chughtai, and C. Raina MacIntyre. 2021. "Estimating the Burden of COVID-19 on the Australian Healthcare Workers and Health System during the First Six Months of the Pandemic." *International Journal of Nursing Studies* 114 (February): 103811. https://doi.org/10.1016/j.ijnurstu.2020.103811.

Quinlan, Michael. 2021. "Covid-19, Health and Vulnerable Societies." *Annals of Work Exposures and Health*. Editorial: 1–5. https://doi.org/10.1093/annweh/wxaa127.

Radio-Canada. 2021. "Le camionnage, une industrie résiliente face à la pandémie." *Votre appel est important pour nous, avec Catherine Perrin*, 29 January 2021. https://ici.radio-canada.ca/premiere/emissions/votre-appel/segments/entrevue/341317/camion-route-temoignage-crise-covid-19-realite.

Reid, Alison, Elena Ronda-Perez, and Marc B. Schenker. 2021. "Migrant Workers, Essential Work, and COVID-19." *American Journal of Industrial Medicine* 64 (2): 7–77. https://doi.org/10.1002/ajim.23209.

Robitaille, David. 2020. "La COVID-19 Au Canada : Le Fédéralisme Coopératif à Pied d'œuvre." In *Vulnerable: The Law, Policy and Ethics of COVID-19*, edited by Colleen Flood, Vanessa MacDonnell, Jane Philpott, Sophie Thériault, and Sridhar Venkatapuram, 79–90. Ottawa: University of Ottawa Press. http://ruor.uottawa.ca/handle/10393/40726.

Ryser, Laura, Greg Halseth, and Sean Markey. 2020. "Dis-Orienting Mobile Construction Workforces: Impacts and Externalities within the Political Economy of Resource-Based Regions." *Labour & Industry: A Journal of the Social and Economic Relations of Work*. https://doi.org/10.1080/10301763.2020.1752353.

Sargeant, Malcolm, and Eric Tucker. 2009. "Layers of Vulnerability in Occupational Safety and Health for Migrant Workers: Case Studies from Canada and the UK." *Policy and Practice in Health and Safety* 7 (2): 51–73. https://doi.org/10.1080/14774003.2009.11667734.

Shan, Desai. 2020a. "People Who Carry Food and Fuel for the World Are Trapped at Sea: A Crewing Crisis in the Context of COVID-19." St John's, NL: *On the Move Partnership*. https://www.onthemovepartnership.ca/people-who-carry-food-and-fuel-for-the-world-are-trapped-at-sea-a-crewing-crisis-in-the-context-of-covid-19/.

– 2020b. "Stranded at Sea in the COVID-19 Pandemic." St John's, NL: *On the Move Partnership*. https://www.onthemovepartnership.ca/stranded-at-sea-in-the-covid-19-pandemic/.

Shan, Desai, and Barbara Neis. 2020. "Employment-Related Mobility, Regulatory Weakness and Potential Fatigue-Related Safety Concerns in Short-Sea Seafaring on Canada's Great Lakes and St Lawrence Seaway: Canadian Seafarers' Experiences." *Safety Science* 121 (January): 165–76. https://doi.org/10.1016/j.ssci.2019.08.017.

Shetty, Aastha. 2021. "ROW Paramedics' WSIB Claims Rejected after Being Exposed to COVID-19 (Update)." *Kitchener Today*, 21 January 2021. https://www.kitchenertoday.com/local-news/row-paramedics-wsib-claims-rejected-after-being-exposed-to-covid-19-3280166.

Simmons, Matt. 2020. "LNG Canada Workers Complained about Unsafe Conditions Prior to COVID-19 Outbreak." *The Narwhal*, 4 December 2020. https://thenarwhal.ca/lng-canada-covid-bc-work-camps/.

Skills for Care. n.d. "Workforce Nationality Figures." Accessed 31 January 2021. https://www.skillsforcare.org.uk/adult-social-care-workforce-data/Workforce-intelligence/publications/Topics/Workforce-nationality.aspx.

Stall, Nathan M., Kevin A. Brown, Antonina Maltsev, Aaron Jones, Andrew P. Costa, Vanessa Allen, Adalsteinn D. Brown, et al. 2021. "COVID-19 and Ontario's Long-Term Care Homes." Science Briefs of the Ontario COVID-19 Science Advisory Table. https://doi.org/10.47326/ocsat.2021.02.07.1.0.

Stannard, Suzanne. 2020. "COVID-19 in the Maritime Setting: The Challenges, Regulations and the International Response." *International Maritime Health* 71 (2): 85–90. https://doi.org/10.5603/IMH.2020.0016.

Statistique Canada. 2021. "Ensemble de données provisoires sur les cas confirmés de COVID-19, Agence de la santé publique du Canada." *Gouvernement du Canada*. 21 January 2021. https://www150.statcan.gc.ca/n1/pub/13-26-0003/1326000320200001-fra.htm.

Syed, Iffath Unissa, and Jesse McLaren. 2021. "COVID-19 Outbreaks in

Long-Term Care Highlight the Urgent Need for Paid Sick Leave." *The Conversation*, 26 January 2021. http://theconversation.com/covid-19-outbreaks-in-long-term-care-highlight-the-urgent-need-for-paid-sick-leave-153538.

The Canadian Press. 2018. "Ontario PCs Roll Back Liberal Labour Reforms in Sweeping New Legislation." *CBC*, 21 November 2018. https://www.cbc.ca/news/canada/toronto/ont-labour-reform-1.4914613.

Tombs, Steve, and David Whyte. 2010. "A DEADLY CONSENSUS: Worker Safety and Regulatory Degradation under New Labour." *The British Journal of Criminology* 50 (1): 46–65.

– 2013. "The Myths and Realities of Deterrence in Workplace Safety Regulation." *The British Journal of Criminology* 53 (5): 746–63. https://doi.org/10.1093/bjc/azt024.

Wallace, Kenyon, and Jenna Moon. 2020. "Toronto Scientists Dug into the Connection between Race, Income, Housing and COVID-19. What They Found Was 'Alarming.'" *Toronto Star*, 12 May 2020. https://www.thestar.com/news/gta/2020/05/12/toronto-scientists-dug-into-the-connection-between-race-income-housing-and-covid-19-what-they-found-was-alarming.html.

Watters, Haydn. 2021. "Public Health Units Can Shut down Ontario Workplaces for COVID. They Rarely Do." *CBC*, 13 January 2021. https://www.cbc.ca/news/canada/hamilton/ontario-public-health-unit-workplace-shutdowns-1.5868512.

Weeks, Carly. 2020. "Ontario, Alberta Change Policy Limiting N95 Masks as Health-Care Workers Demand Greater Access." *The Globe and Mail*, 2 April 2020. https://www.theglobeandmail.com/canada/article-ontario-alberta-change-policy-limiting-n95-masks-as-health-care/.

WSIB Ontario. 2021. "COVID-19 Related Claims Statistics." *WSIB*. 22 January 2021. https://www.wsib.ca/en/covid-19-related-claims-statistics.

Yarr, Kevin. 2020. "How Truckers Driving into 'the Heart of This Pandemic' Are Protecting Themselves." *CBC*, 24 March, 2020. https://www.cbc.ca/news/canada/prince-edward-island/pei-truckers-covid-19-pandemic-1.5508136.

Zarocostas, John. 2020. "UN Leaders Call for Key Worker Recognition for Seafarers." *The Lancet (British Edition)* 396 (10265): 1792. https://doi.org/10.1016/S0140-6736(20)32582-4.

3

Democracy, Law, and Politics in Pandemic Societies

9

The Politics of Populism in an Era of Pandemics: Freedom and Contagion in Brazil

Felix Rigoli

Normality was the Problem (Internet meme)

AN ONGOING APOCALYPSE

The following chapter was written during the COVID-19 pandemic in December 2020. While preparing it, I found that papers published in the third and fourth quarter of 2020 were obsolete. It is then easy to imagine that this text may be laughably out of date even in the near future. Therefore, I will restrict my comments to the aspects that may linger, mainly due to the fact that they were already present before the pandemic took hold.

Apocalypse, a term usually linked to disaster, is the name of the Book of Revelations in the Bible, the uncovering of what was previously veiled. The COVID-19 pandemic, an apocalyptic calamity, acted as a magnifying mirror on our society unveiling the cracks and wrinkles to which the day-by-day life did not allow us the time to pay attention. It exposed the worst defects in the social structure and their uneven impact on different groups; the atavism of collective fears (racism, xenophobia, denial, violence), the cruelty of the destruction of welfare states. It is in this world of job insecurity, where the state is absent, and has already given up its support networks of assistance, public health, and social protection, that the COVID-19 pandemic arises.

At the same time there were emergent samples of solidarity and compassion, some of them skin-deep such as the clapping for health workers, some others coming from the sheer need to eat, shelter, and take care of each other in places forgotten by the governments such as the Indigenous communities[1] and the urban favelas Paraisopolis (one of the largest favelas in Sao Paulo – see Paulo 2020); Ibura, Recife, and Rocinha (the largest favela in Rio de Janeiro; see Teixeira 2020 and #rocinhacontraocorona).

The main argument of this chapter is that this apocalypse cast a potent light on the role of the government, state, and public sector as the key organizer of the society, as opposed to governments that dismantle the public mechanism that keep the people working together. A few decades of "that government is best which governs least," ushered the way for a relatively new paradigm: no government at all is even better.

Contemporary divisions describe governments using polar antinomies: left and right, racism and anti-racism, feminism and patriarchy, even though most analyses show how these divisions are gradually being interweaved, creating the need for multilevel policies and creating priority challenges when choosing sides in the struggle for a better society (Nassif-Pires, Carvalho, and Rawet 2020).

The ways governments chose to react to the once-in-a-generation disaster showed the need of a new dilemma describing their fundamental options: the alternative between chaos and cohesion. A novelty, already existent before the pandemic, was the apparent success of governing by not governing, and that I would call entropic governments.

GOVERNING THROUGH ENTROPY

Entropy is roughly equivalent to disorder. It is also a general law in physics stating that closed systems (through thermodynamic flows) tend to dispersion of their parts in a one-way process. In the biological sphere, life is a permanent anti-entropic struggle to increase the organization of the matter, and when this struggle is abandoned (death), disorganization advances rapidly. There is a reason to say, "it is easy to make fish soup from an aquarium, but just imagine what challenge it is to try to make the aquarium out of the fish-soup" (Walesa 1996). It is in that sense that the new pro-chaos governments inevitably lead to pro-death contents, the so-called necropolitics. Let the aerial pictures of refrigerated morgue trucks and mass graves in the United States and Brazil speak by themselves regarding this concept.

It will be left to historians to decide if this basic trend of governing by letting social entropy run loose is a new breed of political strategies, or simply a new version of former destructive leaders, famous for their casualties' lists. In any case, the COVID-19 pandemic has called attention to the emerging pattern of leaders that govern un-governing, by actively cancelling any efforts to organize and unite society. Bolsonaro's Brazil is a compendium of characteristics that may be encompassed in the ultra-right political program, and the same may be said of Trump's action plan, but there is not necessarily a correspondence between ideology and political entropy.

Until the pandemic began to show its real dimension, many analysts were surprised by the success in electoral terms of this leadership style, in a mixed bunch of anti-democratic or "illiberal" governments.[2] The secret formula of the apparent success of these pro-chaos governments is to let disorder act, an easy promise to make and even easier to accomplish.

BRAZIL: ANATOMY OF CHAOS

In the case of Brazil, Mr Bolsonaro began early in his tenure by promising, jointly with his anti-left discourse, a series of "liberating" initiatives. The first in time and somehow an eccentric one, was to void the use of radar speed surveillance in the federal highways, a promise made to his truck-driver followers. Shortly after, the government went after the Environment Agency (IBAMA) agents that had fined him for illegal sport fishing in the Rio de Janeiro coast, followed by a wider attack on the environment agencies, freezing posts and funding to restrain surveillance and control of wildlife. A much more wide-reaching action was then implemented through public allegations of treason against the Chief Scientist of the National Space Research Institute (INPE) accusing him to be in the payroll of foreign NGO's and working against the Brazilian international image, forging satellite images and numbers to exaggerate the wildfires and deforestation rates. This attack was followed by the dismissal of the INPE authorities, remaining unfilled or with interim third-level staff until today. This was part of a new highly effective "liberation" front: it was the signal given to a large number of illegal settlers, lumbers, and gold diggers telling them that there were no boundaries to deforestation and use of protected lands for profit. The deforestation reached its highest level in over a decade. The

Statista website estimated that even though the COVID-19 pandemic put restrictions on travels and human activities, 11,088 square kilometers of the Brazilian Amazon were destroyed in 2020, up from 10,129 square kilometers in 2019, both the highest deforestation rates since 2008 (Pasquali 2020). The assault is not restricted to trees and fauna: during 2019 there were 160 incidents with invasions and occupations of Indigenous lands (Vick 2020), and many of these incidents ended with Indigenous leaders being killed.

Another area of cancelling collective action was the closure of 99% of the participatory councils that were under Federal authorities. A total of 2,561 councils, advisory boards, ethics committees, and other kinds of formal civil society participation were abolished (Saconi, Aleixo, and Maia 2019). The thirty-two remaining bodies had been created by law, therefore out of presidential authority reach, but their funding was lowered to the minimum. It is worth noting that many powerful stakeholders saluted the massive cancelling of social participation that cut most of the oversight and watchdog activities that wished to keep their activities out of scrutiny. As an example, the pesticides licensed in the country amounted to an average of 163 products per year in 2010–2015, jumping to 392 per year from 2016 to 2020, a 140% increase (Sudré 2019). It was less an intent of extending the autocratic grip on the state machine and more a step towards a modern version of the survival of the fittest, in this case understanding fittest as wealthier, crueler, or with fewer scruples.

Further expanding the "liberation" of the basic instincts of the society, the government assaulted the statistical information system of the country. Once the satellite surveillance was weakened, the government turned its attention to blind the capacity of the country to look inwards, to methodically review indicators of its progress or deterioration. It is already known that Brazil is routinely in the top list of world inequalities, even with ups and downs, and this has always been a matter of concern to scholars and politicians. The Brazilian statistics office, IBGE is a world-class agency with a portfolio of geographic, demographic, and economic activities, and inevitably scans regional, race, and social disparities, showing the status and the effect of social and economic policies. Since the beginning of the Bolsonaro's government, IBGE was the target of multiple criticisms over information regarding poverty, unemployment, and the state of the economy. In the now classic style of twenty-first century populist leaders, the president declared that he trusted more his Facebook questionnaires than population-wide IBGE surveys. The Census to be held in 2020 had (before the COVID-19 pandemic) budget cuts amounting to more than 40%. The guidelines that IBGE received to adapt the Census to the new budget encompassed cuts in questions regarding housing, possession of refrigerators or other household items, rendering it useless to measure changes in housing deficit, poverty, and other key indicators (Hermanson 2019). During the COVID-19 pandemic, after the resignation of the second Minister of Health in a month, the government decided to implement a data blackout regarding COVID-19 cases and deaths, by skipping daily information, updating later with different criteria in order to disrupt the visualization of trends. This blackout prompted the local health authorities and the media to create a consortium to collate and keep track of the cases and deaths. In the same vein, the Ministry of Health blocked and mismanaged the kits for viral tests, making Brazil one of the few countries that do not know the trends of confirmed diagnosis, being also unable to measure key indicators such as test and positivity rates.

During a recorded cabinet meeting on 22 April 2020, the footage released by judicial order showed the intimacy of the entropic government, presided by Bolsonaro. The president pledged to "implode" the national Metrology Institute, due to its obstinate interest in putting GPS trackers in the truck fleet in order to monitor fuel consumption and transit density. Singing the same tune, the Minister of Environment warned his peers that the public opinion was distracted by the pandemic and urged them to hurry up and dismantle as much as possible the regulations protecting nature. In the same meeting, the president exposed his wish to have all citizens armed, fending for themselves, and not trusting in the public services.

Perhaps the most lasting and entropic feature of the Brazilian government, and a common trait of all new populist governments, is the intention to seed distrust in education, science, and scientists. Brazilian public health is well recognized worldwide, led by several cutting-edge teaching and research institutions such as FIOCRUZ and the public universities of Sao Paulo, Bahia and Rio de Janeiro. During the last two years all research agencies were on top of the lists in the budget cuts, and research in social sciences was specially targeted as "with low returns for society" (Passarinho 2019). The political communication regarding the pandemic was characteristically marked by anti-scientific events, mirroring the Trump evolution on that matter: denial, distrust in statistics, magic drugs, and shrugging off responsibilities (The Lancet 2020). Two conservative health ministers were dismissed because they refused to endorse and push the Chloroquine and HCQ treatment through the public health network.

NEGATIONISM AS IDEOLOGY, NEGATIONISM AS TOOL

Populist governments may be divided according to their initial approach to the pandemic into those that decided to use the emergency as an opportunity to show their capacity to rule; and those that opted for showing invulnerability by dismissing the risks.

The former populist governments (e.g., Turkey, Hungary, and Poland) seized the chance of expanding their power and portrayed themselves as captains of a ship in troubled waters, demanding support and obedience. Due to the nature of the pandemic, its unexpected seriousness and long duration, this approach proved to be more competent to manage the population's risk and gained them some support.

The latter governments, in denial of the dangers (notably USA, UK, Brazil), were linked with an a priori option to follow the USA policy related to the virus, and trusting the contents and orientations issued by the ideological entourage of the presidency of that country – albeit not concurrent with the technical agencies of its government (Goolsbee and Syverson 2020). The leadership style in those cases was careless about serious management of crises and eager to move on fast to a fully functioning economy.

This approach failed in two main aspects: the pandemic timeframe was optimistically underestimated, due to wishful thinking and unexpected differences from previous flu, SARS, and MERS pandemics; the economic activity was reduced mainly due to the population's perceived risk and not so much by the stay-at-home orders. Comparing consumer behaviour within the same areas, but across boundaries with different policy regimes suggests that legal shutdown orders account for only a modest share of the decline of economic activity (Goolsbee and Syverson 2020). The results of a macroeconomic study on the economic effects of fear and altruism during a pandemic suggest that stimulating aggregate demand or providing liquidity to businesses have limited capacity to restore employment when consumer spending is constrained by health concerns (Bandler et al. 2020).

As the epidemiologic process evolved, fatal victims mounted and the reality of a deadly catastrophe gained the public opinion. The only escape route left for these populist leaders who chose the wrong alternative, was to stick to their postulates clouded in a smoke screen of negationism. Rochel Camargo et al. (2020) describe five features of the processes to expand negationism, all observed over the last months in public discussions about the pandemic:

1 identification of conspiracies;
2 use of false experts;
3 selectivity, focusing on isolated articles that contradict the scientific consensus ("cherry-picking");
4 creation of impossible expectations for the research;
5 use of misrepresentations or logical fallacies.

The need of watering down the images of excavators performing mass burials demanded an intensification of narratives regarding miracle drugs, distrust in statistics, and blaming the media. The government then recruited a few doctors – oncologists, anesthesiologists, general practitioners, and politicians to act as science advisers, amplifying through social media several theories based in their limited personal experience that contradicted all the evidence. As if to create further confusion, stunts and decoys often seemed to arrive without warning: the president fights with an ostrich over a box of Chloroquine (UOL 2020a); or issue executive orders by Twitter determining that Brazil will never buy a Chinese vaccine that has already been produced by a public lab in Sao Paulo (UOL 2020b). The volume of contents, the dizzying number of narratives and counter-narratives, and the pace of the news cycle were designed to overwhelm people's capacity to process.

THE FAVELA STRIKES BACK

The dissemination of carefully crafted fake news has hampered to an extreme the capacity of bottom-up resilience efforts (Da Empoli 2019), that are now paradoxically blossoming in the favelas of the big cities as the aforementioned initiatives in Paraisopolis, Ibura, Rocinha, and many others. The perception of chaos and its deadly consequences is not exclusive of the scientific community, and many community leaders took matters in their own hands, filling the black hole of information and collective guidance that the government was creating. Most of these communities organized themselves, creating even "Street Presidents" to take care of segments of the neighbourhoods (the largest favelas may have between one hundred thousand and two hundred thousand inhabitants) and organized cooperatives of seamstresses to make masks at home and small home factories to prepare hand sanitizer, cooking basic food to give to isolated persons, and even distributing recycled plastic bottles with water to those homes lacking permanent supply of piped water. It was clear for the community leaders that no help could be expected from above, not from the present government, but also not from previous authorities that usually neglected the design and implementation of policies that take in consideration the favela conditions. For that reason, the #rocinharesiste movement has as its motto: "Rocinha exists, Rocinha insists, Rocinha resists" (InformaSUS UFSCar 2020a).

Even well-organized drug gangs have understood that an epidemic that kills people, and especially poor favela dwellers, is something to be dealt with seriously.

Recently, a social science team studied an extreme case of this phenomenon in Brazil's most emblematic city, Rio de Janeiro, where extreme unequal areas lay just a few meters away one from the other. For some time now, Rio's sociologists have been studying the effects of a city that is no longer divided into rich and poor – the favela and asphalt in the samba-school jargon – as before. There are, already accepted even by the institute of official statistics (IBGE) three regions: the "normal" city of Rio, the regions governed by drug trafficking and the regions under the control of the militias (divided more or less in 60% + 20% + 20% respectively of 9 million inhabitants). The term "militias" is used in Brazil to designate a special type of organized outlaw forces, originally composed of former police or security guards who take control of poorer regions, initially as a form of private protection against drug trafficking. After several decades it degenerated into violent control of important city regions in which they are the law, charging merchants and neighbours for all kinds of services, including transportation, cable TV, and constructing multi-story buildings that are rented out without respect for any legal regulations and, indeed, sometimes collapse, killing all of their occupants (BBC 2019). The phenomenon of the militias is important, because although it is quite restricted to regions of Rio, it is at the same time the basic support of the Bolsonaro family, and therefore is being expanded into other states (Rígoli 2020).

Using the already accepted division of city, in "normal," "drug traffic," and "militia" zones, researchers from several universities in Brazil and Spain reviewed the COVID-19 statistics in terms of cases and deaths in the three regions finding an interesting difference. Using the "normal" city zones as a parameter, the regions controlled by drug traffickers had significantly fewer deaths from COVID-19-related respiratory infections, while in the regions controlled by militia, deaths from the same respiratory infections increased significantly more than in the normal city.

According to testimonies from neighbours, this is due to the opposing attitudes of the leaders of those illegal groups. In the favela Cidade de Deus, the traffickers passed by the streets with megaphones saying: "We are imposing a curfew because nobody is taking it [the coronavirus] seriously. It is better to stay home and relax. Pay attention to this message" while at the same time imposing the use of masks on the street. Meanwhile, a storeowner in a neighbourhood controlled by militia groups commented, "They [the militia] are threatening to kill us all if we keep our businesses closed" (Prado, Nascimento, and Regueira 2020). This is possibly due to the fact that the militias charge, in the style of the Sicilian mafia, a percentage of what is cashed every day. It is also undeniable that militia officers have close connections with the Bolsonaro group in power and they spread the discourse of denial of the pandemic and "going on with their lives" without taking care of the "*gripezinha*" (mild flu).

On the other hand, traffickers are afraid of both themselves and their families (who, unlike militia officers, live in the slums) getting sick. The former health minister, Mandetta acknowledged this fact and tried to negotiate with the traffickers to guarantee health care continuity, shortly before he was forced to resign.

The researchers used a unique approach: they consider the cases and deaths from severe respiratory infections (linked to COVID-19) as the result of two treatments: firstly, Militia control; secondly, drug traffic control. The remaining "normal" areas were used as a control group. This is interesting because both militia-controlled and trafficking neighbourhoods are groups at higher risk for respiratory infections due to poverty, overcrowding, and lack of running water. Comparing 2019 and 2020, the mortality rate due to respiratory infections (as a proxy for COVID-19 deaths) increased a lot throughout the city. However, in militia-controlled neighbourhoods, deaths from respiratory infection increased 29 per cent more than in normal neighbourhoods, while in traffic-controlled regions, deaths from this cause rose 43 per cent less than the average in ordinary neighbourhoods. This paradoxical result – in a country of paradoxes – reveals that, even in extreme cases and out of any normality, the force of cohesive behaviour acts in favour of public health, and inversely, the negative attitudes and "each one for himself" are a factor of death and destruction. It also reveals the chains of transmission that run the death mindset (necropolitics) from the president to the most humble favelas.

THE VACCINES' ENDGAME

The present (end of 2020) act of this tragedy in Brazil – no testing and tracing, pushing magic pills, denial – is a federal versus regional struggle regarding vaccines, their country of origin, if they will be mandatory, who will pay, and who gets them first. The media use terms such as Chinese, Russian, or Oxford to peddle or tarnish several different candidates that are being tested in phase three in Brazil.

The way this issue is being publicly debated is as a matter of distributing and injecting a product as soon as possible. This kind of simplification obscures the fact that the technical efficacy of any vaccine is a component of the wider effort to stop the dissemination of endemic or epidemic diseases. All the epidemiological models of COVID-19 and previous infectious diseases show that no vaccine will be socially effective by itself. In the present case and due to the many unknown pieces of scientific information that are still missing, it is essential to maintain most of the distancing measures, masks, and hygiene until the entire population is vaccinated. An article, discussing the impact of vaccinations and the need to maintain control of the epidemic until the entire population is immunized, concludes that the way vaccination is implemented will contribute more to the success of vaccination programs than the vaccine efficacy determined in clinical trials. The benefits of a vaccine will be substantially diminished if there are discontinuities in either manufacture or distribution, if there is a lack of adherence from the population, or if the epidemic is out of control.

As Cueto (2020) explains:

In these efforts a great deal of hope was placed. The expectation is that by the end of this year or the beginning of 2021, one or more vaccines may be applied in the population. Little attention has been paid to the risks of overvaluing a technology or creating what historians call a "magic bullet." In many stories of previous epidemic outbreaks, technologies emerged that seemed to solve the problem regardless of the social conditions in which people lived (such as DDT against malaria-borne mosquitoes). Generally, little attention was given to the social and institutional factors involved in immunization, or the synergy between a well-structured health team and the population (which enabled the eradication of smallpox in 1980).[3]

Ironically, Brazil is a country with one of the most recognized immunization programs in the world, reaching 90% of the population with an expanded set of vaccines that had until 2013 basically eliminated every major preventable disease. All the international experience shows that community immunity demands common action plans, due to the positive externalities of vaccination. In the case of COVID-19, even the tenuous evidence of immunity given by the present vaccines may be completely voided by the chaotic implementation of different substances, using different timetables, and with different types and degrees of effect, not even counting the nightmare of planning the surveillance of effects (phase 4 evaluation) in a large and disconnected territory.

There is a chilling warning appearing in the landscape of vaccines that until now show efficacy in 60-days trial, in a disease that has exhibited highly variable levels of lasting immunity and even documented cases of second infections. Goldman Sachs investing consulting firm analyzed the case of Hepatitis C, issuing a rhetorical question to the pharmaceutical industry: perhaps creating products that cure patients (in the sense of a definitive cure) is not a sustainable business model? (Mole 2018)

FREEDOM AND CONTAGION: A PERVERSE MEANING FOR "LIBERATION"

To a greater or lesser extent, this type of government claims to "liberate" the individuals, and is now popular in many countries. It is only easier to study in Brazil because of its exaggeration.

It will be left to historians and analysts to say how this idea of dismantling the state affected traditional societies such as the United Kingdom, that may cut its ties from the European Union even breaking the international law (Harris 2020); or India that repealed in one act more than 1,200 regulations, scrapping the planning agency altogether (see Reuters 2015 and Nair 2017). As per the results of the recent elections in the USA, the main champion of governing by chaos, Donald Trump has not succeeded in getting support for his policies. Managing a deadly disease by creating paralysis and havoc is perceivably the worst alternative and it proved fatal for hundreds of thousands of citizens. *Financial Times* chief analyst Martin Wolf wonders if COVID-19 will put an end to populism in the USA, UK, and Brazil due to their extremely poor record in managing the epidemic wave, keeping those three countries in the top list of infection and dead rates. The problem with those leaders, as Wolf puts it is that, "They don't care about government. They don't really understand what government is for. And they're indifferent to it. In some ways and in some cases they're actually trying to dismantle the state" (Wolf 2020).

Populist leadership rule keeps state as formally democratic, but assumes a fierce attitude. The ruling gang aggressively seizes space in the public media and constantly seeks out scapegoats. However, as De Munck states (2020), this type of government does not seek to directly control civil society. It does not deploy an omni-competent government; on the contrary, it destroys the experience and capacity for action of the atate's public services and, instead, seeks to allow corporations to take full control of society.

But probably it is too soon to say that the tide that brought chaos-populist-entropic leaders to power is over. This is a strong current in the world, perhaps revolutionary, that proposes the idea of dynamiting the state, ending the linkages that force society to work in a united way – with exceptions made of the structures that keep financial markets open. In *Seeds of Time* (1994), Fredric Jameson stated that in the current conjuncture it is easier to imagine the end of the world than the end of capitalism. Therefore, this autocratically inclined state supports, as an apparent paradox, economic, health, educational, social, and environmental deregulation on a large scale. It does not seek to control or replace private agents, but to allow them to operate freely at all levels of society. The entropic way of governing is also celebrated by the prophets of disruption, the creed of "move fast and break things" that Facebook preconized, allowing them to contribute to the disruption of democracies all over the world (Teitelbaum 2020).

The use that the Bolsonaro-type populist leaders make of the words freedom and liberation needs to be exposed. The mere idea that there is a "freedom from using a mask," that a person may be free to avoid protection from a virus, that there is a valid freedom for not being vaccinated, all those terms seemed just a decade ago a tale of collective insanity, something that belonged to sci-fi movies. One of the weird features of the pandemic society is the regression of the idea of liberty to the field of primitive pre-Hobbesian societies. The cult for gothic aesthetics and heroes and the return to far past times are a weird component of twenty-first century culture. In the political field it is expressed by a return to a non-state, with no civilization and no obligations, reminiscent of an idealized past with undertones of patriarchy, racism, and inequalities, that Teitelbaum called "Traditionalism" (2020). The idea of liberty is then used in a very particular sense; it is the freedom of not feeling responsible for anything. These seldom called neo-fascist governments are, from a very perverse perspective, governments of liberation. But what kind of liberation is this? They propose the liberation of any obligation of collective solidarity. The pandemic showed us, in a very short period, how this society liberated from the links of solidarity will crumble under any sort of threat that demands joint action. Perhaps waking up to this kind of awareness will be the starting point to work together, as the favelas in Brazil did, to face other long-term global threats to our existence.

NOTES

1 Some of these movements gathered recently in a series of Zoom meetings by the Federal University of Sao Carlos (in Portuguese). See InformaSUS UFSCar (2020b).
2 Among other authors, see Levitsky and Ziblatt (2018) and Mounk (2018).
3 Note: translated from the Portuguese by the author.

REFERENCES

Alfaro, Laura, Ester Faia, Nora Lamersdorf, and Farzad Saidi. 2020. "Social Interactions in Pandemics: Fear, Altruism, And Reciprocity."

National Bureau of Economic Research Working Paper No. 27134. http://www.nber.org/papers/w27134.

Bandler, James, Patricia Callahan, Sebastian Rotella, and Kirsten Berg. 2020. "Inside the Fall of the CDC." *ProPublica*, 15 October 2020. https://www.propublica.org/article/inside-the-fall-of-the-cdc.

BBC. 2019. "Desabamento no Rio: o que dizem investigações e moradores sobre a atuação das milícias na região de Muzema." *BBC*, 12 April 2019. https://www.bbc.com/portuguese/brasil-47917081.

Bruce, Raphael, Alexsandros Cavgias, and Luis Meloni. 2020. "Filling the Void? Organized Crime and COVID-19 in Rio De Janeiro." Working Paper (21 August 2020). http://dx.doi.org/10.2139/ssrn.3678840

Cueto, Marcos. 2020. "Covid-19 e a corrida pela vacina." História, Ciências, Saúde *Manguinhos* 27, no. 3: 715–717. http://www.scielo.br/scielo.php?script=sci_arttext&pid=S0104597020200030071 5&lng=en&nrm=iso.

da Empoli, Giuliano. 2019. "Os engenheiros do caos: Como as fake news, as teorias da conspiração e os algoritmos estão sendo utilizados para disseminar ódio, medo e influenciar eleições." São Paulo: Editora Vestigio.

de Munck, Jean. 2020. "Three Responses to the Coronavirus Crisis." *openDemocracy*, April. https://www.opendemocracy.net/en/democraciaabierta/three-responses-coronavirus-crisis/.

Goolsbee, Austan, and Chad Syverson. 2021. "Fear, Lockdown, and Diversion: Comparing Drivers of Pandemic Economic Decline 2020." *Journal of Public Economics* 193 (January). https://doi.org/10.1016/j.jpubeco.2020.104311.

Harris, John. 2020. "Disruption, destruction and chaos has become the new way of governing." *The Guardian*, 13 September 2020. https://www.theguardian.com/commentisfree/2020/sep/13/tories-new-unscrupulous-politics-misinformation.

Hermanson, Marcos. 2019. "Com novo corte, Censo 2020 pode ser cancelado ou virar contagem populacional." *Brasil de Fato*, 28 August 2019. https://www.brasildefato.com.br/2019/08/28/com-novo-corte-censo-2020-pode-ser-cancelado-ou-virar-contagem-populacional.

InformaSUS UFSCar. 2020a. "Live Do Informasus: Experiências de APS na pandemia: as favelas no enfrentamento da Covid-19." YouTube video, 2:20:24, 15 October 2020, https://youtu.be/hJU3WMSfBvM.

—. 2020b. "Experiências da APS na Pandemia: (re)existência" Kaiowá, Guarani e Terena de Dourados e região." YouTube video, 2:23:02, 25 November 2020. https://www.youtube.com/watch?v=951fOikCF5w&feature=youtu.be.

Jameson, Fredric. 1994. *The Seeds of Time*. Wellek Library Lectures at the University of California, Irvine. New York: Columbia University Press.

Levitsky, Steven, and Daniel Ziblatt. 2018. *How Democracies Die*. New York: Crown Publishing.

Mole, Beth. 2018. "'Is curing patients a sustainable business model?' Goldman Sachs analysts ask." *Ars Technica*, 12 April 2018. https://arstechnica.com/tech-policy/2018/04/curing-disease-not-a-sustainable-business-model-goldman-sachs-analysts-say/.

Mounk, Yascha. 2018. *The People vs. Democracy: Why Our Freedom Is in Danger and How to Save It*. Cambridge: Harvard University Press.

Nair, Harish V. 2017. "Goodbye, old laws: Modi government scraps 1,200 redundant Acts, 1,824 more identified for repeal." *India Today*, 22 June 2017. https://www.indiatoday.in/mail-today/story/narendra-modi-law-ministry-ravi-shankar-prasad-984025-2017-06-22.

Nassif-Pires, Luiza, Laura Carvalho, and Eduardo Rawet. 2020. "Multidimensional Inequality and Covid-19 in Brazil." *Levy Economics Institute of Bard College Public Policy Brief* no. 153. http://www.levyinstitute.org/publications/multidimensional-inequality-and-covid-19-in-brazil.

Paes Manso, Bruno. 2020. *A república das milícias: Dos esquadrões da morte à era Bolsonaro*. São Paulo: Todavia Editora.

Paltiel, A. David, Jason L. Schwartz, Amy Zheng, and Rochelle P. Walensky. 2020. "Clinical Outcomes of a COVID-19 Vaccine: Implementation Over Efficacy." *Health Affairs* 40, no.1 (19 November 2020). https://www.healthaffairs.org/doi/10.1377/hlthaff.2020.02054

Pasquali, Marina. 2020. "Brazil: deforested area in the Amazon rainforest 2004–2020." *Statista*. 3 December 2020. https://www.statista.com/statistics/940696/brazil-amazon-deforestation-rate-area/.

Passarinho, Nathalia. 2019. "Ameaçados por cortes no governo, cursos de humanas cocnentram diversidade." UOL. 5 September 2019. https://educacao.uol.com.br/noticias/bbc/2019/05/09/ameaca-cortes-bolsonaro-cursos-de-ciencias-sociais-humanas-diversidade.htm.

Paulo, Paulo Paiva. 2020. "Paraisópolis contrata médicos e ambulâncias, distribui mais de mil marmitas por dia e se une contra o coronavírus." *Globo*, 7 April 2020. https://g1.globo.com/sp/sao-paulo/noticia/2020/04/07/paraisopolis-se-une-contra-o-coronavirus-contrata-ambulancias-medicos-e-distribui-mais-de-mil-marmitas-por-dia.ghtml.

Prado, Anita, Raphael Nascimento, and Chico Regueira. 2020. "Comércio em área de milícias é obrigado a funcionar durante a quarentena em

Itaboraí." *Globo*, 25 May 2020. https://g1.globo.com/rj/rio-de-janeiro/noticia/2020/05/25/comercio-em-area-de-milicias-e-obrigado-a-funcionar-durante-a-quarentena-em-itaborai.ghtml.

Reuters. 2015. "Modi replaces Planning Commission, aiming to boost growth." *Reuters*, 1 January 2015. https://in.reuters.com/article/india-planningcommission-modi/modi-replaces-planning-commission-aiming-to-boost-growth-idINKBN0KA1NA20150101.

Rígoli, Félix. 2020. "Crimen y Covid (versión carioca)." 25*Siete*, 28 August 2020. https://www.257.uy/post/crimen-y-covid-versi%C3%B3n-carioca.

Rochel Camargo, Kenneth, and Claudia Medina Coeli. 2020. "A Difícil Tarefa de Informar: em meio a uma pandemia." *Physis: Revista De Saúde Coletiva* 30, no. 2: 1–5.

Saconi, João Paulo, Isabela Aleixo, and Gustavo Maia. "Decreto do governo Bolsonaro mantém apenas 32 conselhos consultivos." *Globo*, 29 June 2019. https://oglobo.globo.com/brasil/decreto-do-governo-bolsonaro-mantem-apenas-32-conselhos-consultivos-23773337.

Sudré, Lu. 2019. "Liberação de agrotóxicos no governo Bolsonaro é a maior dos últimos 14 anos." *Brasil de Fato*, 27 November 2019. https://www.brasildefato.com.br/2019/11/27/liberacao-de-agrotoxicos-no-governo-bolsonaro-e-a-maior-dos-ultimos-14-anos.

Teitelbaum, Benjamin R. 2020. *War for Eternity: Inside Bannon's Far-Right Circle of Global Power.* New York: Dey St–HarperCollins.

Teixeira, Marcionila. 2020. "Favelas tomam iniciativa para melhorar o combate à Covid-19." *Diario de Pernambuco*, 4 June 2020. https://www.diariodepernambuco.com.br/noticia/vidaurbana/2020/04/favelas-tomam-iniciativa-para-melhorar-o-combate-a-covid-19.html.

The Lancet Editorial. 2020. "COVID-19 in Brazil: 'So What?'" *The Lancet* 395, Issue 10235, P1461 (9 May 2020).

UOL. 2020a. "Bolsonaro exibe caixa de cloroquina para emas no Palácio da Alvorada." *UOL*. 23 July 2020. https://noticias.uol.com.br/politica/ultimasnoticias/2020/07/23/bolsonaro-exibe-caixa-de-cloroquina-para-emas-no-palacio-da-alvorada.htm.

– 2020b. "Bolsonaro desautoriza acordo de Pazuello e diz que não comprará CoronaVac." *UOL*. 21 October 2020. https://noticias.uol.com.br/politica/ultimas-noticias/2020/10/21/bolsonaro-responde-a-criticas-sobre-vacina-chinesa-nao-sera-comprada.htm.

Vick, Mariana. 2020. "Como a pandemia agrava o risco de invasões em terras indígenas." *Nexo*, 18 April 2020. https://www.nexojornal.com.br/expresso/2020/04/18/Como-a-pandemia-agrava-o-risco-de-invas%C3%

B5es-em-terras-ind%C3%ADgenas#:~:text=As%20invas%C3%B5es%20a%20terras%20ind%C3%ADgenas,janeiro%20e%20setembro%20de%202019.

Walesa, Lech. 1996. "Lech Walesa on the Challenge of Poland's Transformation." *Radio Free Europe: Radio Liberty*, 9 August 1996. https://www.rferl.org/a/1081206.html.

Wolf, Martin. 2020. "Will Covid-19 kill off populism?" *Financial Times*, 13 August 2020. https://www.ft.com/video/1d5916ab-66b9-44ef-8528-804f518837f0.

Borders and the Global Pandemic of COVID-19

Élisabeth Vallet, Mathilde Bourgeon, Laurence Brassard, Gabrielle Gagnon, Julie Renaud

INTRODUCTION

In less than four weeks, in the spring of 2020, the rapid spread of COVID-19 led to a swift closure of borders around the world. At the height of the crisis, in March 2020, 91 per cent of the world's population lived in a country with border restrictions – 39 per cent of them in countries whose borders were completely closed to non-citizens and non-residents (Connor 2020). In Europe, the 25th anniversary of the Schengen Agreement was thus marked by the re-introduction of state border controls (See Wille 2020, 11). At the same time, at the core of the North American zone, Mexico unilaterally closed its border with the United States, while for the second time since the beginning of the twenty-first century, the Canada-US land border – long described as the longest undefended border in the world – was sealed, and the US president announced his intention to deploy the army to the area (see Wille 2020, 11).

These expedient closures, however, did not occur in a vacuum. Indeed, the current movement of border closures must be understood through the evolution that has characterized border regimes since the end of the Cold War. Certainly, the opening of borders combined with the acceleration of globalization following the fall of the Berlin Wall has led to the creation of spaces in which capital, goods and, ultimately, people can move freely – even if these ensembles were themselves ultimately enclosed (Newman 2009). Yet at the turn of each subsequent decade, this process has had significant repercussions. Firstly, the events of September 11 represented the first slowdown in this progression, leading to both the processes of externalizing borders and decelerating flows, with the expressed objective of slowing down the international terrorism contamination. What was initially perceived as only exceptional – a sort of North American epiphenomenon – gradually normalized and extended: the controls put in place following the attacks on American soil ended up redefining regimes, practices, and border crossings around the world, particularly within large regional groups (see, for example, Smith, Ray, Raymond, Sienna, and Lilly 2018). Secondly, a decade later, the Arab Spring of 2011 added to this trend towards selective detention as standards for the right of asylum, or the right to leave one's country as enshrined in the *Universal Declaration of Human Rights* of 1948, were rapidly eroded. Flows have adapted to these decades of evolution while the successive mutations have instead led to the redefinition of territories. Reflecting the fact that globalization is not uniform, borders are now complex, just as the mobilities they are supposed to filter. They are both open and closed, and are meant to be mainly interfaces between two legal regimes.

Consequently, the swift and global movement to close borders to certain types of flows, following the COVID-19 crisis, is consistent with the trend of continuous and increasing border fortification in the world, particularly since the beginning of the twenty-first century (Vallet 2020). While, in the wake of the fall of the Berlin Wall, mobility was clearly the new analytical framework of the global system, symbols of fixity, such as border walls, have emerged from their obsolescence to embrace a growing trend towards a multitude of processes of selective closure and the reticular nature of the border. Thus, in the context of a pandemic for which there was little prospect of spontaneous favourable evolution, no effective medication to reduce the most severe symptoms and for almost ten months no accessible vaccine, borders were quickly considered as a tool that could be rapidly mobilized to reduce mobilities and thus contagion, to the point of dominating public discourse from time to time. But border closures proved to be modular, confirming their role as asymmetric filters. Notably because mobilities, in a globalized and interdependent world, remain one of the keys to the world economy and supply structures, their malleability is therefore the key to a post-pandemic world.

THE PERVASIVE USAGE OF BORDERS IN THE DISCOURSE ON PANDEMICS

The pandemic management process saw the mobilization of a bellicose language based on war and military metaphors to convey the urgency of the situation and to facilitate the deployment of resources; this language quickly gained traction at the borders. This semantic choice defined national borders as the main lines of defence against the virus, restoring border lines to their functions as a means of defining the nation-state: in this context, borders (and their security) became political tools for governments:

> the country is at war with the coronavirus; winning the battle and beating the COVID-19; itching to declare victory over the novel coronavirus; healthcare professionals are on the front line; government ministers meet over Zoom in virtual war cabinets.[1]

As a result, some states have deployed military forces to their national borders, focusing initially on border militarization rather than on tangible measures to curb the spread of the virus. Border fortification, which thus took place rapidly, therefore responds to the confluence of two processes of securitization, one health and the other border-related, through a discursive mechanism that amalgamates the two. Hence: "The practice of naming in this specific case can be understood as a linguistic practice of (re)-border-ing, as 'linguistic (re-)bordering' processes: The disease is assigned to a specific location outside of one's own borders and thus created as something foreign, which is then seen as a threat to the nation from the outside" (Nossem 2020) – identical to the processes observed during the Spanish flu.

The SARS-COV-2 has thus been the subject of such a securitization process: it has been unanimously defined and described as a threat to national security rather than a global issue (Balzacq 2005). Rapidly accepted as such by the people of the various states affected by the pandemic, confronted with worrying figures and the risk of overloading national health systems, the fight against "this enemy" served to legitimize the implementation of exceptional policies, including the hardening of international borders, which were themselves seen as bearers of risk. Indeed, since the virus was deemed to come from outside in connection with flows that were quickly labeled as undesirable or even perceived as a threat to national security, it was only logical, in a rapid securitization process, that borders should become the suitable tool for governments. From this perspective, the border takes the form of a "protective shield" (Berrod and Bruyas 2020), identical to what was done in the eighteenth century to prevent the spread of the last plague epidemic. In fact, "most of our methods of combatting COVID-19 are positively ancient" (Roberts 10): "the best we currently have are medieval measures such as quarantining, travel bans, wearing masks, confinement and social distancing more broadly" (Heisbourg 2020, 7).

Yet history shows that the significance of border fortifications in pandemic situations is often more symbolic than real (Espinoza, Castillo-Chavez, and Perrings, 2020) – as attested by the useless "Mur de la Peste" (Plague Wall; see figures 10.1 and 10.2). Perceived as the line demarcating the interior from the exterior, the "Self" from the "Other," the citizen from the foreigner, the border becomes a buffer space where the opening and closing define an exogenous threat: the closure of the border thus serves the construction of a narrative that differs from this reality. On the one hand, the rapidity of border shutdowns has varied with the level of integration among regional groupings, such as in the European Union, or between Canada and the United States, for example (Fillion 2020; Thiessen 2020). On the other hand, border closure within a dyad has frequently been driven by an increase in the number of cases in the heart of the state that opted to implement border closure, rather than a rise in the cases in the adjacent state. When securing borders as the epidemic worsens domestically, leaders shift the focus and transfer liability for the situation to someone else, without naming him or her. Securitization here is a strategic practice (Balzacq 2005) that goes beyond the implementation of security policies and the mobilization of increased governmental resources. In this respect, the political management of the pandemic is part of an already well-established logic of theatricalization of the border (Vallet 2020): "the symbolic nature of closing the border evoked the sense that something forceful and authoritative was being done" (Scott 2020: 7). The border spectacle (Garrett 2018) obscures more prosaic realities (Simonneau 2020). Evidence of this is that the promptness in identifying national borders as a line of defence has not been followed by a similar movement for sub-national borders, which nevertheless simultaneously contributed to slowing down flows.

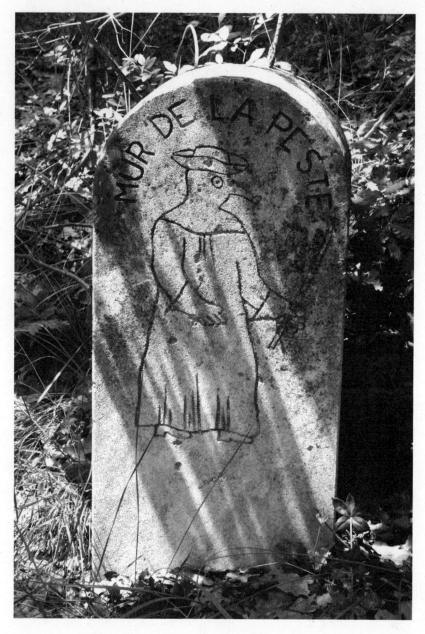

Figure 10.1 | Signalling Post–Wall of Plague / *Borne de signalisation contemporaine Mur de la Peste* (1721). Cabrières-d'Avignon, département du Vaucluse (France).

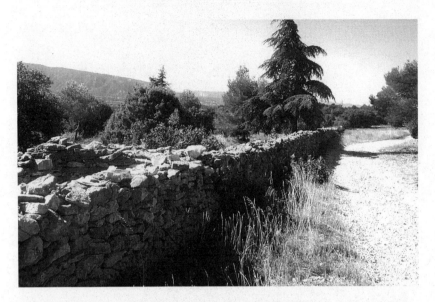

Figure 10.2 | "*Mur de la peste*," wall of dry stone, originally from 1720, under restoration since 1986. The wall was meant to protect the country north of it from the plague which infested the south of France at the time.

In Quebec, even in the early days, commentators were reluctant to include these barriers to sub-national (especially intra-provincial) mobility in the lexical field of limology, despite the fact that international border forms were reproduced within the state, through physical limitations, checkpoints, and flows filtering. Yet, as Alex McPhee's cartographic essay shows below, mobility restrictions across Canada have materialized many societal boundaries.

The management of the pandemic has therefore led to a borderization, a selective frontierization of spaces. Indeed, "in some cases, this has meant the revival of borders that have been long disregarded or backgrounded. In others, this has meant creation of new borders where they previously had not been meaningfully present" (Radil, Castan Pinos, and Ptak 2020). In all cases, borders have become a locus of regulation, "sanitary regulation of population mobility, regulation of capital inflows so as not to fall into economic dependence, regulation of the inflow of goods so that competition is not unfair, regulation to ensure industrial sovereignty, particularly of sanitary products."(Dumont 2020). In the current context, this wave

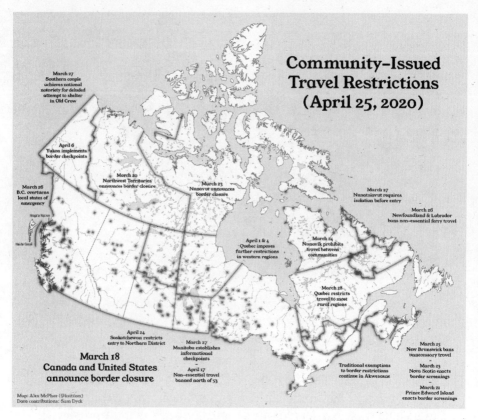

Figure 10.3 | Mapping Experiment: Pandemic Mobility Restrictions in Canada.

of "rebordering due to health issues is taking place in a context of larger political tensions over the effects of globalization, resistance to migration flows, and rapidly shifting geopolitical relationships." (Radil et al. 2020, 4). As such, the pandemic is intensifying the changes that began at the turn of the millennium and which now define the borders of the world.

ACCELERATING BORDER REGIME MUTATIONS

Over the last two decades, border scholars have largely identified contemporary border mutations: thicker, mobile, reticular, pixelated, borders represent kinds of asymmetric membranes that affect flows in a differentiated way (Amilhat and Szary 2020). "Far from deteriorating, weakening, or losing significance in the face of increased flows of capital, information, and commodities, the borders of a nation are reaffirmed as they expand inward and outward, away from the physical demarcation between national territories." (Menjivar 2014, 362). But it has gone further since 2020: "borders are being reconfigured by the politics of pandemics" (Scott 2020, 7). Indeed, the pandemic has both accentuated and generated rapid bordering and debordering processes, so quick in fact that they are in the process of generating profound changes and mutations in what borders now represent, "pointing toward a new multi-layered global border regime which is being reproduced at a variety of scales simultaneously" (Menjivar 2014, 362). (Radil et al. 2020, s4.)

First, Smart Borders have consolidated borders into true asymmetric membranes, where mobilities are filtered according to their desirability. To this end, technology is embedded in the bordering process: it uses contact tracing, just as it did in the case of Ebola (Koch 2016), but this time on a much larger and systemic basis. For instance, in Taiwan, the government "crossed-referenced health and travel databases to identify high-risk individuals and relied on immigration and health services to locate potential at-risk hosts – whether at home, the airport or seaport – to quarantine them systematically" (Wang et al. 2020; Republic of China 2019; Kornreich and Jin 2020). The use of technologies deployed at the border thus makes it possible to filter out undesirable flows in terms of health. Borders thus become a screen, an asymmetrical membrane, which is not watertight but makes it possible to quickly determine the nature and admissibility of flows.

Secondly, mobilities are defined in a more temporary, even ephemeral way and the capacity for bordering and de-bordering is strengthened, thus reinforcing their mobility. For example, in the wake of the appearance of a significant, more contagious, virus mutation in the United Kingdom, the borders of the European Union have rapidly closed to all UK originating flows on the eve of Christmas 2020 (BBC News 2020). This sealing was alleviated in less than forty-eight hours and the flows, filtered more finely, slowly resumed their course. The modular border closures thus apply not only to flows but also to the bodies the state seeks to control. The case of binational couples separated by a border demarcation line is probative. The most documented one concerns: "The couples on the

German-Swiss border, who are no longer able to visit each other due to the border closure but meet at a construction fence that serves as a makeshift form to mark the border. In order to prevent physical contact through the fence between the couples, a second row of fences was set up after a few days, which now keeps the lovers at a distance" (Wille 2020, 12).

The Canada-US border has seen similar mechanisms put in place to prevent binational couples from meeting at the British Columbia border.[2] The social admissibility of border mobility, the promptness of both bordering and de-bordering processes are key here.

Finally, this trend has accentuated the distinction between "national citizens" and "foreigners," demarcating the space and identifying the bodies over which government assumes responsibility and those to which it grants certain rights and protections (Longo 2018, xv).[3] The border response to the pandemic remains based on a threefold hierarchy of rights that defines the border regime: "racial discrimination, whether explicit or not; suspicion against the movement of the poorest; hostility to refugees, when their arrivals, described as 'massive,' are used as a pretext for xenophobic mobilizations" (Blanchard 2018). The Trump government's policy, which has made extensive use of the health issue to reduce immigration to its bare essentials, is consistent with this approach. Also, although they are potential carriers of the virus, undocumented migrants have been included or excluded from national health policies, as if the link of citizenship had an impact on the contagious nature of the virus: the invisibilization of undocumented migrants, even though they are on the "front line," has been a major obstacle to the fight against the virus[4] and has, in some cases, been an increased factor of contagion. Therefore, "demarcation is not only about the lines on the map which are then transformed into physical fences and walls on the ground. It is as much about the way that the societal managers determine the nature of inclusion and exclusion from various social categories and groups" (Newman 2009). The border "is a liminal space" (Vallelly 2020) that "symbolizes a social practice of spatial differentiation" (Van Houtum and Van Naerssen 2001, 126). But in this case, it has expanded to the point of operating deep in the very heart of the national territory, sometimes far from the border line itself: not only is the border thick, but it is viscous and adheres to the bodies that end up carrying it within them (Berrod and Bruyas 2020).

THE STICKINESS OF BORDER EMERGENCY

The change may be long-lasting as the pandemic potentially redefines border regimes, much like the events of September 11 eventually did. For the fact is that "when we see emergency measures passed, particularly today, they tend to be sticky" (Snowden, quoted in Johnson 2020): the longer the pandemic stretches, the more the emergency measures implemented to regulate flows entrench themselves to the point of re-defining the norm. In fact, closing the border, even deemed as a useful means[5] to curtail the effect of the virus, may have set the scene for a permanent state of exception long foreseen by Agamben (see Garrett 2020), especially because border manipulation has been inscribed in globalization anxieties for nearly two decades (Slack et al. 2016). And a crescendo of violence fed, in a way, the state sedentary bias – where "mobility is perceived as a danger" (Chebel and D'appollinia 2012). In this sense, the ground was fertile: "globalization has been widely seen as another significant factor: epidemic outbreaks have been associated with international trade routes since at least the fourteenth century and still are today" (Roberts 2020, 9). The affirmation by the nation-state of its sovereignty seemed to involve the strengthening of the border, a tool for managing globalized flows, even though borders are by definition consubstantial with globalization (Laine 2016) and themselves globalized (Dullin and Forestier-Peyrat 2015). It should be added that "Prior to the COVID-19 crisis, security-oriented narratives had already been used as a pretext by the EU and national governments to introduce emergency measures focused on deterring, containing, criminalizing and/or externalizing migration." (Hut et al. 2020).

First, the pandemic accentuates state control over international migration and further erodes the international refugee protection regime (Simoneau 2020). In the same way the reterritorialization of state authority is part of the rebordering process, it was only logical that "anti-immigration rebordering practices coupled with the national responses to the COVID-19 crisis" (Radil et al. 2020). Hence states, whether in Europe, Asia, or America "have conflated the 'war on the virus' with the 'war on migrants' and imposed drastic new restrictions on international mobility" (Heller 2020).

Secondly, and consequently, several tools mobilized during the pandemic will remain as a permanent feature of new border regimes.

The securitization of a health issue is, according to some analysts, theoretically profitable, since the language of security can be seen "as a means of rallying political support and financial resources to address neglected health issues" while "the impact of particular health challenges is serious enough to warrant the prioritization traditionally accorded to the use of armed force" (Enemark 2009) like it was for AIDS. However, this process runs the risk of taking the fight against the pandemic out of the hands of civil society and into the more elusive territory of military and intelligence – at the expense of human rights and civil liberties (Elbe 2006; see also Ferhani and Rushton 2020, 465). Therefore, the use of technologies such as geosurveillance (to trace for instance border crossers) could very well remain way past the pandemic spikes, notably because "GIS and cartography are important technologies in the production of knowledge for governmentality (i.e., geosurveillance, discipline, and biopower). That knowledge is also subject to normalization that casts people and space as at-risk resources" (Crampton 2003). Moreover, the risk of a hardening of the borders, materialized in the case of the northern demarcation line of the United States by what some see as a Mexicanization of the Canadian border (Dupeyron 2020), is becoming increasingly evident (Boucher and Vallet 2019).

Finally, from the perspective of mobility control, the idea of sanitary passports, which can take several forms, is already in use, as evidenced by the fact that some states require a negative test certificate before boarding a plane – through an externalized control, outside the country of destination and in the hands of the airlines. In doing so, mobility, traditionally facilitated for the North compared to the South, will eventually be subject to additional criteria, such as health controls concomitant with those of the TSA (inherited from the events of September 11 and establishing an additional control between that exercised by the airline and that of the customs authorities) at airports (e.g., taking temperatures) or the existence of travel documents with a health component. Thus, in addition to biometric data, passports (or sub-national travel documents) will include a comprehensive health component integrated with the travel documents. Some countries are already considering an "immunity passport" that would supplement border filters and overlay pre-existing limitations, affecting citizens of the South and the North differently.

At stake, will be the official or implicit reliability rating of health passports or test certificates depending on the location of the authority that established them. This will lead to the re-thinking of the politics of (im)mobility in a post-pandemic era. However, the pandemic has reinforced the inequity of flows and the pixelization of the border. "Paradoxically, those who are today able to confine themselves in good conditions are exactly the same people who had access to freedom of movement in pre-COVID times" (Amilhat and Szary 2020). The notion of mobility and immobility, fixity and fluidity has thus further evolved" (Hut et al. 2020) showing that the evolution of border controls are "more and more differentiated, detached from the territorial logic and more targeted at specific groups" (Jorry 2007, 1).

CONCLUSION

Over the last decade, mobility has become a determining element of global social stratification (Ritaine 2009; Sassen 2014): borders have become mobile (Amilhat, Szary, and Girault 2015), reticular and complex (Dullin and Forestier-Peyrat 2015, 7–9; Canale 2017). Simultaneously open and closed (Delmotte and Duez 2016), they have mutated into asymmetric elastic membranes (Mayor 2011, 661; Hedetoft 2003, 152), forms of biopolitical technological filters. Far from being antonyms of globalization, they are rather consubstantial to the point of defining its contradictory movements themselves. Hence, the identity quest of the nation state through the strengthening of borders presides over the very logic of globalization (Brown 2009; Sassen 1996, 59).

However, this dramatization of the border, far from new, has increased recently. Moreover, the theatralization of the border comes at a cost. In the context of electoral politics, "political parties have driven border issues as political priorities. Identity has trumped trade as a priority issue." (Schain 2019); in the context of pandemic politics, because pandemics are "unique exogenous shocks that generate uncertainty" (Devine et al. 2020), identity has also supplanted health issues. This border mise en scène in the pandemic context is therefore intended to reduce the immediate electoral impact (Welch 1997) and has non-health purposes (Flinders 2020).

Indeed, by emphasizing the need to close borders and adopting a rhetoric emphasizing the risks of their presupposed porosity, leaders have induced a form of mistrust towards the "Other," who lies beyond the line of demarcation. This "pandemic populism" (Dodds et al.) has evolved into a convenient discourse based on borders: "It is not just the closure of physical crossing points between States that has defined COVID-19 responses, but also more symbolic acts of bordering: ground-up and top-down xenophobic discourses – encouraged by fear and security-based narratives – pointed their finger at 'others' as carriers and transmitters of disease" (Hut et al. 2020).

This entrenchment behind border lines thus goes beyond mere border demarcation but represents an erosion of mutual trust and cooperation, the very foundation of the international system (Keohane 1989) and an essential element to the ability to cope collectively with the shock caused by SARS-COV-2 (see Simon and Randalls 2016, 4) – conversely, mobility restrictions can slow down the ability to deal with it (Devi 2020). Behind border changes, (im)mobilities will require rethinking in the light of a post-pandemic era, and with them, the very articulation of the meshwork that holds the international system together.

NOTES

1 Extracted from the database compiled by the authors between March and December 2020, this work was funded by the Minds and SSHRC programs.
2 As *City News 1130* reports show (Renouf and McMahon 2020, Uzda and Hall 2020).
3 See the chapter in this book from Y.Y Chen entitled "Fortress World: Refugee Protection during (and after) the COVID-19 Pandemic" for a discussion on this topic.
4 See, for instance: Chatterjee and Kagwe 2020; Cloutier, Bernier, and Loiseau 2020.
5 Although widely discussed: see Espinoza et al. 2020.

REFERENCES

Amilhat Szary, Anne-Laure. 2020. *Géopolitique des frontières – Découper la terre, imposer une vision du monde*. Paris: Le Cavalier Bleu.
– 2020. "Those Who are Confined, are Also the Most Mobile!" In *Borders in Perspective*, UniGR-CBS Thematic Issue. *Bordering in Pandemic Times: Insights into the COVID-19 Lockdown* vol. 4: 85–7. https://doi.org/10.25353/ubtr-xxxx-b825-a20b.

Balzacq, Thierry. 2005. "The Three Faces of Securitization: Political Agency, Audience and Context." *European Journal of International Relations* 11, no. 2: 171–201.

BBC News. 2020. "Covid-19: More Than 40 Countries Ban UK Arrivals." *BBC News*, 21 December 2020. https://www.bbc.com/news/uk-55391289#:~:text=More%20than%2040%20countries%20have,-Spain%2C%20India%20and%20Hong%20Kong.

Berrod, Frédérique, and Pierrick Bruyas. 2020. "European Union: are Borders the Antidote to the Covid-19 Pandemic?" *The Conversation*, 17 April 2020. https://theconversation.com/european-union-are-borders-the-antidote-to-the-covid-19-pandemic-136643.

Blanchard, Emmanuel. 2018. "La 'libre circulation': retour sur le 'monde d'hier'." *Plein droit* 116, no. 1: 3–7.

Boucher, Vincent, and Élisabeth Vallet. 2019. "Fencing the Border: Balancing Mobility and Security at the Canada-US border." Paper presented at the Association for Canadian Studies in the United States 25th Biennal Conference: Canada: Forces of Inclusion and Exclusion, Montreal, 15 November 2019.

Cantat, Céline, Hélène Thiollet, and Antoine Pécoud. 2020. "Migration as Crisis. A Framework Paper." In *Borders in Perspective*, UniGR-CBS Thematic Issue. *Bordering in Pandemic Times: Insights into the COVID-19 Lockdown* vol. 4. https://www.magyc.uliege.be/wp-content/uploads/2020/04/D3.1-v2-April-2020-1.pdf.

Chatterjee, Siddharth, and Mutahi Kagwe. 2020. "Les travailleurs de la santé sont les soldats de première ligne contre COVID-19." *Afrique Renouveau, Nations Unies*, 24 March 2020. https://www.un.org/africarenewal/fr/a-la-une/les-travailleurs-de-la-sant%C3%A9-sont-les-soldats-de-premi%C3%A8re-ligne-contre-covid-19-prot%C3%A9geons.

Chebel d'Appollonia, Ariane. 2012. *Frontiers of Fear: Immigration and Insecurity in the United States and Europe*. Cornell: Cornell University Press.

Cloutier, Elisa, Jérémy Bernier, and Clara Loiseau. 2020. "Ils se livrent depuis des mois à une guerre sans merci." *Le Journal de Québec*, 29 December 2020.

Connor, Phillip. 2020. "More than Nine-in-Ten People Worldwide Live in Countries with Travel Restrictions amid COVID-19." *FactTank: Pew Research Center*, 1 April 2020. https://www.pewresearch.org/fact-tank/2020/04/01/

more-than-nine-in-ten-people-worldwide-live-in-countries-with-travel-restrictions-amid-covid-19/.

Crampton, Jeremy W. 2003. "Cartographic Rationality and the Politics of Geosurveillance and Security." *Cartography and Geographic Information Science* 30, no. 2: 135–48.

De Gruyter, Caroline. 2020. "Europe Needed Borders. The Coronavirus Built Them." *Foreign Policy,* 4 December 2020.

Devi, Sharmila. 2020. "Travel Restrictions Hampering Covid-19 Response." *The Lancet* 395: 331–2.

Dodds, Klaus, Vanesa Castan Broto, Klaus Detterbeck, Martin Jones, Virginie Mamadouh, Maano Ramutsindela, Monica Varsanyi, David Wachsmuth and Chih Yuan Woon. 2020. "The COVID-19 Pandemic: Territorial, Political and Governance Dimensions of the Crisis." *Territory, Politics, Governance* 8, no. 3: 289–98.

Dullin, Sabine, and Forestier-Peyrat, Étienne. 2015. "*Les frontières mondialisées.*" Paris, Presses Universitaires de France, Collection la Vie des Idées. Available online: ISSN: 2105-3030. https://laviedesidees.fr/Les-frontieres-mondialisees.html

Dumont, Gérard-François. 2020. "La géopolitique des frontières réaffirmée." *Outre-terre. Revue européenne de géopolitique.* Ghazipur Publications: 75–88.

Dupeyron, Bruno. 2020. "Why Trump Tried to Use the Coronavirus Crisis to 'Mexicanize' the US-Canada Border." *The Conversation,* 2 April 2020.

Enemark, Christian. 2009. "Is Pandemic Flu a Security Threat?" *Survival* 51, no. 1: 191–214.

Espinoza, Baltazar, Carlos Castillo-Chavez, and Charles Perrings. 2020. "Mobility Restrictions for the Control of Epidemics: When Do They Work?" *PLOS ONE* 15, no. 7: e0235731. https://doi.org/10.1371/journal.pone.0235731.

Ferhani, Adam, and Simon Rushton. 2020. "The International Health Regulations, COVID-19, and Bordering Practices: Who Gets In, What Gets Out, and Who Gets Rescued?" *Contemporary Security Policy* 41, no. 3: 458–77.

Fillion, Stéphanie. 2020. "In Canada, Patience Wearing Thin Over Trump's Antics." *Foreign Policy,* 14 April 2020.

Garrett, Terence M. 2020. "COVID-19, Wall Building, and the Effects on Migrant Protection Protocols by the Trump Administration: The Spectacle of the Worsening Human Rights Disaster on the Mexico-US Border." *Administrative Theory & Praxis* 42, no. 2: 240–8.

Goussot, Michel. 2020. "Les frontières de l'Amérique du Nord. Enjeux et perspectives." *Population & Avenir* 749, no. 4: 17–19.

Hamez, Grégory, Frédérique Morel-Doridat, Kheira Oudina, Marine Le Chavez, Mathias Boquet, Nicolas Dorkel, Nicolas Greiner, and Sabrina de Pindray d'Ambelle. 2020. "La frontière 'nationale' brouillée par le COVID-19." In *Borders in Perspective*, UniGR-CBS Thematic Issue. *Bordering in Pandemic Times: Insights into the COVID-19 Lockdown* vol. 4: 63–7.

Heller, Charles. 2020. "De-Confine Borders: Towards a Politics of Freedom of Movement in the Time of the Pandemic." *Centre on Migration, Policy and Society (COMPAS) Series* Working Paper no. 20-147, 25.

Heisbourg, François. 2020. "From Wuhan to the World: How the Pandemic Will Reshape Geopolitics." *Survival* 62, no. 3: 7–24.

Hut, Elodie, Caroline Zickgraf, Francois Gemenne, Tatiana Castillo Betancourt, Pierre Ozer, Céline Le Flour. 2020. "COVID-19, Climate Change and Migration: Constructing Crises, Reinforcing Borders." *IOM Environmental Migration Portal*. http://hdl.handle.net/2268/248812

Johnson, Stephen. 2020 "Edward Snowden Warns 'Bio-Surveillance' May Outlast Coronavirus." *Big Think*, 27 March 2020. https://bigthink.com/politics-current-affairs/coronavirus-tracking.

Laine, Jussi P. 2016. "The Multiscalar Production of Borders." *Geopolitics* 21, no. 3: 465–82.

Longo, Matthew. 2018. *The Politics of Borders: Sovereignty, Security and the Citizen after 9/11*. Cambridge: Cambridge University Press.

Menjívar, Cecilia. 2014. "Immigration Law Beyond Borders: Externalizing and Internalizing Border Controls in an Era of Securitization." *The Annual Review of Law and Social Science* 10: 353–369.

Newman, David. 2009. "Contemporary Research Agendas in Border Studies: An Overview." In *The Routledge Research Companion to Border Studies*, edited by Doris Wastl-Walter. London: Ashgate Publishers.

Nossem, Eva. 2020. "Linguistic Rebordering: Constructing COVID-19 as an External Threat." In *Borders in Perspective*, UniGR-CBS Thematic Issue. *Bordering in Pandemic Times: Insights into the COVID-19 Lockdown* vol. 4: 77–80. https://doi.org/10.25353/ubtr-xxxx-b825-a20b.

Owen, David. 2020. "Open Borders and the COVID-19 Pandemic." *Democratic Theory* 7, no. 2: 152–9.

Parker, Noel, and Nick Vaughan-Williams. 2012. "Critical Border Studies: Broadening and Deepening the 'Lines in the Sand' Agenda." *Geopolitics* 17, no, 4: 727–33.

Radil Steven M., Jaume Castan Pinos, and Thomas Ptak. 2020. "Borders Resurgent: Towards a Post-Covid-19 Global Border Regime?" *Space and Polity*. 9 July 2020. https://doi.org10.1080/13562576.2020. 1773254.

Renouf, Ria, and Martin MacMahon. 2020. "Fence Built Along Canada-US Border South of Aldergrove." *City News 1130*, 19 August 2020.

Ricciardi, Toni. 2020. « Pandémies et frontières : à la recherche du coupable ». In Gamba COVID-19: *le regard des sciences sociales*, edited by Fiorenza Gamba, Marco Nardone, Toni Ricciardi, Sandro Cattacin, 301–316. Zürich: Seismo. https://archive-ouverte.unige.ch/unige:137598

Roberts, Adam. 2020. "Pandemics and Politics." *Survival* 62, no. 5 (23 September 2020). https://www.tandfonline.com/doi/full/10.1080/00396338.2020.1819641.

Roche, Jean Jacques. 2014. "Walls and Borders in a Globalized World: The Paradoxical Revenge of Territorialization." In *Borders, Fences and walls: State of Insecurity?*, edited by Elisabeth Vallet, 105–115. Aldershot: Ashgate Publishing Limited.

Saunders, Doug. 2020. "Why Travel Bans Fail to Stop Pandemics: Hasty Border Closures Invite Chaos – and Can Seed New Outbreaks." *Foreign Affairs*, 15 May 2020. https://www. foreignaffairs.com/articles/canada/2020-05-15/why-travel-bans-fail-stop-pandemics.

Schain, Martin A. 2019. *The Border: Policy and Policies in Europe and the United States*. New York: Oxford University Press.

Scott, James W. 2020. "Introduction to *A Research Agenda for Border Studies*." In *A Research Agenda for Border Studies*, edited by James W. Scott, 3–24. Cheltenham: Elgar Research Agendas.

Shafer, Ronald G. 2020. "Spain Hated Being Linked to the Deadly 1918 Flu Pandemic. Trump's 'Chinese Virus' Label Echoes That." *The Washington Post*, 23 March 2020.

Simonneau, Damien. 2020. "Gérer les frontières par temps de pandémie." *L'Économie politique*, 87, no. 3: 91–8.

Smith, Matthew J., Sayan Basu Ray, Micah Sienna, Meredith B. Lilly. 2018. "Long-Term Lessons on the Effects of Post-9/11 Border Thickening on Cross-Border Trade between Canada and the United States: A Systematic Review." *Transport Policy* 72 (December): 198–207.

Sohn, Cristophe. 2014. "Modelling Cross-Border Integration: The Role of Borders as a Resource." *Geopolitics* 19, no. 3: 587–608.

Thiessen, Tamara. 2020. "Coronavirus: Some of These 24 European Countries Have Closed Their Borders to Tourists." *Forbes*, 14 March 2020.

Tran, Van C. 2020. "The Borders Around Us: Forced Migration and the Politics of Border Control," *City & Community* 19, no. 2: 323–9.

Uzda, Liza, and Mike Hall. 2020. "Peace Arch Park closing temporarily as number of visitors doubles." *City News 1130*, 18 June 2020.

Vallelly, Neil. 2020. "The Border and the Pandemic." *Social Anthropology (Anthropologie sociale): The Journal of the European Association of Social Anthropologists* (18 May 2020). doi:10.1111/1469-8676.12860.

Vallet, Élisabeth. 2020. "State of Border Walls in a Globalized World." In *Borders and Border Walls: In-Security, Symbolism, Vulnerabilities*, edited by Andréanne Bissonnette and Élisabeth Vallet. London: Routledge.

Van Houtum, Henk, and Ton van Naerssen 2002. "Bordering, Ordering and Othering." *Tijdschrift voor Economische en Sociale Geografie* 93, no. 2: 125–36.

Welch Larson, Deborah. 1997. "Trust and Missed Opportunities in International Relations." *Political Psychology* 18, no. 3: 701–34.

Wille, Christian. 2020. "Bordering in Pandemic Times: Insights into the COVID-19 Lockdown." In *Borders in Perspective*, UniGR-CBS Thematic Issue. *Bordering in Pandemic Times: Insights into the COVID-19 Lockdown* vol. 4. http://cbs.uni-gr.eu/en/resources/publications/thematic-issues/borders-perspective-vol-4.

Wolman, David. 2020. "Amid a Pandemic, Geography Returns with a Vengeance." *Wired*, 14 April 2020.

Youde, Jeremy. 2020. "How 'Medical Nationalism' is Undermining the Fight Against the Coronavirus Pandemic." *World Politics Review*. https://www.worldpoliticsreview.com/articles/28623/how-medical-nationalism-is-undermining-the-fight-against-the-coronavirus-pandemic

New Zealand's Scale-Free Response to a Scale-Free Pandemic

Tim Tenbensel

I: INTRODUCTION

From an international perspective, New Zealand has been lauded as one of the most successful societies in dealing with COVID-19. While the societal experience in New Zealand in the first half of 2020 was very similar to other high-income countries, both the number of cases and the fatality rates were miniscule. As such, New Zealand has a great chance of minimising the dreadful impact of the pandemic. Nevertheless, the pandemic has been by far the most significant shock New Zealand society has experienced since the 1940s. New Zealand experienced many similar policy debates to other countries regarding the nature of policy responses, the same heightened concerns about the possible impact on health systems, and similar clamouring to hold political leaders responsible for failures in implementation of government responses.

This essay is a reflection on the dynamics of scale, and the challenges of comparing New Zealand's experience and response to those of other countries. Insights about scale, fractals and "indexicality" are drawn from the work of the sociologist Andrew Abbott to illustrate the scale-free nature of COVID-19 problem definitions and policy responses. The chapter begins with my own attempt to tell the story of how the COVID-19 epidemic and the governmental response to it played out during 2020. I then highlight how various elements of this response contradicted the image of New Zealand as a highly liberal society in terms of both economic policy and social values, and the associated minimal role of the state in regulating behaviour. This then sets up a series of broader reflections on proportionality and scale. In particular, I develop the argument that there is no stable vantage point from which to judge the "proportionality" of New Zealand's response relative to other jurisdictions, and that by exploring the scale-free features of COVID-19, it is possible to glimpse the scale-free nature of more established policy issues and debates.

II: THE AOTEAROA NEW ZEALAND COVID-19 STORY – A COMBINATION OF LUCK AND GOOD MANAGEMENT

At the time of writing (late December 2020), the experience of living in New Zealand is simultaneously "normal" and utterly extraordinary. It is normal in the sense that day-to-day life is much like it was in 2019. If someone had woken up from a twelve-month coma, perhaps the only thing they would notice is the fact that all public transport passengers were wearing protective masks. They would also be likely to notice the widespread practice of scanning QR codes on entering shops and offices. While these changes are clearly noticeable, they would not seem in a different league to changes in other years, such as the sudden proliferation of e-scooters.

To be sure, our recovering coma patient would probably be highly surprised if she attempted to book an international flight. Her travel agent would likely be unemployed. If she booked her own flight it would likely be significantly more expensive. On top of that, the airline would inform her that she would need to stay isolated in a hotel room for fourteen days on her return to New Zealand and pay around $3,000 NZD for the privilege of doing so.

Nevertheless, in terms of day-to-day life in New Zealand, the sense of relative normality experienced by its residents is utterly extraordinary in many respects. It is not a situation that New Zealanders take for granted. New Zealand residents know only too well that it is a situation that can be and has been subject to abrupt change.

This relative normality is due to the fact that there is currently no community transmission of the COVID-19 coronavirus. The number of total recorded cases is a tick over two thousand (420 cases per million), and the death toll stands at twenty-five (five cases per million). To put this in recent historical perspective, nearly that number of people died in a volcanic eruption in December 2019, and twice that number were victims of a lone gunman in the attack on two mosques in March 2019.

New Zealand is in this situation due to a combination of good luck and good management. On the good luck side, we are an island nation which makes borders easier to manage, the virus arrived relatively late on our shores (28 February 2020 was the first official case, although it may have actually been a little earlier), and it did not arrive in winter. Our system of government is comparatively simple – there are no layers of federalism to negotiate. Another piece of good fortune is that the Director General of the Ministry of Health, Dr Ashley Bloomfield was a public health medicine specialist.

New Zealand was poorly prepared for a pandemic of any kind; ranked thirty-fifth, it was well below most high-income countries (GHS Index 2021). In this context, the story of good management is founded on the exceptional political communication skills of Prime Minister Jacinda Ardern and the calm reassurance of Dr Bloomfield. Swift political decision-making also allowed the under-resourced and under-prepared public health infrastructure time to get up to speed. The border was closed on 15 March (day seventeen). After a brief transition, the country was placed in "Level 4" lockdown from 26 March to 28 April (Days 28–60). This lockdown was amongst the most stringent enacted anywhere in the world (Blavatnik School of Government 2020). Under Level 4, all schools and most workplaces were closed. People could only maintain contact and proximity to others in their immediate household (their bubble). The only reasons for leaving one's residence were for grocery shopping, exercise, or if one was designated as a worker providing essential services.

With regards to other policy responses, New Zealand's adopted similar approaches to many other countries in terms of economic stimulus packages (Mazey and Richardson 2020). The economic contraction was short and sharp, followed by a strong rebound in the second half of 2020 (Statistics New Zealand 2020b). There has been profound economic dislocation for those working in travel and tourism, but most parts of the economy have survived relatively unscathed thus far. The largest burden has been borne by those in the casualized labour force – the vast majority of whom are women (Statistics New Zealand 2020a).

Implementation of COVID-19 policy responses was anything but smooth, and many significant faults and weaknesses became apparent in the early days of establishing community testing, border controls, and quarantine management (Mazey and Richardson 2020).

Inevitably, this account of New Zealand's experience invites comparisons with the experiences elsewhere in the world. Although the country "went hard and went early," did we go too hard, or not hard enough? Could we have gone earlier, or did we jump the gun? Compared to other possible courses of action, did we choose the right one? Many other questions also arise – how does COVID-19 compare to other policy problems (such as climate change)? How does it compare to other historical examples of crisis management? These sorts of questions are always worth asking, but seem more pressing because of the profound sense of disorientation that the pandemic has engendered.

III: HOW COVID-19 HAS CONFOUNDED US – THE POWER OF THE STATE AND POLITICAL ACCOUNTABILITY

This profound disorientation has pervaded almost every corner of experience, albeit in very different ways for different people. At a national political level, the experience of the Level 4 and Level 3 lockdowns between March and May 2020 highlighted many disconnects between New Zealand's image of ourselves and the new reality.

Many commentators have observed that the countries that took the most stringent approach to containing or suppressing COVID-19 were East Asian countries in which cultural and social norms both reflected and enabled a more authoritarian approach. New Zealand, arguably, outdid them all, yet in the eyes of its citizens, it does not fit that cultural mould. How was it that a country that has prided itself on both its economic liberalism (in relation to trade barriers, openness of the economy, relatively low taxes, and pro-business labour laws) and more recently on its social liberalism (witness the themes of inclusivity that characterized the collective response to the mosque shootings of March 2019), managed to top the index in terms of authoritarian responses to the pandemic? For the first nine days of Level 4 lockdown, a court subsequently determined that the government's response was not even lawful (Nightingale 2020). Legislation to grant special government powers was passed retrospectively in early April 2020.

Nevertheless, this effective suspension of liberal democracy under the guise of public health was widely accepted as necessary in the sense of the ends justifying the means, and the unconstitutional use of state power barely raised a murmur of discontent. From late March to early June 2020, it appeared as if Thomas Hobbes' elaborate fantasy expounded in *Leviathan* (and famously depicted on its cover) suddenly materialised in the form of "the team of 5 million" personified in the figure of Jacinda Ardern.

A second profound reversal pertained to the relative centrality of public health advice and expertise compared to other inputs into governmental decision-making processes. While the centrality of public health is common to all governmental responses to COVID-19, arguably it rose faster and further in New Zealand than in most comparable countries. In the decade prior to 2020, funding for public health functions had deteriorated substantially. Under the previous National Party-led government, public health experts in universities and the public sector had been marginalised from policy processes regarding non-communicable diseases. But in the COVID-19 response, public health problem definitions and responses held sway to such an extent that other sources of policy advice from Treasury and other economic portfolios were subordinated (Trevett 2020).

One notable casualty of the COVID-19 response was New Zealand's self-image as a society that is built on a Treaty partnership between the Indigenous Māori and the Crown which stands for the system of government established by British settlers in the nineteenth century. Under crisis conditions, the nature of the policy response emphasised the disparity of power between Crown and Māori, and a notable lack of partnership or involvement in decision-making (Jones 2020). The fact that Māori (and other population groups) were not subject to the full force of COVID-19's iniquitous health outcomes was widely acknowledged. However, many indirect effects of the COVID response, including the differential impact of job losses and social hardship, were real and severe.

The governmental response to COVID-19 has also produced some disorientation around political accountability. According to a well-known political aphorism "success has a thousand fathers, failure is an orphan," New Zealand's experience in 2020 simultaneously confirms and undermines this. The political messaging that accompanied the lockdown between March and May was that of collective effort. The "team of 5 million" messaging served as a rhetorical device that minimised the distinctions between state and society, elites and the relatively powerless. In doing so, it diffused the attribution of success in eliminating community transmission of COVID from the government to the whole country.

Even though it appeared that the government was acting against type by not loudly claiming credit, it did reflect a more powerful political strategy that played to Ms Ardern's strengths. She has consistently projected an image of a political leader who is "above the fray" of divisive partisan politics, and this perception had been well-established before the pandemic. This non-partisan approach paid big electoral dividends. Having been in a three-way coalition prior to the October election, Ardern's Labour party returned to government as the sole governing party with an outright majority. Its vote topped 50 per cent, an achievement that was unprecedented in the eight previous elections under New Zealand's proportional representation electoral system. This result was widely interpreted as reflecting the electorate's gratitude for the government's performance in successfully steering the country towards elimination of community cases.

But with such success, one of the most profound ironies of New Zealand's COVID-19 situation is the increased political risk for political leaders. This situation was most clearly illustrated by the fate of Dr David Clark, the Minister of Health until 2 July 2020. In April, Dr Clark breached the Level 4 restrictions put in place by the government he was a key member of, by taking his mountain bike to a local park (Manch and Cooke 2020). The nature of his egregious misjudgment was that he was engaging in an activity (biking) that heightened the risk of personal injury, which might lead to contact with individuals outside his bubble, and that he was more than 2 km from home (2.3 km to be precise).

Furthermore, in mid June, two recent international arrivals were granted a compassionate quarantine exemption so that they could visit a dying relative. Rather than self-isolating, they drove from Auckland to Wellington (a nine-hour drive) and stopped to ask directions when leaving Auckland (Small 2020). Coming one week after most of the restrictive conditions had been relaxed, this too was considered by the political opposition and the media as a sackable offence for a minister of health. This story hit the news on the same day that Dr Clark released a major report prefiguring significant change to New Zealand's health system, perhaps a once-in-a-generation health policy event. Coverage of these proposed reforms was drowned out by the outrage that accompanied the news that New Zealand's community-free transition status may be in jeopardy. The minister hung on by his fingernails for a further two weeks before eventually resigning.

The Opposition National Party also portrayed a small August 2020 outbreak as evidence of government failure. Nevertheless, the government was able to draw on established healthy reserves of political credit and was able to ride out a series of early implementation failures in its border control and quarantine management system (Mazey and Richardson 2020). Although the source of the August outbreak was never pinpointed, this had been successfully contained within three weeks. By the end of 2020, the fate of Dr Clark was a blip on the radar.

However, the story of Dr Clark illustrates something highly paradoxical. The more successful a government is in containing COVID, the easier it is to pinpoint the blame for any COVID-related failures to the individual actions, decisions, and control exercised by executive government. Compare this to the situation in the UK where the far more serious systemic failures are less easily sheeted home to a minister or the head of the Ministry of Health. Whereas Dr Clark's mountain biking 2.3km from home led to an eventual resignation, British Prime Minister Johnson's chief adviser, Dominic Cummings, survived much longer after travelling 400km from London while taking in a bit of sightseeing while the rest of his country was locked down.

Compared to any other ministerial resignation in recent (or distant) New Zealand history, the controversy surrounding Dr Clark may well seem "over the top." More broadly, readers who may have been complementary and supportive of New Zealand's COVID-19 strategy may now be wondering, "was this reaction really proportionate to the problem?" In so many respects, what has happened in New Zealand (as in most other countries) is "off the scale" in terms of the reference points and bearings that are normally used to judge such things. So, if we have lost our bearings, is it possible to regain them? Is it possible to pinpoint the criteria of judgment, the measures and indicators, and the standards and benchmarks that could give us our bearings?

IV: PROPORTIONALITY AND SCALE

Any judgment of proportionality, over-reaction, and under-reaction depend on establishing a baseline of comparison that incorporates both the extent of the policy problem and the effects of the solutions.

For defining the nature of COVID-19 as a policy problem, the degree of uncertainty, and the enormous width of confidence intervals in modelling any of the key parameters including infection rates, death rates, and economic effects, has meant that there is a vast range of problem definitions and estimates of the scale of the problem.

At one end of this spectrum, it is possible to juxtapose the most optimistic epidemiological estimates of prevalence, transmission, and mortality with the most pessimistic economic projections. Using such a combination, proponents of "Plan B" in New Zealand have vehemently put the case that the policy response has been highly disproportionate, and akin to killing a flea with a sledgehammer (Thornley 2020).

At the other end of the scale, there are also academic commentaries that have chastised New Zealand's approach for taking "a less vigorous response to this pandemic during its early stages" compared to Taiwan (Summers et al. 2020). The relative deficiencies outlined in this article focus primarily on the unpreparedness of New Zealand's public health response system. The authors argued that the stringency of a Level 4 lockdown could have been avoided had New Zealand acted more quickly and been better prepared – a valid argument if one's comparator is Taiwan. New Zealand's case rate per million is sixteen times as high as Taiwan's, whose superior performance was achieved with a far less drastic measures.

This attempt to judge government responses in terms of proportionality is also prominent in policy studies literature. These are part of a long tradition stretching back to Anthony Downs (Downs 1972), and including the famous work of Baumgartner and Jones (Baumgartner and Jones 1993), that seeks to explain why the attention of governments and their policy responses are rarely proportionate. The most recent extension of this work has been in the analyses of Israeli political scientist Moshe Maor of policy over-reaction and under-reaction (Maor 2018). Together with Mike Howlett, Maor has applied this analysis to government responses to COVID-19 (Maor and Howlett 2020).

In doing so, they draw attention to psychological factors and make the argument that the Norwegian government panicked and that the Israeli government instigated harsh lockdown measures as a politically-calculated over-reaction (Maor and Howlett 2020). Taking our cue from these assessments, it seems plausible to characterize New Zealand's response as an over-reaction as well, even without attributing motivations of panic or political expediency.

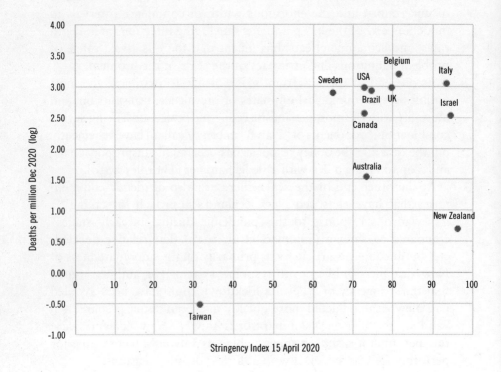

Figure 11.1 | Plotting COVID-19 health outcomes (deaths per million) against the stringency of policy responses.

However, assessing the proportionality of responses to COVID-19 is rather fraught with difficulty. Deploying a highly restrictive set of social controls to deal with a disease that has to date accounted for twenty-five deaths can easily be characterized as "using a sledgehammer to kill a flea." But in COVID-19's cartoon-like world, that flea can quickly become an elephant which is impervious even to sledgehammers.

In order to illustrate the difficulties of international comparisons, I present a brief (and very selective) mapping of the stringency of policy responses against the number of deaths attributed to COVID (Figure 1). The figures are taken from Oxford University's Blavatnik

School of Government's COVID Response tracker (Blavatnik School of Government 2020). This website provides daily measurements of government responses across the world, aggregated into a series of indices, one of which is the "stringency index" which compares government responses in terms of the degree of restrictions placed on citizens.

Looking at the data from the "first wave" of COVID-19 responses in mid-April 2020, Figure 11.1 shows that New Zealand is clearly an international outlier, but it also shows that the comparisons we make with other countries are extremely diverse. If New Zealand is compared with Australia by looking "north-west," we can tell a story that by having more stringent policy responses New Zealand was able to achieve better outcomes. If we look to the north and compare New Zealand to Israel – substantially better outcomes were achieved consequent to a similar scale of response. But in relation to Taiwan to the south west, we look considerably worse on both dimensions. A different range of countries, other timeframes, other indexes of government responses, a non-logarithmic scale, and other measures of outcomes could have been chosen, but it is likely that these would all result in similar challenges of interpretation about the proportionality of New Zealand's (or any country's response).

Any attempt to define proportional responses is rather fraught for many reasons. The first reason is that getting a true sense of the scale of COVID and its potential effects remains a highly elusive enterprise. We know that internationally, comparing the magnitudes of cases and deaths between countries is challenging. This does not mean one cannot make any comparisons, but just that they are inevitably coarse-grained rather than fine-grained.

Secondly, if and when finer-grained measurements become feasible, the comparisons would likely look different. It is highly likely that the international league tables of COVID cases and deaths will change substantially if and when the accepted forms of measurement change. The problem is analogous to the task of comparing the measurement of coastlines between different countries. Depending on what scale we use, the relativities between countries can change substantially. This is because some coastlines are "crinklier" than others (West 2017). Therefore, Russia's coastline is significantly longer than Norway's if the scale of resolution is coarse (say 1km) but Norway's coastline is lengthier than Russia's if a finer-grained increment (1 metre) is used.

The coastline paradox was first articulated by Lewis Richardson in the 1950s, and was something of a mathematical curiosity until the development of fractal mathematics and geometry a generation later (West 2017). The concept of fractals originated in the pioneering work of French mathematician Benoit Mandelbrot. A fractal pattern is one in which the phenomena of interest is scale-free, which means that the same pattern is apparent at large scales, small scales, and everything in between. This is known as "self-similarity." The most accessible example of a fractal is to look at a broccoli or cauliflower. If you detach a small stem from the outside of the vegetable, and then magnify it, it would look virtually identical to the whole. This also illustrates the connection between a cauliflower and the coastline paradox. If you attempted to measure the surface area of a cauliflower, your measurements would vary considerably according to the measurement increment used. A measurement in increments of microns will come up with a significantly larger figure than if the increment were centimetres.

These concepts of fractals, self-similarity, and scale can also be applied more metaphorically. The key pioneer of this approach has been the American sociologist Andrew Abbott. Abbott's work in many areas has been widely influential, although his approach to sociology and social science frequently draws heavy (and often justified) criticism (Wilterdink 2018). Where Abbott is most useful is in his generation of metaphors that are useful to think with. His exploration of the metaphor of fractals is outlined in his book *The Chaos of Disciplines* which was published in 2001 (Abbott 2001).

In this book he begins by describing the nature of debates within academic disciplines in general, and sociology in particular, in terms of the simplest fractal pattern – the branching of one line into two (see Figure 11.2).

Any major difference in theoretical assumptions, methodological preferences or ideological position can be represented by this bifurcation. Abbott develops the metaphor by charting the process of bifurcation unfolding at multiple levels and time periods, or both. So in social scientific disciplines, an initial bifurcation between sociology and history occurs (in the US at least) when one sub-tribe of social scientists (sociologists) take an asynchronous approach to explaining change, distinguishing themselves from the historians who are interested in chronological narratives of change. But in the subsequent iteration, historians branch into "pure" historians and

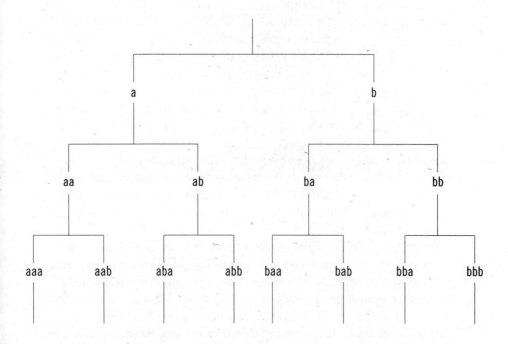

Figure 11.2 | A simple fractal structure.

those with a more sociological bent, while the original generation of sociologists bifurcates into historical sociology and "pure" sociology. Debates and disputes at different levels of the fractal structure are self-similar. The important implication of this is that to the protagonists in sub-disciplinary debates, the distance between historical sociologist and their "opponent" is far more significant (and proximate) in their world than the broader difference between social scientists and natural scientists.

Other examples include methodological debates between qualitative and quantitative approaches (Knappertsbusch 2020), or value debates drawing on the distinction between equality and freedom. The fractal metaphor in these is applied in a very simple way, but Abbott shows how even the most basic fractal branching (a one-dimensional differentiation of two positions) can produce complex dynamics over time.

Where the fractal metaphor becomes most useful is in thinking about distance between things. This distance could be about differences between occupational and class positions, or between theoretical and methodological positions, or between political positions. In this way, a seemingly trivial doctrinal dispute about the nature of the Holy Trinity can become the major schism that propels the development of Christianity in the fourth century. A radical egalitarian cult could splinter according to whether its leader should be able to sleep on a raised mattress, or on the floor like all the other members. While these differences appear insignificant to those outside these debates, they become the principal markers of differentiation and distance to those on the inside. Abbott uses the term "indexicality" to describe these variations in frames of reference.

Indexicality fundamentally shapes social perceptions, and clearly applies to policy debates. To most international health policy experts, the arcane arguments about regulation of mandatory health insurance schemes under the USA's Affordable Care Act may seem trivial compared to the overarching issue of universality of healthcare entitlements, yet these arguments had enormous significance in the US context (Tuohy 2018).

One could interpret the fractal metaphor as a source of distortion of "true" perception, but this is not what Abbott is arguing at all. Instead, there is no fundamental standpoint from which to view the dynamics of a fractal system. What fractal thinking offers, according to Abbott, is the imperative of making judgments (including comparative judgments) in situated contexts that are shaped by past histories. This is in contrast to positing a helicopter view from which an objective observer can judge the proportionality of policy responses by measuring them in terms of a fixed scale of reference. Different scales of reference therefore produce quite different comparative judgments. Political and policy judgment (indeed judgment of any sort) entails an awareness of the range of scales and frames of reference, and the capacity to move between them.

Comparative judgments therefore require a great deal of contextual information. One cannot meaningfully make comparisons without taking into account country-specific conditions and features. Although the nature of the COVID-19 virus and of the threat it presents may be universal, their filtering through local contexts creates different effects even when debates look superficially similar across contexts. It is important to have a sense of where the debate sits within the overall fractal system.

Importantly, New Zealand debates regarding responses to COVID-19 did not map on to pre-existing and deep political cleavages as occurred in the USA and many other countries. While there are many superficial similarities in debates about topics such as mandatory mask-wearing, border control measures, and school closures, these debates were principally generated as responses to emergent issues and situations rather than as symbols of a broader socio-political cleavage.

V: CONCLUSION

Thinking in terms of scale, fractals and indexicality helps to make intelligible the various ways in which COVID-19 confounds us in New Zealand and elsewhere. The emergence of the pandemic has catapulted us into a new and strange territory in which our taken-for-granted ways of making sense of the world have been disrupted. This applies most definitely to the frames, or scales of reference, by which we take bearings of where we are. In this new territory we are, at least initially, scrambling to work out who we should compare ourselves to, on what dimensions, and at what scale.

The disruption to an image of New Zealand as a country in which the state has a relatively light touch is most palpable if our comparison is historical, but less stark if the comparisons are with other liberal democracies in 2020. With regards to the dynamics of electoral politics and notions of political accountability, New Zealand's frames of reference have become highly paradoxical. Alongside the historical vote of approval for an incumbent governing party for its success in keeping the virus out, the flipside is a more laser-like attribution of blame and responsibility should anything happen to jeopardise our hard-won status.

In this new and unnerving territory, the frames and scales by which we judge success, failure, over-reaction, and under-reaction are unstable and complex. Judgments of New Zealand's successes and failures in dealing with COVID-19 cover multiple scales, but there is simply no way to objectively determine what the right scale is. In this respect, COVID-19 is far from unique. The same plethora of different scales and criteria of judgment apply to any policy issue where there are differences about what should be done and how things should be done. The same scale-free (or multiple scale) dynamics apply to debates around economic inequality, climate change, and prison systems.

What is different is that the COVID-19 territory in 2020 was unfamiliar. In more established policy debates, protagonists develop a keen sense of where they are situated in relation to other actors and make various calls regarding which differences and distances matter, and which do not. What is more, the territory is different in different ways across different settings. Learning to navigate the contours of the COVID-19 policy territory might not help us do so in Brazil and vice versa. Thus, in trying to get our bearings we are doubly disoriented. This stage of disorientation will most likely be superseded by adjustment to a new normal. However, it does provide a window into some of the features of policy problem definitions and solutions that are often hidden in plain sight.

REFERENCES

Abbott, Andrew. 2001. *Chaos of Disciplines*. Chicago: University of Chicago Press.

Baumgartner, Frank R., and Brian D. Jones. 1993. *Agendas and Instability in American Politics*. Chicago, University of Chicago Press.

Blavatnik School of Government. 2020. "Coronavirus Government Response Tracker." Oxford University. https://www.bsg.ox.ac.uk/research/research-projects/coronavirus-government-response-tracker.

Downs, Anthony. 1972. "Up and Down with Ecology – The 'Issue-Attention' Cycle." *Public interest* 28 (Summer): 38–50.

GHS Index. 2021. "Global Health Security Index." https://www.ghsindex.org/.

Jones, Rhys. 2020. "Covid-19 and Māori health: 'The Daily 1pm Briefings Have Been an Exercise in Whiteness.'" *The Spinoff*, 13 May 2020.

Knappertsbusch, Felix. 2020. "'Fractal Heuristics' for Mixed Methods Research: Applying Abbott's 'Fractal Distinctions' as a Conceptual Metaphor for Method Integration." *Journal of Mixed Methods Research*, 14, no. 4: 456–472.

Manch, Thomas, and Henry Cooke. 2020. "Health Minister Drives to Local Park to Ride His Mountain Bike, amid Coronavirus Lockdown." *Stuff*, 2 April 2020.

Maor, Moshe. 2018. "Rhetoric and Doctrines of Policy Over-and Underreactions in Times of Crisis." *Policy & Politics* 46, no. 1 (January): 47–63.

Maor, Moshe, and Michael Howlett. 2020. "Explaining Variations in State COVID-19 Responses: Psychological, Institutional, and Strategic Factors in Governance and Public Policy-Making." *Policy Design and Practice* 3, no. 3: 1–14.

Mazey, Sonia, and Jeremy Richardson. 2020. "Lesson-Drawing from New Zealand and Covid-19: The Need for Anticipatory Policy Making." *The Political Quarterly* 91, no. 3 (July–September): 561–570.

Nightingale, Melissa. 2020. "Covid 19 Coronavirus: Lockdown Unlawful for First Nine Days, High Court Finds, but Says Action was Justified." *New Zealand Herald*, 19 August 2020.

Small, Zane. 2020. "COVID-19: Government Suspends Compassionate Exemptions from Managed Isolation." *Newshub*, 16 June 2020.

Statistics New Zealand. 2020a. "COVID-19's Impact on Women and Work." *Statistics New Zealand*. 3 November 2020. https://www.stats.govt.nz/news/covid-19s-impact-on-women-and-work.

– 2020b. "Gross Domestic Product." *Statistics New Zealand*. 17 December 2020. https://www.stats.govt.nz/indicators/gross-domestic-product-gdp.

Summers, Jennifer, Hao-Yuan Cheng, Hsien-Ho Lin, Lucy Telfar Bernard, Amanda Kvalsvig, Nick Wilaon, and Michael G. Baker. 2020. "Potential Lessons from the Taiwan and New Zealand Health Responses to the COVID-19 Pandemic." *The Lancet Regional Health-Western Pacific* 4, no. 100044 (1 November 2020).

Thornley, Simon. 2020. "Do the Consequences of this Lockdown Really Match the Threat?" *Stuff*, 31 March 2020.

Trevett, Claire. 2020. "Covid 19: Ministry of Health Criticised for Covid-19 Handling." *New Zealand Herald*, 18 December 2020.

Tuohy, Caroline Hughes. 2018. *Remaking Policy: Scale, Pace, and Political Strategy in Health Care Reform*. Toronto: University of Toronto Press.

West, Geoffrey. 2017. *Scale: The Universal Laws of Growth, Innovation, Sustainability, and the Pace of Life in Organisms, Cities, Economies, and Companies*. New York: Penguin.

Wilterdink, Nico. 2018. "Driving in a Dead-End Street: Critical Remarks on Andrew Abbott's Processual Sociology." *Theory and Society* 47 (1 August 2018): 539–557.

4

Health, Science, and Public Policy During and After COVID-19

12

Science and Public Policy in a Post-Pandemic World

Nicholas B. King

It is tempting to divide history into times "before" and "after" the COVID-19 pandemic, and to ask how the pandemic has changed things. For it unquestionably has. Millions have died; millions more have contracted the disease and will live with its long-term and still largely unknown consequences. The pandemic has triggered a global economic downturn that will likely last for years. It is still an open question when and even whether social life will return to "normal," with handshakes and hugs, social gatherings, and maskless mass events. There is a good chance that, like the four other endemic human coronaviruses, SARS-COV-2 is here to stay (Roberts 2021).

We can, however, also see continuity amidst upheaval. Many of the changes that we ascribe to the pandemic were set in motion long before 2020, and it is better to ask how the pandemic has arrested or accelerated those changes. Such is the case with the role of science in public life. Amidst the pandemic, scientists, science advisers, scientific knowledge, and scientific activity have occupied the public spotlight to an unusual degree. Epidemiologic models predicting the spread of the COVID-19 virus with and without public health interventions directly informed decision-makers and are hotly debated on social media. American science adviser Dr Anthony Fauci, director of the National Institute of Allergy and Infectious Diseases, is a household name, alternately venerated as a voice of scientific reason and vilified as a fear-mongering bureaucrat. Millions of people have developed opinions, however informed, on the effectiveness of different types of masks, the potential of treatments like hydroxychloroquine, and the timeline of vaccine development. And in many countries, one's position on scientific facts (are masks effective? are vaccines safe?), and the trustworthiness of science in general, are deeply intertwined with politics and personal identity.

While the intensity of the pandemic has lent it exceptional urgency, it would be a mistake to presume that it has fundamentally changed the production and consumption of scientific knowledge – yet. The COVID-19 pandemic has accelerated and surfaced long-term trends in the ways that scientific knowledge is produced, circulated, interpreted, and acted upon. How we collectively respond to these trends in a post-pandemic world will depend in large part on our implicit models of what science is and its appropriate role of science in public life.

SCIENCE AND THE WEAPONIZATION OF UNCERTAINTY

The COVID-19 pandemic has been a double-edged sword for the scientific enterprise. On one hand, and from an historical perspective, science has unquestionably triumphed. The virus was identified, its basic biology and epidemiology understood, countermeasures implemented, and vaccines developed with exceptional speed. Notwithstanding notable exceptions, decision-makers have generally heeded the warnings and advice of scientific advisers, and successful pandemic response appears to be correlated with willingness to act on scientific advice. New Zealand's effective containment of the virus has been credited to Prime Minister Jacinda Ardern's decisive, science-informed leadership and close working relationships with the scientific community (Baker, Wilson, and Anglemyer 2020). Despite being hit by the virus comparatively early, Taiwan, Vietnam, Singapore, and Thailand mounted quick and effective science-informed public health responses. By contrast, catastrophically slow responses in the United States, United Kingdom, and Brazil have corresponded with refusals to heed the advice of science and public health advisers.

On the other hand, in the public arena science has suffered. Individual scientists have been maligned and harassed on social media; political leaders have publicly denounced science and sidelined scientific advisers; and public mistrust of science appears to be growing. A flood of scientific preprints – articles that are publicly posted without undergoing peer review – has been cited as contributing to the spread of COVID-related misinformation. But peer-review is no panacea: two of the world's premier medical journals, *The Lancet* and *The New England Journal of Medicine*, retracted widely-publicized studies of potential COVID-19 treatments on the same day (Joseph 2020). These developments and more have shaken the traditionally unassailable authority of science in public policy.

Of particular note is the role of uncertainty in the interface between science and public life. A principal weapon in the populist arsenal is to proclaim absolute certainty, celebrating the authority and personal charisma of a powerful leader, while demeaning other sources of evidence. Certainty is an indication of power and control, uncertainty a risible sign of weakness rather than an indication of an honest appraisal of the situation. One of the Trump administration's first public acts was to repeatedly double down on claims that his inauguration was the largest in history, despite decisive photographic evidence to the contrary (Swaine 2018). This display of power over subordinates and willful ignorance of the facts was simply the first in a long series of steps towards the Trump's administration's catastrophic handling of the COVID-19 pandemic (Levy 2016).

Along with the celebration of certainty comes a demonization and weaponization of uncertainty. A principal tactic in the weaponization of uncertainty is to insist on impossible levels of certainty to justify changes to the status quo, and disparage one's opponents when they cannot provide it. While tobacco companies, climate change deniers, and other "merchants of doubt" have covertly employed this tactic for decades (Oreskes and Conway 2010), during the COVID-19 pandemic it has been employed openly and repeatedly in attacks on epidemiologists who revise their COVID-19 mortality estimates in light of new information about current interventions (Wan and Blake 2020).

THREE WAYS FORWARD

What is the best way to respond to the apparent crisis of confidence in science and attendant weaponization of uncertainty? The answer to this question depends upon one's implicit model of science and its proper role in public life.

One model, which is arguably the most prevalent among scientists themselves, holds that science is a set of principles and methods to accurately describe, explain, and predict what will happen in the world – and policy must be made on the basis of accurate descriptions, explanations, and predictions. A recent US National

Academies of Science, Engineering and Medicine report thus defines science as "a mode of inquiry that aims to pose questions about the world, arriving at the answers and assessing their degree of certainty through a communal effort designed to ensure that they are well grounded. Scientific inquiry focuses on four major goals: (1) to describe the world (e.g., taxonomy classifications); (2) to explain the world (e.g., the evolution of species); (3) to predict what will happen in the world (e.g., weather forecasting); and (4) to intervene in specific processes or systems (e.g., making solar power economical or engineering better medicines)" (National Academies of Science, Engineering and Medicine 2019).

Under this model, scientists are distinguished not by particular attributes or dispositions, but rather by sharing a set of common assumptions (that the world is consistent and governed by discernable and quantifiable rules) and adhering to common methods of producing knowledge (hypothesis formulation and testing, continual modification of theories in light of new evidence, characterization and communication of confidence and uncertainty, aggregation and synthesis of knowledge, and working towards consensus). Scientists are accorded special authority because these assumptions and methods produce accurate, reliable, objective, and useful knowledge. This is the basis of the "evidence-based policy" approach which, as one Canadian government report argues, "levers the best available objective evidence from research to identify and understand issues so that policies can be crafted by decision makers that will deliver desired outcomes effectively, with a minimal margin of error and reduced risk of unintended consequences. Compared to subjective values, the factual interpretations of special interests and advocacy groups, and selective or ideologically-driven viewpoints informing the policy development process, an evidence-based approach has as its great advantage neutrality and authoritativeness. This stems from sound, rigorous, comprehensive and unbiased policy research" (Townsend and Kunimoto 2009).

A second model holds that scientists are objective, neutral, unbiased, and able to distinguish that which is a matter of "fact" from that which is one of perspective, ethics, or emotion – and policy must be unbiased, objective, and unemotional. As political economist William Davies notes:

> According to the ideal of modern science, scientists are unlike members of a crowd or political figures, because they are able

to separate their feelings from their observations. They are able to distinguish that which is a matter of "fact" from that which is one of perspective, ethics or emotion. They can do so because they are able to park their own identities when they enter the laboratory or field, and act merely as neutral mediators between the data that they collect and the documents that end up in journals ... Scientists seek our trust and respect because they promise to represent things accurately ... To trust in science is to trust in the capacity of people to report and record things in an adequate fashion, and to leave their own biases and emotions at the door. (Davies 2018)

While it shares the first model's emphases on objectivity, neutrality, and accuracy, this model shifts the emphasis from the methods of producing knowledge to the attributes and dispositions of the people who produce and disseminate it. This distinction is crucial when considering the role of science in public life. Under the first model, decision-makers should accord science a special role because it produces the most reliable and accurate information for policy purposes, thus reducing the biases inherent in human judgment. Under the second model, decision-makers should accord scientists a special role because they are special kinds of people, able to free themselves from the biases and emotions that cloud others' judgments.

The COVID-19 pandemic has demonstrated the limitations of each of these models of science. While in the long term the scientific method may produce knowledge that is relatively more accurate, reliable, and useful, in the short-term it has to wrestle with the same uncertainties that all forms of knowledge-production confront. Legitimate disagreements over the effectiveness of different kinds of masks, the R-naught of the virus, the effectiveness of different interventions, and the appropriate assumptions for modelling the spread of infections have all illustrated the fact that at any one time, even the best scientific methods may fail to produce knowledge so reliable that it makes policy decisions self-evident. This is a feature, not a bug of the scientific method: it recognizes the inherent instability of knowledge, and thus the necessity of subjecting all models, theories, and claims to continuous scrutiny and updating. Yet if public trust in science depends upon the absolute infallibility of the knowledge that it produces, then it will always be open to the charges of fallibility that are central to the weaponization of uncertainty. Model One is unsupportable.

Model Two fails for the simple fact that we cannot and should not anoint individuals as infallible, unbiased purveyors of fact. Scientists may indeed aspire to "park their own identities" when they enter the lab, engage in public debate, or advise decision-makers on the best response to the pandemic; but in practice this is an unattainable ideal. Again, this is a feature rather than a bug: at their best, scientific methods seek to reduce bias and characterize uncertainty precisely because humans are fallible and uncertainty is ubiquitous. And, as with Model One, if public trust in science depends upon the absolute infallibility and objectivity of scientists themselves, then they will always be open to legitimate and illegitimate charges of bias and fallibility that are central to the weaponization of uncertainty.

It is commonplace to lament the "politicization of science" during the COVID-19 pandemic. Authoritarian rulers like Trump and Bolonaro have indeed politicized science by demonizing scientists and scientific institutions, promulgating misinformation and disinformation, and promoting themselves as infallible and authoritative sources of information, often directly contradicting established scientific and public health authorities. Yet the lamentation is best read as a sign that Models One and Two are not (or are no longer) sustainable. Ultimately, the demystification of science during the COVID-19 pandemic presents an opportunity rather than a barrier to advancing the role of science in public life.

A third model of science and its role in public life holds that science is a value-laden, historically-contingent, context-dependent form of producing knowledge, which has no special claim to infallibility, objectivity, or efficacy – but whose values are the best foundation for policy. This model insists on recognizing the scientific enterprise both as it is and as it aspires to be, without mistaking the latter for the former. The scientific enterprise can be lauded for its aspirations to objectivity and infallibility, and the values that guide those aspirations, without believing that the scientific method or individual scientists perfectly embody those aspirations. As historian of science Naomi Oreskes has argued, "in suppressing their values and insisting on the value-neutrality of science, scientists have gone down a wrong road. They have made the mistake of thinking that people would trust them if they believed that science was value-free" (Oreskes 2019). Similarly, sociologists

Harry Collins and Robert Evans insist on "looking at science as an institution that can give moral leadership [...] democracies need science because science is, or can be, a fountainhead of good values. Science's understandings are continually disputed, but science's values are eternal. Thus, whatever position one takes on the value of science's outputs – and most people will still reach for truth and utility when justifying science – the argument from science's values will stand" (Collins and Evans 2017).

The values most closely associated with science were first elucidated by sociologist Robert K. Merton in the mid-twentieth century. Merton identified four "institutional imperatives": "communism" (scientific knowledge is the property of the scientific community as a whole, in order to promote active sharing and cooperation); "universalism" (science may be practiced by anyone, regardless of race, nationality, gender, or culture, and adjudication of knowledge-claims should be entirely impersonal); "disinterestedness" (scientists and scientific institutions should act for the common benefit, rather than for personal gain); and "organized skepticism" (scientific knowledge should be subject to continuous scrutiny and robust debate; Merton 1973). To these institutional norms we may add "transparency and openness" (scientific knowledge, and the processes by which it is produced, should be fully available for public review); and "comfort with uncertainty" (scientific knowledge should characterize and communicate confidence and uncertainty).

Taken together, these values accord well with broader democratic ideals of inclusion, openness, and transparency, and can inform the institutional design of science, justify the place of science in public life and policymaking, and offer one means of counteracting the weaponization of uncertainty. We should embrace as a virtue science's unique commitment to understanding, quantifying, and communicating uncertainty. The best predictive models provide best- and worst-case scenarios, and are revised as new information comes to light; the most trustworthy sources of information transparently and unflinchingly communicate uncertainty; and the best decisions flow from understanding and embracing uncertainty rather than denigrating it and proclaiming false certainty (Manski 2013). Democratic institutions in the post-pandemic world should take these values as central organizing principles.

REFERENCES

Baker, Michael G., Nick Wilson, and Andrew Anglemyer. 2020. "Successful Elimination of Covid-19 Transmission in New Zealand." *New England Journal of Medicine* 383, no. 8: e56. https://www.bbc.com/news/world-asia-52344299.

Collins, Harry, and Robert Evans. 2017. *Why Democracies Need Science*. Malden: Polity Press.

Davies, William. 2018. *Nervous States: Democracy and the Decline of Reason*. New York: W.W. Norton and Company.

Joseph, Andrew. 2020. "Lancet, New England Journal Retract Covid-19 Studies, Including One that Raised Safety Concerns about Malaria Drugs." *Stat*, 4 June 2020. https://www.statnews.com/2020/06/04/lancet-retracts-major-covid-19-paper-that-raised-safety-concerns-about-malaria-drugs/.

Levy, Jacob T. 2016. "Authoritarianism and Post-Truth Politics." *Niskanen Center*, 30 November 2016. https://www.niskanencenter.org/authoritarianism-post-truth-politics/.

Manski, Charles F. 2013. *Public Policy in an Uncertain World*. Cambridge: Harvard University Press.

Merton, R. K. 1973. *The Sociology of Science: Theoretical and Empirical Investigations*. Chicago: University of Chicago Press.

National Academies of Science, Engineering and Medicine. 2019. *Reproducibility and Replicability in Science*. Washington, DC: National Academies Press.

Oreskes, N. 2019. *Why Trust Science?* Princeton NJ: Princeton University Press.

Oreskes, Naomi, and Eric M. Conway. 2010. *Merchants of Doubt: How a Handful of Scientists Obscured the Truth on Issues from Tobacco Smoke to Global Warming*. New York: Bloomsbury Press.

Roberts, Grace C. 2021. "Coronavirus Might Become Endemic – Here's How." *The Conversation*, 5 February 2021. https://theconversation.com/coronavirus-might-become-endemic-heres-how-153572.

Swaine, John. "Trump Inauguration Crowd Photos Were Edited after He Intervened." *The Guardian*, 6 September 2018. https://www.theguardian.com/world/2018/sep/06/donald-trump-inauguration-crowd-size-photos-edited.

Townsend, Thomas, and Bob Kunimoto. 2009. *Capacity, Collaboration and Culture: The Future of the Policy Research Function in the Government of Canada*. Ottawa: Government of Canada.

Wan, William, and Aaron Blake. 2020. "Coronavirus Modelers Factor in New Public Health Risk: Accusations Their Work is a Hoax." *Washington Post*, 27 March 2020. https://www.washingtonpost.com/health/2020/03/27/coronavirus-models-politized-trump/.

13

Wise Government and Wise Science in Times of Crisis

Jean-Louis Denis, Clara Champagne, Justin Waring

THE CHALLENGE

In the era of post-truth, science denial, fake news, and conspiracy theories, it is surprising – ironic, even – that billions of people across continents have turned to science for a solution, vesting their hopes in scientists: in the time of COVID-19, science is, as Carl Sagan (1995) would say, the "candle in the dark."

Scientific communities have answered that call. A survey of 2,500 American, Canadian, and European scientists conducted by Kyle Myers at Harvard Business School reveals that 32 per cent have reoriented their research to focus on COVID-19 (Yong 2020). The science journalist Ed Yong reports that on *Web of Science*, there are twice as many articles about COVID-19 as there are for polio, measles, cholera, and dengue, "diseases that have plagued humanity for centuries" (Yong 2020, 50). Multiple safe and efficient vaccines are already being administered, with many others in the last phases of testing. This intense research "pivot," as Yong calls it, is unprecedented.

The COVID-19 pandemic is a crisis. Crises call for immediate, decisive action. Under intense time pressures, with uncertainties characterizing nearly every aspect of this crisis, policy-makers must implement extraordinary measures: restrictions of liberties via lockdown measures, border closures, quarantines, face covering mandates, compulsory closings of businesses, school on Zoom. More than ever, governments are a symbol, the mirror of a people's fears, hopes, and values, and the conductor of an ensemble of moving parts that must be coordinated into an efficacious and agile response. Politicians have often justified their actions by a familiar phrase: "We are following the science" (Stevens 2020, 560). Of course, this is an oversimplification. The policy-science interface has perhaps never been so complex.

Politics, policy, and science are strange bedfellows, a peculiar alliance. They act upon different imperatives, and yet when it comes to a crisis like COVID-19, they are interdependent. Over the last two hundred years, science and government have worked together as part of a complex assemblage to govern the productive health of contemporary societies both through and beyond the "State" (Foucault 2007). The technologies of this bio-power for the classification, measurement, and governing of health operate beyond the "State" and disciplinary expertise to become internalized by individuals; governing health becomes a project for oneself. The relationship between "State," science, and citizens is key to governing the productive well-being of society, and the COVID-19 pandemic has arguably destabilized this interface, requiring a return to more disciplinary forms of control and sovereign authority.

Science is by nature and by design a slow, meandering, contentious, communal enterprise. None of these characteristics are suited for a swift response to a pandemic. How to mix political, policy-making, and scientific capacities and leadership in a productive and legitimate way poses a wicked policy problem.

In this chapter, we will examine the government-science interface in the COVID-19 context. What structures were created or mobilized to ensure the utilization of scientific knowledge in the pandemic response? How did structural legacies impact the mobilization of scientific assets? What kind of expertise was considered? What was expected of science during the pandemic, and how did these expectations run counter to good, normal science? What can we learn from COVID-19 about communicating science in the face of uncertainty? And what will be the long-term impact of the pandemic on the interface between politics, policy, and science?

1 – Government and Science

In 2004, Philip Davies published a paper that caught the attention of many policy-makers. In it, Davies reflects on the possibility of an evidence-based government. The paper starts with a quote by John Maynard Keynes: "There is nothing a government hates more than to be well-informed; for it makes the process of arriving at decisions much more complicated and difficult."

The COVID-19 pandemic offers a window of choice to explore the prospects and practicalities of an evidence-based government. The pandemic – a sanitary crisis the likes of which had not been seen in a century – culminated in amazing pressures and expectations for public and political leaders (Boin et al. 2017). Governments needed to act quickly despite uncertainties; not acting was hardly an option. The epidemiological projection released by Neil Ferguson of the Imperial College London in March 2020 predicted tens of millions of deaths worldwide if strict measures were not implemented. This model, despite its flaws, sprung leaders across continents to action (Kreps and Kriner 2020). Governments turned to scientific experts for guidance on how to mitigate the damage of the pandemic.

The Merriam-Webster dictionary defines an interface as "the place at which independent and often unrelated systems meet and act on or communicate with each other"; the word comes to us from *inter* – between – and *face*, as in *surface*: an interface is the "surface regarded as the *common boundary* of two bodies." The Canadian philosopher and media theorist Marshall McLuhan is said to be the first to have used "interface" in its now common meaning, the place of interaction between two systems. Science and government are two such bodies, two independent and often unrelated systems which act on different imperatives, follow different logics.

The idea that science can be called to duty to help resolve major societal challenges is not new. Over the last two hundred years, science and government have worked together as part of a complex assemblage to govern the productive health of contemporary societies. Although science and government might act upon different imperatives, they have aligned in ways that render phenomena or subjects known and governable. While this remains the case with COVID-19, it is also true that the relationship between policy and science has at times looked fragile, where the demands and expectations of one has not been matched by the other.

Governments can and should be learners. Science is a privileged means by which governments can assess the foundations and potential consequences of their decisions. The relatively new area of research known as "knowledge utilization" (also referred to as knowledge mobilization, exchange, transfer, or translation, although there are conceptual differences between these terms) analyzes how science can best inform policies and decisions. To put it another way, it is the study of the science-government interface.

Knowledge utilization developed as a response to a growing demand for partnerships between governments and researchers in the creation and utilization of knowledge (Estabrooks et al. 2008). Research funding agencies have also espoused the ideal of a knowledge-based society by adopting policies and programs to strengthen the connections between researchers and decision-makers and doers of all sorts (Tetroe et al. 2008).[1] These aspirations are still very contemporary with raising awareness of emerging major societal and global challenges and the recognition that science could – and should – play a role in facing large-scale problems (Hällgreen, Rouleau, and De Rond 2018). The publication in November 2020 of the UN *Research Roadmap for the* COVID-19 *Recovery* is a clear example of this desire to put science to contribution.

Notwithstanding the many serious environmental risks and "bads" that have been made possible through scientific breakthroughs (Beck 1992), science is often considered an antidote to protect societies and people from unwise leaders or irrational decisions. However, turning science into an instrument to resolve collective problems is a challenging task. Research in the field of knowledge utilization has led to the development of complex models of knowledge production and exchange. For example, Ian D. Graham and his colleagues developed a model of the knowledge-to-action process that presents ideal phases of knowledge creation and action (Graham et al. 2006). Such models expressly recognize the complex, dynamic, fluid, and often strenuous process of getting research from academic campuses and research laboratories to government buildings. In fact, knowledge utilization processes are in many ways like science itself: slow, meandering, contentious, communal. In other words: far from ideal when swift, decisive, unilateral government action is needed.

Thus, while some scientists may perform high-impact research, the pathways between usable knowledge and knowledge utilization remain serendipitous (Weiss 1979). This is especially true in times of crisis, when the imperative of quick decision-making is not conducive to good science or complex exchanges between scientists and policy-makers (Van Dooren and Noordegraaf 2020). As H. Holden Thorp, the editor-in-chief of *Science*, writes: "science is being asked to provide a rapid solution to a problem that is not completely described [...] This is not just fixing a plane while it's flying – it's fixing a plane that's flying while its blueprints are still being drawn" (Thorp 2020, 1405). The response to COVID-19 called for evidence- and decision-making in a highly uncertain and evolving situation. In such a context, "unambiguous evidence" is "an unachievable ideal"; "the effectiveness of response measures is situated and emergent" (Lancaster, Rhodes and Rosengarten 2020).

II – Inheritance

A variety of contextual factors, including factors related to structural aspects of government, inevitably influences the way knowledge was used for government decisions in the time of COVID-19 (Yan et al. 2020). Indeed, institutional frameworks and capacities within governments influence the role played by science in policy-making. As Van Dooren and Noordegraaf write, "[t]he use of science is not merely rhetorical. Scientific expertise is institutionalized in decision-making procedures" (Van Dooren and Noordegraaf 2020, 611).

Despite assurances from some leaders that they "followed the science," the response to COVID-19 did not start as a blank slate waiting to be filled by scientific knowledge. The structural apparatus mobilized to respond to the crisis was years in the making. The organization of health care and public health systems had an impact on governments' ability to respond effectively to the crisis, sometimes making it hard for them to actually implement measures following "the science." For example, the Canadian government certainly regretted the exodus of pharmaceutical companies and manufactures, propelled over the years by political and economic decisions, when faced with the problem of producing vaccines and personal protective equipment in a timely fashion – a key measure to protect health care workers and the general population from infection. By comparison, in the United Kingdom, a well-developed pharmaceutical sector and the government's willingness to proactively fund drug research and advance purchase prospective treatments enabled it to respond with pace to subsequent vaccination roll-out (Iacobucci 2020; Exworthy, Mannion, and Powell 2016; Dixon, Edwards, and Murray 2020). In the province of Quebec, chronic underfunding and budget cuts in public health research and institutions also surely affected these institutions' ability to do what "the science" warranted. Contact tracing and isolation were evidently shoddy in Quebec, where the regional public health sector recently suffered the cut of a third of its annual budget in a health reform with many faults, including horrible timing. At the federal level, Canada also had weak capacities in its national agency of public health at the onset of the pandemic. This situation proved to be a hurdle to the development of a coherent, rapid, and well-developed federal response in the early stages of the crisis (Desson et al. 2020).

A similar situation can be seen in the UK, especially in England. A decade of constrained funding for the health care sector, together with profound structural reforms that fragmented the organization of care services (Exworthy and Mannion 2016) and diminished the role of public health as a distinct and significant area of national and regional policy-making, clearly framed the response to COVID-19. This situation was arguably worsened by the UK government's enthusiasm for outsourcing and contracting out many of the key functions of the COVID response, such as the test and trace IT infrastructure. Further still, during the pandemic, the English government announced the dissolution of its national body Public Health England with the creation of a new agency targeted explicitly at pandemic response and test-and-trace facilities, the National Institute for Health Protection (Iacobucci 2020). Although possibly better suited to the reactive response to a major public health crisis, this change may have diverted attention from underlying public health issues and health disparities, which have been starkly brought to light by the pandemic.

These are just a few examples to show that "the science" may have something to say about which measures to favour, but governments' leeway to actually implement these measures is restricted by the structures it already has in place; by the institutional fragility it tolerated or created.

Moreover, past collaboration between the executive power of a government and its public agencies clearly influenced the propensity to mobilize and rely on internal scientific capacities. A history of tension between a government and its own agencies, a political culture with a low tolerance for controversies, or limited scientific capacities within the government might have frustrated policy-makers' ability to rely on and benefit from the scientific expertise within these agencies. These factors may explain the spread of ad hoc scientific advisory structures and committees to advise governments during the pandemic.[2] Faced with the pandemic, some governments relied mostly on available scientific capacities found in public agencies while others relied mostly on these new ad hoc advisory scientific committees; some adopted a mix of both approaches (Gaille et al. 2020). Advisory scientific structures set up by governments were more or less independent and were more or less characterized by political consanguinity (Moatti 2020). Challenges to the SAGE (Scientific Advisory Group for Emergencies) committee in the UK, with the creation of an alternate SAGE, exemplified how suspicion of cold politicization had an impact on the credibility and potential role of science in the management of the pandemic (Horton 2020).

An analysis of the case of France also underlines how concentration of political authorities, coupled with an inherent and inevitable risk of crisis politicization, posed a challenge to the mobilization of scientific evidence to tame the pandemic (Hassenteufel 2020). Indeed, Hassenteufel argues that, in France, programmatic elites have a hold on policy-making, with consequences on which experts will be mobilized to provide scientific advice during the pandemic. This is not unique to France; issues around the capacity of governments to mobilize the best scientific assets to contain the pandemic and think about post-pandemic issues plagued many jurisdictions.

Another example is Quebec, where a high level centralization of power at the hands of technocrats may have hampered large-scale mobilization of external experts, with the exception of those close to power. Technocrats are, in a sense, in-house experts that may feel threatened by outside expertise or may not have the institutional channels and autonomy to connect with the broader scientific community; thus, in highly technocratic systems, there could be a lower tendency to seek external advice and expertise (Gleave 2021). There are "insiders" and "outsiders" within the science-policy interface. Further, there are inherent tensions within and between the scientific communities about who has influence, who is recognized as an "expert," and who is awarded funding; questions reminiscent of the boundary disputes between science and non-science (Gieryn 1983).

There is a growing recognition in policy science literature that governments are inhabited by people, instruments, and organizations with various levels of skills, expertise, knowledge, material resources, and political acumen (Wu, Ramesh, and Howlett 2015). The pandemic has revealed how securing capacities is a challenge for most countries and how their experience with previous pandemics and their current capacities condition responses to the crisis (Capano et al. 2020; Desson et al. 2020; Béland and Marier 2020). Capacities are fundamental to frame and support government interventions, yet they are often neglected before, during, and after crises. The ideal of an evidence-based government is not one of an absolute appearance of rationality in policy-making but a matter of having the capacities to relate in a productive and collaborative way with science.

We need to further investigate the political and institutional factors that help governments adopt a nuanced but rich view on the benefits of science in uncertain times and influence the development and mobilization of capacities. These factors include political regimes, formal political institutions, the state of social policies, and the prevalent political culture, including scientific networks (Béland et al. 2021; Greer et al. 2020; Quegly 2020). In many jurisdictions, an unusual level of political consensus eased the dialogue between science and government (Merkley et al. 2020; Detsky and Bogoch 2020; Olagnier and Mogensen 2020). Meanwhile, extreme political polarization in other jurisdictions such as Brazil and the United States impeded responses to the pandemic and hindered reliance on scientific advice.[3]

III – Perspectives and Blind Spots

Analysis of decision-making in health policy also reveals the complexity of deriving sound and clear advice from a heterogeneous and complex body of evidence (Brown 2012). In this regard, Davies (2004) refers to the distinction between normal science, where a significant body of knowledge seems relatively stable and offers more clarity to support policy-making, and science based on novel or contested knowledge and unexplored ground. Davies gave global governance and e-government as examples of the latter; it seems clear that COVID-related science also falls in this category. The COVID-19 context was characterized by high uncertainties and velocity in the scientific knowledge available to classify, survey, and mitigate risks (Quegly 2020). Informing policy decisions with an unstable stock of knowledge is a tough scientific dilemma, and while scientific communities are aware of the risks relating to the validity of published studies and knowledge syntheses produced in such a febrile context, policy-makers and the general public might not be.

In his paper, Davies also underlined that an evidence-based government should ground its decisions in the integration of a complex mix of the expertise, experience, and judgments of policy-makers with the best available scientific evidence. Scientific knowledge is never enough; it should inform but cannot dictate decisions because of necessary trade-offs among a constellation of considerations. It is more appropriate, perhaps, to talk about evidence-*informed* – rather than evidence-*based* – policy-making. In the COVID-19 context, we can also refer to Martin, Hannah, and Dingwall's (2020) notion of *eminence*-based policy-making. Indeed, debates around issues such as whether to mandate mask-wearing, when to enact and release lockdown measures, how to enforce social distancing, and how to best roll-out vaccines revealed considerable tensions both within the scientific communities and between scientists and policy-makers. Without evidence that warrants unequivocal policy guidance, past expertise, pre-eminence in the field, and public profile influenced policy as much as – and perhaps more than – the science itself.

Policy decisions have to achieve a reasonable balance among competing policy dilemmas such as protecting health and limiting social and economic deprivation. The duty of governments is to develop and implement strategies and incentives to promote a reasonable consideration of science in political and public decisions. And, as Lancaster, Rhodes, and Rosengarten (2020) point out: "In emergencies, it becomes difficult to hold onto the notion that evidence generated to inform decision making can somehow stand apart and separate itself from the social and political worlds in which it is made and will be put to use. When evidence and decision making are proceeding simultaneously, these matters of concern are even more obviously inescapably conjoined, requiring processes of reflexive dialogue and engagement which work to actively incorporate these concerns and values quickly and decisively, rather than maintaining a veneer of scientific objectivity."

Decisions about the pandemic were influenced by the way politicians and policy-makers frame problems and solutions. A growing body of literature sees policy discourses and decisions as rhetorical devices that are engaged in a political contest around meanings (Jones and Exworthy 2015). The way problems and solutions are framed is associated with patterns of interests and values that necessarily exclude or pay less attention to some policy options. For example, the distinction in health policy between producing healthcare and producing health represents very different approaches to what should be prioritized in policy decisions (Evans and Stoddart 1990). During the pandemic, there was no easy answer to inevitable policy trade-offs. We should pay more attention to how scientific disciplines contributed to an idiosyncratic framing of the pandemic if we want to have more comprehensive and balanced responses in the future. Similarly, we have to consider the role of political ideologies like populism in framing problems and solution within governments if we want to better grasp the role that is attributed to science in policy developments. These considerations call for dialogue and reflexivity at the government-science interface and they are challenging for both institutions.

A study on the composition of advisory scientific committees to manage the pandemic across various countries shows that they replicate a narrow view of science. These structures are characterized by a pre-eminence of scientific medical leaders and epidemiologists, with almost no participation of scientists from the social sciences and humanities (Rajan et al. 2020). These structures also tend to be poorly inclusive in their membership. While medical specialties and epidemiology are natural suspects to understand the "hard side" of the pandemic (such as models of virus propagation, risks distribution among a population, and the consequences of the virus for human health), they offer very limited insights on the social dimensions and consequences associated with the evolution, management, and recovery from a pandemic. Strategies for economic and social recovery, behavioural and communication challenges associated with the acceptability of public health measures, strategies to reorganize care, and protection of human rights are just a few examples of pandemic issues where social sciences and humanities can provide key insights. As Yong writes: "To study COVID-19 is not only to study the disease itself as a biological entity [...] What looks like a single problem is actually all things, all at once. So what we're actually studying is literally everything in society, at every scale, from supply chains to individual relationships" (Yong 2020, 58).

Governments should value a more comprehensive view of science. In addition, internal scientific capacities of governments and ad hoc advisory scientific structures might be too limiting in the end. Broader partnerships between universities, research centres, and governments could bring more pluralism in knowledge that is considered to inform policy decisions during the pandemic (Daviter 2019).

IV – *Choices*

One must also recognize the limitations of science and the limited role of evidence in structuring policy choices. Appeals to science such as the familiar phrase "we are following the science" obscure the fact that many choices were implicitly made when governments implemented certain measures to respond to COVID-19, and that these were inherently political choices that "science" had nothing to do with. Choices have to be made; competing priorities weighed. Science cannot decide for us if we should prioritize the safety of seniors at the expense of the education of children. It cannot choose what, between culture, trade, job security, mental health, and respect of individual rights, should matter most. It cannot tell us whether we should keep museums and libraries open despite risks, or who should get the vaccine first, or if the number of new daily cases is few enough to reopen small businesses and restaurants. Epidemiological models can inform decision-makers on the potential consequences, from a public health point of view, of implementing one measure over another one, at one particular moment rather than earlier or later, but science cannot decide what our societal concerns, priorities, and values are. Science cannot dictate how policy-makers should, in their response to the crisis, weigh considerations which are fundamentally moral and political, and which, in a democracy, rest with elected leaders: "to govern is to choose" (Maani 2021).

As Alex Stevens (2020) states, "different approaches were informed by scientific findings, but they resulted from political decisions, not science." When decision-makers justify their choices by stating that they "followed the science," they stifle debate on these political exercises of prioritization. Voices for more transparent decision-making during the pandemic illustrated social demands for such political arguments and debates on priorities.

Moreover, science is not monolithic. Science is not, as Stevens puts it, "an apolitical and indisputable tablet of stone." Different experts in different fields hold different views on which public policies must be implemented in the time of COVID-19. Experts in the same field often disagree. This is an integral part of science, not a problem to be fixed: "Science works by researchers coming up with different ideas. They then test them and find many of them to be wrong. There are some ideas [...] that have been tested so thoroughly that they are beyond reasonable dispute. The best way to deal with a rapidly developing viral pandemic is not one of them" (Stevens 2020, 560). This complexity of the body of scientific knowledge that can inform COVID-19 policies is rarely acknowledged when politicians state that they are "following the science." As underlined previously, prioritizing one expert over another, one expertise over another, when many different considerations are relevant to COVID-19 decision-making, is also a choice: "There is not just one 'scientific' approach to dealing with COVID-19." (Stevens 2020, 560)

The phrase "we are following the science" misleads as to what science can actually offer public policy-making.[4] Science is above all a process; it is the choice to go about discovering the world by following certain norms and processes to reduce bias, increase the likelihood that we are right, and adapt or revise if necessary. Science is by nature and by design complex and incomplete; it cannot offer up absolute truths or fail-proof solutions, especially in a crisis marked by uncertainty: "A provisional and contested set of statements about how the world is cannot be used directly as a rule for what governments should do" (Stevens 2020, 560). Pretending otherwise is a perversion of science: of its role, its process, its strengths, and its limits. Yet it is precisely the clear acknowledgment of its limits and of the uncertainty that is inherent to the scientific enterprise that gives science its epistemic strength. Scientists know this but, as Thorp writes, "the general public – who are agonizing over how long this pandemic will last, how it will affect the economy, and whether they and their loved ones will be safe – are looking for hope wherever they can find it" (Thorp 2020, 1405). If politicians magnify these hopes, and science fails to deliver, the consequences could be disastrous (Kreps and Kriner 2020). Van Dooren and Noordegraaf rightly and eloquently observe that "[w]hen scientific advice and expertise are expected to "get rid" of problems, then science cannot deliver. The staging of science as the savior of society leads to a depoliticization of policy and a politicization of science [...] It leads to expectations that normal science cannot meet" (Van Dooren and Noordegraaf 2020, 614).

As noted by Jamieson, science is trustworthy because it adheres to its norms and processes, which "increases the reliability of the resulting knowledge and the likelihood that the public views science as reliable" (Jamieson et al. 2019, 19231). Science holds a privileged cultural status that "vests its claims with special rhetorical force" in public debates (Jamieson 2017, 15). Although science and politics might be regarded as inter-linked parts of a broader apparatus of governing (Foucault

2007), there is at the very least a symbolic boundary between science and politics, where the "rules" of scientific debate offer claims of "truth" that are distinct from the "judgments" of political debate (Gieryn 1983). By distinguishing itself from politics, science "retains its privileged cultural status it has earned as a result of its commitment to knowledge-producing and -protecting norms and institutionalized structures that have over time generated reliable knowledge" (Jamieson 2017, 17). When governments encourage unreasonable expectations as to what science can deliver, deception is sure to follow, thus putting this privileged status in peril: "the science itself is called into question and science communication is vulnerable to attack as veiled political communication," (Jamieson 2017, 18) thus "eroding the capacity of custodians of scientific knowledge [...] to ground debate" (Jamieson 2017, 22). Science may be self-correcting, but public communication of science is not. When science and politics become undistinguishable – when their interface is a merge rather than a crossroads – science risks losing its cultural specificity and authority.

WISE GOVERNMENT AND WISE SCIENCE

Although science and government act upon different imperatives, they often align in ways that render phenomena or subjects known and governable. The pandemic showed how politics and science melted together, creating various levels of expectation and mutual understanding between these two worlds. There are other examples of this melting of the science-government interface, such as the global climate emergency, but perhaps unlike these other issues, COVID-19 involved such urgency and uncertainty that it further complicated the interface between politics and science. What can we learn from this extreme context on the prospect and meaning of an evidence-informed government?

Science and government can and must work together to respond effectively to threats such as the COVID-19 pandemic. However, wisdom calls for reasonable expectations about what science can contribute in such contexts. Not so long before his death, Foucault shared his reading of a text by Kant on the historical meaning of the Enlightenment (Foucault 1984). He proposed to think of the Enlightenment less as a historical period and more as a present disposition of the self that values the act of reasoning in context. Being wise and responsible is a matter of predisposition and judgment; it is a demonstration of careful and attentive reasoning in a context where valuable knowledge and facts are considered. Being reasonable is a disposition where governments work hard to frame and assess problematic situations and define necessary constraints in an explicit and deliberate way. Reasoning in context is the duty of politicians and public leaders.

Science too must be wise. It is important for researchers to calibrate expectations and value the cardinal rules of skepticism and nuance when they share findings and communicate evidence. Pressures for rapid scientific discovery and advice made the respect of such principles difficult in the COVID-19 context. The pandemic showed that science communication is as much about communicating the nature of science – what it can and cannot deliver – as it is about communicating scientific "facts." Evidently, "following the science" proved to be an unsatisfactory justification for government action when the science was in many ways emerging, lost, contradictory, and unclear.

In addition, scientists must promote a broad view of the knowledge claims that are appropriate to consider for the wide range of problems associated with a major crisis such as COVID-19. It is a puzzling challenge for science to reconcile social demands for usable knowledge in a pressing context like the pandemic with a relevant and legitimate role of research-based evidence in dealing with collective problems.

Recovery from the pandemic is a predominant theme these days with the prospect of mass vaccination. We suggest that serious thinking on institutions and strategies that help connect science and government should be a priority in the recovery phase. One condition is nurturing a political culture that embraces uncertainty and complexity, and that adheres to a more comprehensive and inclusive view of scientific knowledge. Furthermore, certain political conditions need to be met to achieve the project of a wise government and wise science. For example, political polarization may limit the ability of adopting a balanced and productive view on the value and use of scientific knowledge for political leadership in times of uncertainty. The recovery period could be a moment of reconciliation between the worlds of science and government. What is clear is that wise government should both rely on and protect science. How to best perform this balancing act is much less certain.

NOTES

1 A critical interpretation of the knowledge translation agenda is that governments have aligned publicly-funded research, with wider economic and societal imperatives, with the necessity for researchers to demonstrate "impact" or "return on investment"; but at the same time risking disciplines, such as the arts and humanities, that struggle to demonstrate such knowledge exchange.
2 For example, the Conseil Scientifique in France: https://solidarites-sante.gouv.fr/IMG/pdf/reglement_interieur_cs.pdf.
3 Our colleague Felix Rigoli addresses this issue in chapter 9 of this book: "The Politics of Populism in an Era of Pandemics."
4 Our colleague Nicolas B. King addresses this issue in chapter 12 of this book: "Science and Public Policy in a Post-Pandemic World."

REFERENCES

Balog-Way, Dominic H.P., and Katherine A. McComas. 2020. "COVID-19: Reflections on Trust, Tradeoffs, and Preparedness." *Journal of Risk Research* 23, no. 7-8: 838–48.

Beck, Ulrich. 1992. *Risk Society: Towards a New Modernity*. Translated by Mark Ritter. London: Sage Publications.

Béland, Daniel, Gregory P. Marchildon, Anahely Medrano, and Phillip Rocco. 2021. "COVID-19, Federalism, and Health Care Financing in Canada, the United States, and Mexico." *Journal of Comparative Policy Analysis: Research and Practice*: 1–14.

Béland, Daniel, and Patrik Marier, P. 2020. "COVID-19 and Long-Term Care Policy for Older People in Canada." *Journal of Aging & Social Policy* 32, no. 4-5: 358–64.

Boin, Arjen, Paul t'Hart, Eric Stern, and Bengt Sundelius. 2017. *The Politics of Crisis Management: Public Leadership Under Pressure*. Cambridge, UK: Cambridge University Press.

Bol, Damien, Marcos Giani, André Blais, and Peter John Loewen. 2020. "The Effect of COVID-19 Lockdowns on Political Support: Some Good News for Democracy?" *European Journal of Political Research* (19 May 2020).

Brousselle, Astrid, Emmanuel Brunet-Jailly, Christopher Kennedy, Susan D. Phillips, Kevin Quigley, and Alasdair Roberts. 2020. "Beyond COVID-19: Five Commentaries on Reimagining Governance for Future Crises and Resilience." *Canadian Public Administration* 63, no. 3: 369–408.

Brown, Lawrence D. 2012. "The Fox and the Grapes: Is Real Reform

Beyond Reach in the United States?" *Journal of Health Politics, Policy and Law* 37, no. 4: 587–609.

Campbell, Donald T. 1969. "Reforms as Experiments." *American Psychologist* 24, no. 4: 409–29.

Capano, Giliberto, Michael Howlett, Daryll S.L. Jarvis, M. Ramesh, and Nihil Goyal. 2020. "Mobilizing Policy (In)capacity to Fight COVID-19: Understanding Variations in State Responses." *Policy and Society* 39, no. 3: 285–308.

Davies, Phillip. 2004. "Is Evidence-Based Government Possible?" Jerry Lee Lecture 2004. *4th Annual Campbell Collaboration Colloquium*, Washington, DC, 19 February 2004.

Daviter, Falk. 2019. "Policy Analysis in the Face of Complexity: What Kind of Knowledge to Tackle Wicked Problems?" *Public Policy and Administration* 34, no. 1: 62–83.

Desson, Zachary, Emmi Weller, Peter McMeekin, and Mehdi Ammi. 2020. "An Analysis of the Policy Responses to the COVID-19 Pandemic in France, Belgium, and Canada." *Health Policy and Technology* 9, no. 4: 430–46.

Detsky, Allan S., and Isaac Bogoch. 2020. "COVID-19 in Canada: Experience and Response." *Jama*, 10 August 2020.

Dixon, Jennnifer, Nigel Edwards, and Richard Murray. 2020. "Dismantling PHE in the Midst of a Pandemic Carries Serious Risks." Joint letter to the *Sunday Telegraph* from the Health Foundation, Nuffield Trust, and The King's Fund. *The Health Foundation*. https://www.health.org.uk/news-and-comment/news/dismantling-phe-in-the-midst-of-a-pandemic-carries-serious-risks.

Estabrooks, Carole A., Linda Derksen, Connie Winther, John N. Lavis, Shannon D. Scott, Lars Wallin, and Joanne Profetto-McGrath. 2008. "The Intellectual Structure and Substance of the Knowledge Utilization Field: A Longitudinal Author Co-Citation Analysis, 1945 to 2004." *Implementation Science* 3, no. 1: 1–22.

Evans, Robert G., and Stoddart, Gregory L. 1990. "Producing Health, Consuming Health Care." *Social Science & Medicine* 31, no. 12: 1347–63. https://doi.org/10.1016/0277-9536(90)90074-3.

Exworthy, Mark and Russell Mannion. 2016. "Evaluating the Impact of NHS Reforms – Policy, Process and Power." In *Dismantling the NHS? Evaluating the Impact of Health Reforms*, edited by Mark Exworthy, Russell Mannion, and Martin Powell, 3–16. Policy Press.

– 2016. *Dismantling the NHS? Evaluating the Impact of Health Reforms*, edited by Mark Exworthy, Russell Mannion, and Martin Powell. Policy Press.

Foucault, Michel. 1984. "Qu'est-ce que les Lumières?" *Magazine Littéraire*, 207: 35–39.
– 2007. *Security, Territory, Population: Lectures at the Collège de France, 1977–78*. New York: Springer.
Gaille, Marie, Philippe Terral, Philippe Askenazy, Regis Aubry, Henri Bergeron, Sylvia Becerra, et al. 2020. *Les sciences humaines et sociales face à la première vague de la pandémie de Covid-19-Enjeux et formes de la recherche*. Doctoral dissertation, Centre National de la Recherche Scientifique: Université Toulouse III – Paul Sabatier.
Gibbons, Michael, Camille Limoges, Helga Nowotny, Simon Schwartzman, Peter Scott, and Martin Trow. 1994. *The New Production of Knowledge: The Dynamics of Science and Research in Contemporary Societies*. London: Sage.
Gieryn, Thomas F. 1983. "Boundary-Work and the Demarcation of Science from Non-Science: Strains and Interests in Professional Ideologies of Scientists." *American Sociological Review* 48, no. 6: 781–95.
Gleave, R. 2021. "Whose Science are the Government Following? The Organization of Scientific Advice to Government in the COVID-19 Response." In *Organizing Care in the Time of COVID-19*, edited by Justin Waring, Jean-Louis Denis, Anne Reff Petersen, and Tim Tenbensel. Forthcoming. New York: Palgrave.
Graham, Ian D., Jo Logan, Margaret B. Harrison, Sharon E. Straus, Jacqueline Tetroe, Wenda Caswell, and Nicole Robinson. 2006. "Lost in Knowledge Translation: Time for a Map?" *The Journal of Continuing Education in the Health Professions* 26: 13–24.
Greer, Scott L., Elizabeth J. King, Elize Massard da Fonseca, and Andre Peralta-Santos. 2020. "The Comparative Politics of COVID-19: The Need to Understand Government Responses." *Global Public Health* 15, no. 9: 1413–16.
Hällgren, Markus, Linda Rouleau, and Mark De Rond. 2018. "A Matter of Life or Death: How Extreme Context Research Matters for Management and Organization Studies." *Academy of Management Annals* 12, no. 1: 111–53.
Hassenteufel, Patrick. 2020. "Handling the COVID-19 Crisis in France: Paradoxes of a Centralized State-Led Health System." *European Policy Analysis* (10 December 2020).
Horton, Richard. 2020. *The COVID-19 Catastrophe: What's Gone Wrong and How to Stop It Happening Again*. Hoboken: John Wiley & Sons.

Iacobucci, Gareth. 2020. "Public Health England is Axed in Favour of New Health Protection Agency." *BMJ* 370 (18 August 2020). https://doi.org/10.1136/bmj.m3257.

Jamieson, Kathleen Hall. 2017. "The Need for a Science of Science Communication: Communicating Science's Values and Norms." In *The Oxford Handbook of the Science of Science Communication*, edited by Jamieson, K.H., Dan M. Kahan, and Dietram Scheufele, 15–25. Oxford: Oxford University Press.

Jamieson, Kathleen Hall, Marcia McNutt, Veronique Kiermer, and Richard Sever. 2019. Signaling the Trustworthiness of Science." *Proceedings of the National Academy of Sciences* 116, no. 39: 19231–6.

Jones, Lorelei, and Mark Exworthy. 2015. "Framing in Policy Processes: A Case Study from Hospital Planning in the National Health Service in England." *Social Science & Medicine* 124: 196–204.

Kreps, Sarah E., and Douglas L. Kriner. 2020. "Model Uncertainty, Political Contestation, and Public Trust in Science: Evidence from the COVID-19 Pandemic." *Science Advances* 6, no. 43 (21 October 2020).

Lancaster, Kari, Tim Rhodes, and Marsha Rosengarten. 2020. "Making Evidence and Policy in Public Health Emergencies: Lessons from COVID-19 for Adaptive Evidence-Making and Intervention." *Evidence & Policy* 16, no. 3: 477–90.

Maani, Nason, and Sandro Galea. 2021. "What Science Can and Cannot Do in a Time of Pandemic." *Scientific American*, 2 February 2021. https://www.scientificamerican.com/article/what-science-can-and-cannot-do-in-a-time-of-pandemic/

Makri, Anita. 2021. "What Do Journalists Say About Covering Science During the COVID-19 Pandemic?" *Nature Medicine* 27, no. 17-20 (13 January 2021).

Greenhalgh, Trisha, Manuel B. Schmid, Thomas Czypionka, Dirk Bassler, and Laurence Gruer. 2020. "Face Masks for the Public during the Covid-19 Crisis." *BMJ* 369 (9 April 2020). https://doi.org/10.1136/bmj.m1435.

Martin, Graham P., Esmée Hanna, Margaret McCartney, and Robert Dingwall. 2020. "Science, Society, and Policy in the Face of Uncertainty: Reflections on the Debate around Face Coverings for the Public During COVID-19." *Critical Public Health*, 30, no. 5: 501–8.

Merkley, Eric, Aengus Bridgman, Peter John Loewen, Taylor Owen, Derek Ruths, and Oleg Zhilin. 2020. "A Rare Moment of Cross-Partisan Consensus: Elite and Public Response to the COVID-19 Pandemic in Canada." *Canadian Journal of Political Science/Revue canadienne de science politique* 53, no. 2: 311–18.

Moatti, Jean-Paul. 2020. "The French Response to COVID-19: Intrinsic Difficulties at the Interface of Science, Public Health, and Policy." *Nature* 579 (7 April 2020): 319–20.

Mohammed, Anwar, Regan M. Johnston, Clifton van der Linden. 2020. "Public Responses to Policy Reversals: The Case of Mask Usage in Canada during COVID-19." *Canadian Public Policy* 46, no. S2: S119–26.

Olagnier, David, and Trine H. Mogensen. 2020. "The Covid-19 Pandemic in Denmark: Big Lessons from a Small Country." *Cytokine & Growth Factor Reviews* 53: 10–12.

Pollitt, Christopher, and Geert Bouckaert. 2017. *Public Management Reform: Comparative Analysis – Into the Age of Austerity*. Oxford: Oxford University Press.

Rajan, Dheepa, Kira Koch, Katja Rohrer, Csongor Bajnoczki, Anna Socha, Maike Voss, Marjolaine Nicod, Valery Ridde, and Justin Koonin. 2020. "Governance of the Covid-19 Response: A Call for More Inclusive and Transparent Decision-Making." *BMJ Global Health* 5, no. 5: e002655.

Ritchie, Stuart. 2020. *Science Fictions: Exposing Fraud, Bias, Negligence and Hype in Science*. New York: Metropolitan Books.

Ruano, Juan, Francisco Gómez-García, Dawid Pieper, and Livia Puljak. 2020. "What Evidence-Based Medicine Researchers Can Do to Help Clinicians Fighting COVID-19?" *Journal of Clinical Epidemiology* 124: 183–5.

Sagan, Carl. 1995. *The Demon-Haunted World*. New York: Penguin Random House.

Stevens, Alex. 2020. "Governments Cannot Just 'Follow the Science' on COVID-19."
Nature Human Behaviour 4: 560–1.

Tetroe, Jacqueline M., Ian D Graham, Robbie Foy, Nicole Robinson, Martin P. Eccles, Michel Wensing, Pierre Durieux, et al. 2008. "Health Research Funding Agencies' Support and Promotion of Knowledge Translation: an International Study." *The Milbank Quarterly* 86, no. 1: 125–55.

Thorp, H. Holden. 2020. "Underpromise, Overdeliver." *Science* 367, no. 6485: 1405.

Van Dooren, Wouter, and Mirko Noordegraaf. 2020. "Staging Science: Authoritativeness and Fragility of Models and Measurement in the COVID-19 Crisis." *Public Administration Review* 80, no. 4: 610–15.

Weiss, Carol H. 1979. "The Many Meanings of Research Utilization." *Public Administration Review* 39, no. 5: 426–31.

Wu, X., M. Ramesh, and M. Howlett. 2015. "Policy Capacity: A Conceptual Framework for Understanding Policy Competences and Capabilities." *Policy and Society* 34, no. 3-4: 165–71.

14

Rewriting the Story of How the World Developed COVID-19 Vaccines: A Work of Fiction on Responsible Health Innovation Path Creation

Pascale Lehoux, Renata Pozelli Sabio, Hassane Alami, Lysanne Rivard, Hudson Pacifico Silva

INTRODUCTION: REINVENTING THE HEALTH INNOVATION PATH FOR PANDEMIC SOCIETIES

Health innovation development is a multi-sectoral endeavour that is highly regulated, institutionalized, and globalized. The health innovation development pathway typically entails a careful, if not slow pace. Indeed, scientific and regulatory institutions aim to ensure the effectiveness and safety of new technologies before they can be implemented in health systems and this requires time, effort, and money.

At the time of writing this chapter, that is, barely ten months after the World Health Organization (WHO) declared SARS-COV-2 a pandemic, three COVID-19 vaccines had obtained market approval in the United States of America (USA), Canada, and the European Union (EU) and vaccination campaigns had begun. The pandemic thus seems to have accelerated innovation, representing an unparalleled large-scale institutional phenomenon. One may ask, however, were we not facing already known economic and political dynamics with largely predictable outcomes? While rich governments had purchased billions of doses before any vaccine had even come into existence, critics asked whether Low- and Middle-Income Countries (LMICs) were going to get their share and at what price.

Focusing on COVID-19 vaccines, the aim of this chapter is to reflect on how health innovation development processes may be realigned towards a more responsible innovation pathway, one generating equitable, affordable, and sustainable innovations (Silva et al. 2018). To do so, we took the liberty of producing a theoretically-informed work of fiction. Drawing from the literature on path dependence, anticipatory governance, and Responsible Innovation in Health (RIH), we tell a story in which the world succeeded in developing and distributing COVID-19 vaccines in a more responsible way. Though our story deliberately deviates from what actually happened, it sheds light on key twenty-first century challenges for public institutions: firstly, determining what innovation paths are best aligned with the public goods pandemic societies must protect; and secondly, governing the work of public, private and non-governmental actors along such new trajectories.

PROLOGUE

The Conceptual Underpinnings of Our Work of Fiction

At the onset of the pandemic, experts and journalists repeatedly stressed that the future is uncertain. Surveillance data and study results on SARS-COV-2 were shared day after day and the need for various health technologies such as personal protection equipment, diagnostic tests, mechanical ventilators, drugs, vaccines, telehealth, or contact tracing apps was emphasized. Such unprecedented media attention brought innovation development processes to the forefront and contributed to what foresight scholars would call "future-making" (Fuerth 2009). Yet, paths "in the making" (Boon et al. 2015) typically face inertia as well as lock-ins that characterize path dependence where "the suite of possible future evolutionary trajectories" is contingent on both the past and the current state of the innovation system and where the "present controls what possibility is to be explored" (Martin and Sunley 2006).

Despite what path dependence theory would predict, several scientific and regulatory changes took place during the pandemic to speed up health innovation development and use. These changes were made possible thanks to a series of more or less concerted efforts at the national and international levels. Some of them were prompted by lockdowns that "unlocked" financial resources and lifted regulatory barriers for physicians to provide telehealth services or by medical equipment shortages and other vulnerabilities in our globalized supply chains. Such changes may be understood as a slight deviation from the existing path or a point of departure in the creation of a novel path (Boon et al. 2015). Though path dependence scholars recognize that lock-ins do not necessarily happen on the most optimal path, they cannot identify ex post "what should have been different in the past to have a different future" and "whether human agency could have made that critical course of events different or not" (Vergne and Durand 2010). Path dependence theory suggests, however, that "exogenous shocks" can shake an innovation system free of its trajectory (Vergne and Durand 2010), deeply transform structural relationships among agents, and, eventually, keep them away from "places everyone would wish to have been able to avoid" (David 2001).

Our alternative story thus posits SARS-COV-2 as an external shock of sufficient magnitude to trigger the creation of a new path. It also recognizes the multiple roles public institutions play in health innovation such as financing research and development (RandD), regulating market approval, and purchasing healthcare products (Mazzucato 2018). They are thus "central figures" in path creation, bringing in their cognitive resources, policy instruments, institutional frames, and responsibilities in serving the public interest (Boon et al. 2015). Their agency in path creation is likely to be conditioned by "preconfigured selection environments" that may restrict possibilities (Boon et al. 2015). At the same time, public institutions have the capacity to identify, nurture, and shield certain niches (Lehoux et al. 2019) where particular innovative efforts, for instance those addressing climate change or food security, may "serve as laboratories" that are a prelude to more profound changes because they make visible the consequences of current lock-ins (Vanloqueren and Baret 2009).

We thus developed our story by considering plausible drivers and inhibitors (Wright et al. 2020), the central role multilateral organizations could play as well as the global public goods the COVID-19 crisis puts at stake (Torreele et al. 2021).

Global Public Goods in Pandemic Societies: Global Health, Climate Change, and Intellectual Property

While a public good refers to "a commodity that an individual can consume without reducing its availability to others (non-rival in consumption) and of which no one is deprived (non-excludable)"

(Abi Younes et al. 2020), global public goods "refer to programmes, policies, and services that have a truly global reach" even though their benefits may be unevenly distributed across countries (WHO 2002). Calling for a solution that goes beyond a biomedical commodity, COVID-19 requires articulating three global public goods: global health, climate change, and intellectual property (IP).

The zoonotic nature of SARS-COV-2 was recognized early, but the interactions between human health, animal health, and the environment were rapidly tossed aside as governments were too busy deciding on their respective courses of action. The pandemic highlighted inequalities within and across countries, but also how global health and climate change are deeply intertwined. While the carbon emissions of rich countries continue to rise, health problems associated to climate change disproportionality affect LMICs. According to the *Lancet* Countdown on health and climate change, "if the response to COVID-19 is not fully and directly aligned with national climate change strategies," the Paris Agreement commitments will not be met and this will damage "health systems today, and in the future" (Watts et al. 2020). Underscoring the socioeconomic inequalities in mortality due to COVID-19, Horton (2020a) called for a "syndemic" understanding of the disease and ways to address it: "Syndemics are characterised by biological and social interactions between conditions and states, interactions that increase a person's susceptibility to harm or worsen their health outcomes. ... The vulnerability of older citizens; Black, Asian, and minority ethnic communities; and key workers who are commonly poorly paid with fewer welfare protections points to a truth so far barely acknowledged – namely, that no matter how effective a treatment or protective a vaccine, the pursuit of a purely biomedical solution to COVID-19 will fail" (Horton 2020a).

Beyond the many lock-ins the World Trade Organization (WTO) agreements impose on the current innovation path, the power to determine who can own and exploit technoscientific knowledge is key. At the time of writing this chapter, the vaccines developed by Oxford-AstraZeneca, Pfizer/BioNTech, and Moderna had received accelerated market clearance. Though some of these pharmaceutical firms did not "want to be seen to be profiting from the global crisis" (Hooker and Palumbo 2020), Pfizer's stock value "soared more than 7 per cent" when it announced that its vaccine was 90 per cent effective and this coincided with Pfizer CEO Albert Bourla selling his

"$5.6 million worth of shares" (Agence Science Presse 2020). Such lucrative transactions are predictable because they are embedded in the value extraction strategies of today's highly financialized pharmaceutical firms that operate on a monopolistic basis thanks to IP protection (Torreele et al. 2021). For Baker et al. (2017), healthcare, food security, and climate change are sectors where the WTO IP system has been proven inadequate, inefficient, and a "hindrance to welfare."

Our story thus opens up an innovation path that mitigates the environmental impacts of COVID-19 vaccine development, production, and distribution and unleashes scientific knowledge and technical know-how to support a global distributed long-term capacity building strategy.

AN ALTERNATIVE STORY OF COVID-19 VACCINE DEVELOPMENT, PRODUCTION, AND DISTRIBUTION

Following the work of Boon et al. (2015) on path creation, we describe three "moments" that prompted global institutions to take specific actions, keeping at the core of their future-oriented vision the global public goods described above.

Readers should keep in mind that though the quotations we use below are real, our story is not and the chronology of the sources we quote is not respected.

April 2020 Emergency Special Session of the UN General Assembly: Opening Up a New Innovation Path

The story begins when the Security Council of the United Nations (UN) convened an emergency General Assembly in April 2020. This decision echoed the call of *The Lancet's* Editor-in-Chief for whom COVID-19 was the "greatest threat to peace and security" since World War II and a meeting under the auspices of the UN the "only means available to construct a global response" (Horton 2020b).

The General Assembly gathered experts from around the world whose first task was to summarize what was known and unknown about SARS-COV-2 (e.g., propagation, infectivity, immunity after infection, mutation, response to treatments). The discussion clarified that vaccines that could prevent severe manifestations of COVID-19 and reduce hospitalization would have a substantial public health impact and should be deployed in conjunction with other measures to reduce community transmission (Pollard and Bijker 2020). The second task for experts was to take stock of the failures and successes of previous vaccine development initiatives for infectious diseases, including those from zoonotic origins (e.g., MERS, Zika, Ebola). Here, the knowledge and know-how of representatives from LMICs proved particularly informative. They insisted on vaccine candidates that did not require a cold chain and could avoid the use of syringes and needles. Industrialized countries also recognized the need to anticipate the logistical challenges raised by the distribution of vaccines in smaller cities, rural, or hard-to-reach areas. These combined demands led to prioritize RandD efforts around single-dose vaccine candidates that could be administered orally or through microneedle patches (Sullivan et al. 2010) and others that may require two doses but could be manufactured more quickly such as those using RNA antigen encoding (Pollard and Bijker 2020). Aiming for a set of vaccines with complementary strengths and limitations was seen as a key element of an integrated strategy that took into consideration their global production and distribution.

During the General Assembly, the role of the WTO was discussed because of the importance of anticipating up front how the Trade-Related Aspects of Intellectual Property Rights (TRIPS) agreement could affect global vaccine development efforts and the ways infrastructures and knowledge-based capacities in multiple countries could help produce the vaccines in an efficient and environmentally sustainable manner (Bruni 2016). Tensions were of course palpable. Some countries asked the WTO for a waiver from specific provisions of TRIPS because they wondered whether the vaccines would be made available in "sufficient quantities and at an affordable price" (Communication to WTO 2020). From their perspective, the "rapid scaling up of manufacturing" around the world was "an obvious crucial solution to address the timely availability and affordability" of vaccines for all (Communication to WTO 2020). The WTO argued that TRIPS, "the most comprehensive multilateral agreement on IP," provides enough flexibilities to accommodate the needs of LMICs (WTO 2020b). This view was challenged by members for whom these flexibilities serve "corporate interests in developed countries disproportionately," underscoring that only Brazil, India, or China are sufficiently influential to use them (Baker et al. 2017). The WTO conceded that some developing countries faced "periodic shortages of specific products" (WTO 2020a), but opposed the idea that economic pressures, threats, or "diplomatic lobbying" took place among WTO member countries (Baker et al. 2017).

At that point in the discussion, the General Assembly members were invited to pause and reflect on two very different post-COVID-19 futures: "one grounded in a new-found commitment to collaboration to seek stability, safety, and security" and "one where nation states fall into nationalistic self-interest, protectionism, and remain blind to new and emerging threats" (Cairns and Wright 2020). Then, aligning with their commitment to the Sustainable Development Goals 2030 agenda, members supported a decisive motion – where no veto could be applied – according to which the WTO IP system impeded the production of the solutions needed to overcome COVID-19. The UN General Assembly closed the April 2020 Emergency Special Session by appointing a set of high-level committees who were tasked to adopt a mission-oriented innovation governance approach where the risks and rewards of the global COVID-19 vaccine development efforts would be shared by all member states and with the aim of reducing inequalities within and across countries (Mazzucato 2018; Torreele et al. 2021).

May–July 2020: Setting in Place Responsible Anticipatory Governance

In May 2020, the committees adopted a collaborative governance framework wherein "public and private actors work collectively in distinctive ways, using particular processes, to establish laws and rules for the provision of public goods" (Ansell and Gash 2008). To orchestrate COVID-19 vaccine development efforts around the world, the chairs of each committee set in place interdisciplinary and intersectoral deliberative processes that brought "anticipation" and "governance" together (Guston 2014). The goal was to develop collective anticipatory capacities by bringing together different views on how public institutions and the private sector can approach scientific uncertainties and jointly resolve practical issues, ranging from clinical studies to supply chains. To envision various possible trajectories, the committees deployed "anticipatory sense-making, creativity and learning capabilities" (Kimbell and Vesnić-Alujević 2020). This was meant to avoid the "parochial" assumptions and "failure of imagination" (David 2001) that may have prevented them from freely envisioning an unprecedented path to design and deliver safe, effective, affordable, and eco-friendly COVID-19 vaccines. This anticipatory governance approach was reinforced by adopting the four "Responsible Research and Innovation" (RRI) process requirements (Stilgoe et al. 2013):

1. To anticipate the risks and unintended consequences of different vaccine candidates, their modes of production, delivery, and distribution;
2. To reflect on the values, biases and social norms that underlie and shape each of these options;
3. To include a variety of stakeholders, including the publics, potential users, and other concerned parties when developing these options; and
4. To respond to the emerging issues associated to these options and their shifting contexts in a swift and efficient manner.

To support their collaborative governance framework, the committees were specifically empowered to counteract "self-interested actions" by more influential countries (Cairns and Wright 2020). The aim was to acknowledge, explicitly, the boundaries, legacies and financial incentives of the pre-pandemic ways of developing and commercializing vaccines that could have plagued their work (David 2001). The committees were expecting value conflicts to emerge, especially in view of the public goods they were tasked to nurture. To this end, all committee members were trained and equipped to handle "steep power gradients" (Genus and Stirling 2018), identify lock-ins that could hinder their path creation process, and access the "keys" to reopen any of these locks (Beyer 2010). This capacity building strategy was accompanied by a transparent information sharing mechanism that was crucial to avoid duplication of efforts or irreversible resource commitments, and establish efficient learning loops (David 2001).

In June 2020, the committees were briefed on "Responsible Innovation in Health" (RIH), which would help define the tangible responsibility features the COVID-19 vaccines should possess in view of the contexts where they would be researched, manufactured, and distributed (Silva et al. 2020). RIH emphasizes, among others, the need to reduce health inequalities, adopt responsible business models and mitigate environmental impacts as much as possible, a vision that all committee members endorsed at this point.

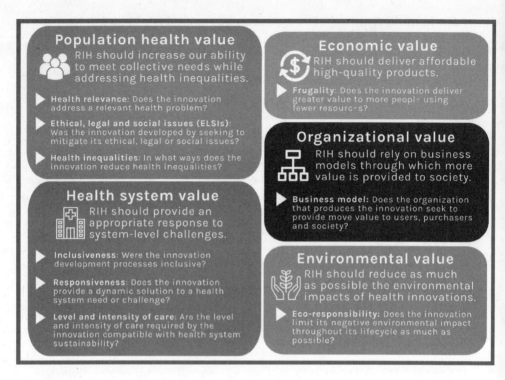

Figure 14.1 | The RIH value domains and attributes.

In July 2020, the committees launched a series of parallel decentralized workshops with experts and civil society representatives. The aim was to generate as many scenarios as possible grounded in the knowledge and know-how of multiple countries (Cairns and Wright 2020; Wright et al. 2020). The workshops were set to ponder whether and how the vaccines could meet the nine RIH attributes (see Figure 14.1). For participants to fully explore various scenarios, a "fair forecasting" logic prevailed (Vanloqueren and Baret 2009). Aiming for diversity in these workshops was key since participants had to consider the very different locations where the vaccines would be developed, manufactured, and delivered. Because designers' key strength is to envision new kinds of relationships between people and the material world that can "disrupt institutional logics and social norms" (Kimbell and Vesnić-Alujević 2020), it is under the guidance of design experts that close to a thousand participants brainstormed to create various vaccine scenarios and identified their respective merits and risks (Stemerding et al. 2018).

Though not all workshops generated actionable avenues, the key characteristics of the most promising and diverse scenarios were communicated at the end of July 2020 to the committees whose task was now shifting from path creation to path-making.

August 2020–January 2021: Affordable, Frugal, and Eco-Responsible Vaccine Production and Distribution

The six month-period that followed was intense and productive: in January 2021, three vaccines obtained market approval by a temporary central authority that continuously analyzed the scientific data generated throughout the pre-clinical and clinical research phases. This was made possible because hundreds of scientists and innovation management experts from the public and private sectors in all WTO member states were supported by thousands of volunteers with complementary skills together with undergraduate and graduate students who could complete their course requirements through dedicated "COVID-19 internships." These operational teams focused on the most promising scenarios that emerged from the workshops, which had in common three RIH features we describe below. Rather than narrowly focusing on the biomedical solution itself, the operational teams adopted a holistic view to consider how these RIH features could influence the RandD process, administration route, manufacturing, and delivery of each vaccine candidate. As Figure 2 illustrates, key scientific and regulatory steps had been optimized through a transparent quality assurance system that covered the whole process, from vaccine development to "last-mile" delivery, which had to fit with a range of locations where vulnerable groups could be reached in priority.

The first RIH feature – business model – draws attention to the tension between the redistribution of financial returns to shareholders and the provision of a high-quality solution that provides value not only to users and purchasers (governments in the case of COVID-19 vaccines), but also to society. Rather than relying on a "patent race" amongst the most powerful pharmaceutical firms, a prize-based approach was put in place because it is the "best system to influence the direction of RandD" (Abi Younes et al. 2020). In exchange of a prize and worldwide public notoriety, the operational teams

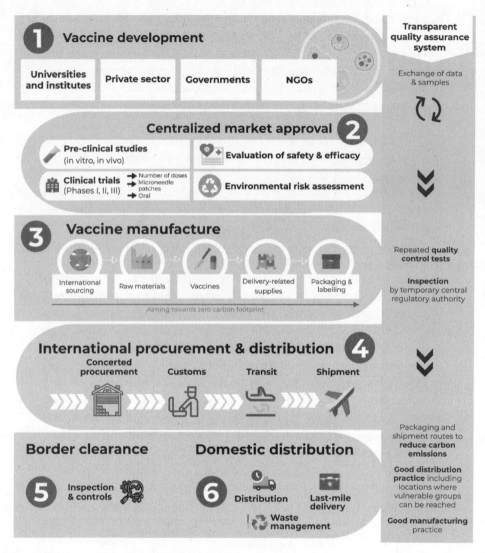

Figure 14.2 | Key steps in vaccine development, production and delivery.

that came up with an effective and safe vaccine with "verifiable" results had to put it into the public domain (Abi Younes et al. 2020). The RandD efforts were paid upfront, mostly by governments and NGOs through a centralized mechanism that pooled global resources equitably (Baker et al. 2017). This innovation strategy, where both cooperation and competition co-existed, substantially reduced the overall RandD costs and enabled the timely transfer of knowledge and know-how required to prepare and expedite manufacturing processes in a large number of countries.

The second RIH feature – frugality – refers to the ability to deliver greater value to more people by using fewer resources such as capital, materials, energy, and labour time. Frugality directed the teams' attention not only to the affordability of the vaccines, but more importantly to the resources required by their production, distribution, and delivery (Silva et al. 2020). The teams who successfully developed RNA-messenger vaccines recognized key logistical challenges: the very low temperature their stability requires and the limited timeframe within which they can be administered (Pollard and Bijker 2020). However, their production could be supported in emerging economies such as South Africa, Brazil, India, and China. The research platforms needed to scale up vaccine manufacturing in these countries were integrated within longer-term domestic policies where technoscientific capacity building is of "critical importance for welfare" (Baker et al. 2017). Knowing that the health and economic impacts of COVID-19 would be "felt for years to come," improved regulation and manufacturing capacities could contribute to rebuild national economies (Watts et al. 2020). The teams who successfully developed vaccines administered through microneedle patches relied on decades of research on live attenuated vaccines where lifelong protection with a single dose is more often observed (Pollard and Bijker 2020). These teams were particularly interested in reducing "last-mile" delivery hurdles and the material, cultural, and linguistic barriers that affect large-scale vaccination campaigns where a mix of rural, isolated, or less populated areas have to be reached.

They developed and pre-tested creative science-based communication tools in multiple languages that were meant not only to combat misinformation (Cairns and Wright 2020), but also to empower local communities in overcoming health literacy barriers and making sure the vaccine patches would be administered safely.

The third RIH feature – eco-responsibility – refers to the reduction of the negative environmental impacts of an innovation (Silva et al. 2020). The operational teams' eco-friendly decisions were motivated by the fact that the health sector contributed in 2017 "to approximately 4·6% of global greenhouse gas emissions, a rise of 6·1% from 2016" and less than a quarter of healthcare companies had "signed up to sustainable business practices" (Watts et al. 2020). Working under the auspices of the UN General Assembly gave them the legitimacy to impose eco-responsible principles. Though countries with high per-capita carbon emissions, such as EU countries and the USA, rarely if ever connected health and climate change "in their speeches at the UN's major global forum," the public interest and the science connecting health and climate change substantially increased in the last decade (Watts et al. 2020). The use of microneedle patches was seen as a sensible strategy to mitigate environmental impacts. ARN-messenger vaccines required syringes and vials, which are considered biomedical waste in many countries and must be handled by specific facilities to be properly incinerated. The sheer number of vials needed to provide two-dose vaccines created an unprecedented demand for sand, the second most consumed natural resource after water (Blais 2020). The teams thus optimized the size of the vials and the number of doses they could contain. A careful attention was devoted to packaging and shipment routes to reduce carbon emissions. Lastly, the new facilities where all vaccines were manufactured aimed to fulfil "Net Zero" principles, for example, high energy efficiency, renewable sources (Pencheon and Wight 2020).

Overall, the operational teams discovered that "significant increasing returns" could be realized along the novel path they had created (Vanloqueren and Baret 2009). Their local yet globally coordinated small-scale experiments contributed to materialize a flexible trajectory that brought them closer to where they wish they had been before the SARS-COV-2 pandemic.

EPILOGUE: FROM PATH DEPENDENCE TO PATH CREATION

Written within "a world that is changing almost by the minute" (Cairns and Wright 2020), the above work of fiction is not devoid of conflicts, but does end on a happy note. Our story deliberately circumvented key health innovation constituencies such as pharmaceutical firms and capital investors who typically define the path that all others follow. This is especially true in innovation systems where entrepreneurial drivers and what firms and shareholders can do to increase profits are deep-rooted (Martinuzzi et al. 2018) and where "granting civil society much more influence in future making efforts" is warranted (Stemerding et al. 2018). Setting a new innovation path – defining both its direction and socio-material characteristics – thus entails major power shifts: who gets to decide what political and economic interests shall be protected or not?

One of our story's assumptions is that a global anticipatory governance approach that pulls in the knowledge and skills of diversified groups can open up such a path. Beyond valuable achievements (e.g., sophisticated forms of collective problem solving), collaborative governance can generate problematic results as well (e.g., manipulation, distrust; Ansell and Gash 2008). Hence, a better understanding of how such governance can shift the distributed responsibilities and powers of the various actors involved would be very valuable (Ribeiro and Shapira 2018). While "basically anything can be argued to be path-dependent" (Vergne 2013), the path creation literature provided us with useful complementary concepts to structure our story. To path dependence key elements – initial conditions, contingencies, exogenous shocks, self-reinforcing loops, and lock-ins – Garud et al. (2010) add the much needed concept of agency. Path dependence posits actors as "creatures buffeted" by events and "resigned" to remain locked-in through self-reinforcing mechanisms over which they have no control (Garud et al. 2010). For Garud et al. (2010), "initial conditions are not given, but rather constructed" by agents, contingencies offer them "the possibilities to pursue certain courses of action while making others more difficult," what is considered exogenous or endogenous depends on how they (re)draw boundaries and self-reinforcing mechanisms do not simply exist, but are "cultivated." Path creation is thus likely to occur when actors fully recognize their own agency and responsibilities and can no longer exclude those who are deliberately left out of the established pathway.

A second assumption in our story lies with the idea that financial resources can be pooled and redistributed equitably when the urgent need is to orchestrate concerted RandD efforts and direct their outcomes towards a single global mission: making vaccines affordable for all, while building sustainable knowledge-based infrastructures around the world (Torreele et al. 2021). Though it may seem ingenuous, it would be equally naïve not to recognize that we currently "tolerate and sanction" the known economic inefficiencies of an IP regime that supports monopolies in rich countries and produces environmental externalities that are never factored in the price of products (Baker et al. 2017; Bruni 2016). According to Abi Younes et al. (2020), a vaccine cannot "strictly speaking" be understood as a public good because its consumption reduces its availability to others. However, the knowledge that underlies COVID-19 vaccine development and production as well the herd immunity they provide are public goods (Abi Younes et al. 2020). Our story thus aligns with Baker et al. (2017) for whom a "substantial recalibration" of the WTO approach to IP is required to improve standards of living in LMICs and to support innovations that "have the highest value in terms of their contribution to addressing the challenges facing our global society."

A final assumption is that a biomedical solution to COVID-19 can only fail (Horton 2020a). Treating COVID-19 as a syndemic would have forced leaders and policymakers to broaden their repertoire of policy tools and address animal health, human health, and the environment as one single twenty-first century challenge. Though we concur with Pollard and Bijker (2020) who stress that the "biggest challenges" to immunization programs have to do with the "strong headwinds" against their deployment, such as poor infrastructure, lack of funding, or vaccine hesitancy, we disagree with their assertion that "these are not classical scientific challenges." They are clearly beyond the epistemic grasp of basic scientists, but rather well known to social scientists who conduct applied health research. Because it typically takes more than ten years to develop a vaccine, it is true that the COVID-19 pandemic demonstrated the value of vaccine technologies that "facilitate rapid development, production and upscaling" (Pollard and Bijker 2020). Yet, the pandemic concurrently showed the urgency of transforming an innovation path that materializes these vaccines only when governments are ready to pay twice: for private firms to develop them and for these same firms to supply them. Overall, choosing one's preferred innovation path amounts to choosing one's political economy (Vanloqueren and Baret 2009). Before making such decisions, the "generic wisdom that history has to offer to public policy makers" is to keep open options "for a longer period than impatient market agents would wish" (David 2001).

CONCLUSION

When the goal is to steer innovation in a more desirable direction, Fuerth (2009) argues that the past can be seen as a prologue, but not a destiny. Likewise, this chapter suggested that visions of the future have to be provoked to raise awareness and instill willingness to change.

Yet, much remains to be achieved if the goal is to provoke a societal transformation. Are there "normal" pre-pandemic societies to which we can get back? And, if yes, normal for whom? (Cairns and Wright 2020). Alternatively, are pandemic societies here to stay? In any case, academics should debunk current understandings of how "things are" that support the status quo (Boon et al. 2015). This seems warranted when established paths and their lock-ins reinforce historical power imbalances and persistent inequalities within and across countries. We are facing too many challenges that require a global concerted response. Responsible innovation is one tangible means to help us tackle such challenges by asking: "for whom shall pandemic societies innovate?" We are at "an inflection point" where global recovery efforts must be "synergistic with the long-term public health imperative of responding to climate change" (Watts et al. 2020). Strong political will and mission-oriented investments that empower public institutions in serving the public interest are needed now.

We would like to thank Robson Rocha de Oliveira who provided us with helpful comments on a previous version of the chapter and Catherine Hébert for her comments and for having created the visuals that accompany this chapter.

REFERENCES

Abi Younes, George, Charles Ayoubi, Omar Ballester, Gabrielle Cristelli, Gaétan de Rassenfosse, Dominique Foray, Patrick Gaulé, et al. 2020. "COVID-19: Insights from Innovation Economists." *Science and Public Policy* (1 July 2020).

Agence Science Presse. 2020. "Le PDG de Pfizer a vendu des actions le jour de l'annonce." *La Presse*, 11 November 2020.

Ansell, Chris, and Alison Gash. 2008. "Collaborative Governance in Theory and Practice." *Journal of Public Administration Research and Theory* 18: 543–71.

Baker, Dean, Arjun Jayadev, and Joseph E. Stiglitz, J. 2017. "Innovation, Intellectual Property, and Development: A Better Set of Approaches for the 21st Century." *AccessIBSA*: Innovation and Access to Medicines in India, Brazil, and South Africa.

Beyer, Jürgen. 2010. "The Same or Not the Same – On the Variety of Mechanisms of Path Dependence." *International Journal of Social Sciences* 5: 1–11.

Blais, Stéphan. 2020. "Le risque de pénurie de fioles à vaccin est réel." *La Presse Canadienne,* 13 December 2020.

Boon, Wouter P., Eric Aarden, and Jacqueline E. Broerse. 2015. "Path Creation by Public Agencies – the Case of Desirable Futures of Genomics." *Technological Forecasting and Social Change* 99: 67–76.

Bruni, Pietro. 2016. "Impacts of Pharmaceutical Pollution on Communities and Environment in India." Researched and prepared for Nordea Asset Management by Changing Markets and Ecostorm.

Cairns, George, and George Wright. 2020. "A Reflection on the Mass Production of Scenarios in Response to COVID-9." *Futures and Foresight Science* 2, no. 3-4 (7 June 2020).

Communication to WTO Council for Trade-Related Aspects of Intellectual Property Rights. 2020. "Waiver from Certain Provisions of the TRIPS Agreement for the Prevention, Containment and Treatment of COVID-19." *Communication from India and South Africa* (2 October 2020).

David, Paul A. 2001. "Path Dependence, its Critics and the Quest for 'Historical Economics.'" In *Evolution and Path Dependence in Economic Ideas: Past and Present*, edited by Pierre Garrouste and Stavros Ioannides, 40. Cheltenham: Edward Elgar Publishing.

Fuerth, Leon S. 2009. "Foresight and Anticipatory Governance." *Foresight* 11, no. 4: 14–32.

Garud, Raghu, Arun Kumaraswamy, and Peter Karnøe. 2010. "Path Dependence or Path Creation?" *Journal of Management Studies* 47, no. 4: 760–74.

Genus, Audley, and Andy Stirling. 2018. "Collingridge and the Dilemma of Control: Towards Responsible and Accountable Innovation." *Research Policy* 47, no. 1: 61–9.

Guston, David H. 2014. "Understanding 'Anticipatory Governance.'" *Social Studies of Science* 44, no. 2: 218–42.

Hooker, Lucy, and Danielle Palumbo. 2020. "Covid Vaccines: Will Drug Companies Make Bumper Profits?" *BBC News*, 18 December 2020.

Horton, Richard. 2020a. "Offline: COVID-19 is Not a Pandemic." *The Lancet* 396, no. 10255 (26 September 2020): 874.

– 2020b. "Offline: It's Time to Convene Nations to End this Pandemic." *The Lancet,* 396, no. 10243 (4 July 2020): 14.

Kimbell, Lucy, and Lucia Vesnić-Alujević. 2020. "After the Toolkit: Anticipatory Logics and the Future of Government." *Policy Design and Practice* 3, no.2: 1–14.

Lehoux, Pascale, Geneviève Daudelin, G., Jean-Louis Denis, Phillipe Gauthier, and Nicola Hagemeister. 2019. "Pourquoi et comment sont conçues les innovations responsables? Résultats d'une méta-ethnographie." *Innovations* 2, no. 59: 15–42.

Martin, Ron, and Peter Sunley. 2006. "Path Dependence and Regional Economic Evolution." *Journal of Economic Geography* 6, no. 4: 395–437.

Martinuzzi, André, Vincent Blok, Alexander Brem, Bernd C. Stahl, and Norma Schönherr. 2018. "Responsible Research and Innovation in Industry – Challenges, Insights and Perspectives." *Sustainability* 10, no. 3: 702.

Mazzucato, Mariana. 2018. "Mission-Oriented Innovation Policies: Challenges and Opportunities." *Industrial and Corporate Change* 27, no. 5: 803–15.

Pencheon, David, and Jeremy Wight. 2020. "Making Healthcare and Health Systems Net Zero." *BMJ* (30 March 2020): 368.

Pollard, Andrew J., and Else M. Bijker. 2020. "A Guide to Vaccinology: From Basic Principles to New Developments." *Nature Reviews Immunology* 21: 83–100.

Ribeiro, Barbara, and Phillip Shapira. 2018. "Anticipating Governance Challenges in Synthetic Biology: Insights from Biosynthetic Menthol." *Technological Forecasting and Social Change* 139: 311–20.

Silva, Hudson P., Andrée-Anne Lefebvre, Robson R. de Oliveira, and Pascale Lehoux. 2021. "Fostering Responsible Innovation in Health: An Evidence-Informed Assessment Tool for Decision-Makers." *International Journal of Health Policy and Management* 10, no. 4: 181.

Silva, Hudson P., Pascale Lehoux, Fiona Alice Miller, and Jean-Louis Denis. 2018. "Introducing Responsible Innovation in Health: A Policy-Oriented Framework." *Health Research Policy and Systems* 16, no. 90.

Stemerding, Dirk, Wieke Betten, Virgil Rerimassie, Zoë Robaey, and Frank Kupper. 2018. "Future Making and Responsible Governance of Innovation in Synthetic Biology." *Futures* 109: 213–26.

Stilgoe, Jack, Richard Owen, and Phil Macnaghten. 2013. "Developing a Framework for Responsible Innovation. *Research Policy* 42, no. 9: 1568–80.

Sullivan, Sean P., Dimitrios G. Koutsonanos, Maria del Pilar Martin, Jeong

Woo Lee, Vladimir Zarnitsyn, Seong-O Choi, Niren Murthy, Richard W. Compans, Ioanna Skountzou, and Mark R. Prausnitz. 2010. "Dissolving Polymer Microneedle Patches for Influenza Vaccination." *Nature Medicine* 16: 915–20.

Torreele, Els, Mariana Mazzucato, and Henry Lishi Li. 2021. "Delivering the People's Vaccine: Challenges and Proposals for the Biopharmaceutical Innovation System." UCL *Institute for Innovation and Public Purpose*. Policy Brief series (IIPP PB 12).

Vanloqueren, Gaëtan, and Phillippe V. Baret 2009. "How Agricultural Research Systems Shape a Technological Regime that Develops Genetic Engineering but Locks Out Agroecological Innovations." *Research Policy* 38, no. 6: 971–83.

Vergne, Jean-Phillippe. 2013. "QWERTY is Dead, Long Live Path Dependence." *Research Policy* 42: 1191–4.

Vergne, Jean-Phillippe, and Rodolphe Durand. 2010. "The Missing Link between the Theory and Empirics of Path Dependence: Conceptual Clarification, Testability Issue, and Methodological Implications." *Journal of Management Studies* 47, no. 4: 736–59.

Watts, Nick, Markus Amann, Nigel Arnell, Sonja Ayeb-Karlsson, Jessica Beagley, Kristine Belesova, et al. 2020. "The 2020 Report of The Lancet Countdown on Health and Climate Change: Responding to Converging Crises." *The Lancet* 397, no. 10269: 129–70.

World Health Organization (WHO) Commission on Macroeconomics and Health. 2002. Working Group 2. *Global Public Goods for Health: The Report of Working Group 2 of the Commission on Macroeconomics and Health*. Geneva, Switzerland: World Health Organization.

World Trade Organization (WTO). 2020a. "How WTO Members Have Used Trade Measures to Expedite Access to Covid-19 Critical Medical Goods and Services." *Information Note*. World Trade Organization (WTO). 16 September 2020.

– 2020b. "The TRIPS Agreement and COVID-19." *Information Note*. World Trade Organization.

Wright, David, Bernd Stahl, and Tally Hatzakis. 2020. Policy Scenarios as an Instrument for Policymakers. *Technological Forecasting and Social Change* 154 (May): 11997.

5

Global Health and International Relations in a Pandemic Context

15

The Future of Health and Human Rights in Pandemic Societies

Lisa Forman

INTRODUCTION

Health and human rights scholars have long argued the theoretical proposition first advanced by Jonathan Mann and others that health and human rights are inextricably interrelated and mutually constitutive (Mann et al. 1999). The COVID-19 pandemic has reinforced the validity of this idea at almost every turn: pandemic control measures around the world have frequently veered into human rights violation; ostensibly universal health systems in high-income countries have struggled to provide adequate COVID-19 testing, tracing, and treatment; lockdowns have frequently been unmatched by the socio-economic supports to enable all to shelter in place; and Black and Indigenous people of colour (BIPOC) in many places have shown greater susceptibility to COVID-19 exposure infections and death given the health impacts of long-standing systemic racism and discrimination (Sekalala, Forman, Habibi, and Meier 2020; Forman and Kohler 2020). In doing so, the pandemic has underscored the imperative for strong, integrated protections of all human rights related to health to enable people to fully comply with COVID control measures. At the same time the pandemic has illuminated the limitations of international human rights law when it comes to key aspects of COVID responses, including the nature of the criteria governing the legitimate restriction of human rights related to health and the duties governing interstate cooperation. The disparity in COVID-19 vaccine access in low and middle-income countries is a testament to the jarring lack of solidarity and cooperation in this key domain. So too is the relatively limited adherence of states to the larger international law framework governing pandemic response contained in the World Health Organization's (WHO) *International Health Regulations* (IHR).[1]

Yet inasmuch as COVID-19 is illustrating the weaknesses of international law related to health, it may conversely animate another proposition about this body of law. This is the idea that major shifts in international law and human rights practice have often occurred because of "[m]ajor shocks to the system [which] provide limited windows of opportunity for effecting large changes in the system" (Hathaway 2002, 2002–3). This is a dynamic deeply rooted within the genesis of the United Nations and international human rights law following the atrocities of World War II (Forman 2020). To the extent that the COVID-19 pandemic places tremendous stress on the international law framework for health, it may also reinforce a longer standing challenge for this body of law and the right to health in particular, to more effectively and expeditiously evolve to meet the health challenges of our time (Forman 2020).

In this chapter, I will consider both these theories in the context of the COVID-19 pandemic in the following way: I will first flesh out the human rights dimensions of the pandemic, and the ways that global responses are bringing to light the strengths and weaknesses of the international law framework related to health and human rights. I will turn to consider the IHR from a human rights perspective, and ways in which it could be reformed to better reflect this body of law. I will conclude with thoughts about the way that the "shock" of COVID-19 could impact on both international human rights law and the IHR, and what the shock-response nature of international law suggests about the inattention of this legal regime to the quotidian structural inequities that sustain and deepen human rights violations in the health domain.

HUMAN RIGHTS AND COVID-19 GLOBALLY

A recent historical account of COVID-19 suggests that "[p]andemics are central to global history. They have global impact and create anchor points in time. They also interrogate the foundations of society, the sustainability of its material basis, the role of expertise, our social codes, and behavioural norms" (Frankema and Tworek

2020, 333). This interplay between pandemics and social norms and responses is evident through the multiple endemic and epidemic disease outbreaks of the past century, from the 1918 Spanish Flu, the 1968 Hong Kong influenza, the 2003 SARS, and 2014 Ebola outbreaks, to the ongoing HIV and AIDS pandemic. Indeed, many of these outbreaks have provoked the development of international law related to human rights and health. For example, HIV and AIDS strongly motivated the evolution of the right to health in international law to more explicitly protect access to essential medicines and to regulate state conduct in political economic and trade domains that impact on health and drug pricing (Forman 2008). Similarly, the early 2000s SARS outbreak provoked the 2005 revisions of the WHO's IHR.[2]

The COVID-19 pandemic is likely to act as a similar "anchor point" that tests our laws, policies, and social codes when it comes to the fairness and equity of domestic and global responses to COVID-19, from the treatment of people made marginal and vulnerable by long-standing systemic discrimination and inequity, to the ability of low and middle-income countries to access COVID-19 vaccines. Historians remind us that these tensions are ever-present in plagues, which are marked both by blame, stereotyping and othering, and by "coercive, racialized and hierarchical governance," both domestic and imperial (Birn 2020, 342). These dimensions are all too apparent in COVID-19 where race, income, age, and disability are proving in many places to be key determinants of both COVID morbidity and mortality and of human rights violations associated with COVID-19 policies and enforcement.[3]

Since March 2020, almost every country in the world has implemented comprehensive and stringent COVID responses from containment and closure measures, such as states of emergency, lock-downs, quarantines and travel restrictions, closing of workplaces, schools, and public transport; to public health measures, such as public information campaigns, testing, contact tracing, face-covering policy; to economic responses, such as income support and debt relief (Hale, Boby, Angrist, et al. 2020, 4). Many such measures have justifiably restricted individual rights to free movement, assembly, privacy and economic activity, to the extent that they have been time-limited, necessary to achieve public health goals, proportionate, and non-discriminatory. These are the criteria established in "The Siracusa Principles" to guide policy-makers in what constitutes legitimate restrictions of human rights (UN Commission on Human Rights 1984). Yet a significant number of countries have misused the pandemic to justify police violence, authoritarian power grabs, and corruption, and many other countries have implemented COVID responses that fail to meet the human rights criteria set out in "The Siracusa Principles" (Forman and Kohler 2020). A global monitor of COVID measures found that by November 2020, more than 61 per cent of all the countries in the world had implemented COVID-19 measures that were concerning from a democracy and human rights perspective because they were "either disproportionate, illegal, indefinite or unnecessary in relation to the health threat" (International Institute for Democracy and Electoral Assistance [IDEA] 2020, 1). In Hungary, the prime minister enacted a state of emergency without a clear time limit, allowing him to essentially rule by decree (Sekalala, Forman, Habibi, and Meier 2020, citing Quinn 2020). In the Philippines, lockdown enforcements have resulted in the citation of over one hundred thousand people with fifty thousand arrested (Alindogen 2020). In Uganda, the president who has been in power for thirty-five years used COVID-19 as a pretext during the 2020 election to break up political gatherings and clamp down on the opposition and the media (Human Rights Watch Uganda 2020).

As these examples suggest, COVID-related human rights abuses are often opportunistic attempts to tighten already autocratic control, with the majority of such abuses in countries that were already non-democratic prior to the pandemic (IDEA 2020, 1). Yet COVID has also fuelled a pre-existing global trend away from democracy (Freedom House 2019), and human rights abuses have been widespread in democracies too (IDEA 2020, 1), with evidence in multiple countries of disproportionate and coercive enforcement of COVID-19 measures against racialized and marginalized communities (Morales and Joseph 2020; Human Rights Watch India 2020; Human Rights Watch Uganda 2020).

Yet there has been less focus in these accounts of the extent to which the pandemic is placing pressure on the right to health, which is centrally implicated in both state duties to appropriately respond to a public health emergency and in individual entitlements to receive appropriate COVID-19 related health care as well as the social determinants of health. Health systems in high-income countries have struggled to provide adequate COVID-19 testing, tracing, and treatment (Cousins 2020; Alonso-Zaldivar 2020), with non-COVID-19 health-care restricted (RTL News 2020), vulnerable populations at high risk of infection and negative health and social impacts, and lockdowns exacerbating poverty, domestic violence, and mental health problems (Human Rights Watch 2020; WHO Europe 2020; Forani 2020; Forman and Kohler 2020). These impacts are expected to get worse with estimates that COVID will push almost 150 million people, 1.4 per cent of the global population, into extreme poverty by the end of 2021 (World Bank 2020). Moreover, the socioeconomic pressures are expanding with COVID-19 variants of concern on the rise and successive waves of infections sending countries globally back into lockdowns and states of emergencies.

The pandemic thus creates or at least highlights major weaknesses within international law related to health. First, is the need to clarify and strengthen the criteria that govern restrictions of rights during a pandemic. "The Siracusa Principles" were drafted to address the civil and political rights contained in the International Covenant on Civil and Political Rights (ICCPR) rather than those in the International Covenant on Economic, Social, and Cultural Rights (ICESCR; UN Commission on Human Rights 1966), and these treaties have considerably different limitations provisions. These rules were thus not drafted in order to address a health crisis, albeit that public health is a recognized ground on which to limit certain ICCPR rights. Yet "The Siracusa Principles" say little about public health other than indicating that its invocation must be restricted to serious threats to individual or population health, be specifically aimed at preventing disease or injury or providing care for the sick and injured, and give due regard to the WHO's IHR which prescribe state duties with regard to disease outbreaks.[4] The general criteria regarding restrictions are repeated in the United Nations Committee on Economic, Social, and Cultural Rights (UNCESCR's) General Comment 14 which interprets the Covenant's right to health (UNCESR 2000). General Comment 14 specifies that restrictions must be in accordance with international human rights law (not simply domestic law), and that there must be strict necessity for such restrictions (UNCESR 2000, paras. 28 and 29). Yet there is not sufficient guidance in General Comment 14 or elsewhere as to how public health restrictions should apply to the right to health and to health needs falling within core obligations under this right, nor does it outline the appropriate and varying standards of scrutiny that should attach to such restrictions. The need for such clarity is evident in how COVID lockdowns are placing far-reaching restrictions on the right to health and on core obligations such as non-discrimination. These impacts are likely to amplify if the pandemic generates austerity cutbacks like those adopted after the 2008 financial crisis which saw significant health budget cuts in high and low-income countries (Nolan 2014, 2–3; Ortiz and Cummins 2013, i; Kyrili and Martin 2010, 38). COVID underscores the importance of assuring far more clarification of the criteria for restricting human rights in the context of public health threats like pandemic.

Second, is the need to bolster the duties of cooperation and assistance within international human rights law. The pressures on realization of the right to health are reinforced by the limited and highly inequitable access to COVID-19 vaccines in low and middle-income countries, with many national responses characterized by "vaccine nationalism" or "my nation first" approaches (Forman and Kohler 2020). For example, the Serum Institute India, the world's largest producer of vaccine doses, issued a statement that the majority of its products "would have to go to our countrymen before it goes abroad" (Forman and Kohler 2020). Under former US President Trump, Operation Warp Speed adopted an America-first vaccine policy that explicitly rejected international cooperation (Cohen 2020). The European Union has threatened to slow vaccine exports after production delays in the Pfizer vaccine (Rabson 2021). Such approaches undercut social norms of solidarity as well as state duties under economic, social, and cultural rights like health to engage in international cooperation and assistance.[5] More pressingly, the threat is that low and middle-income countries will be excluded from the public health benefits of COVID-19 vaccines for years to come, amplifying for such countries, the public health threat faced by COVID infections and the socio-economic impacts of continued travel and trade restrictions as access to vaccines grows in high income countries. COVID, like HIV and AIDS before it, is underscoring that wealthy countries are fairly comfortable with allowing and exacerbating deep health inequities in low and middle-income countries including during a major global health crisis. Social movement campaigns for affordable antiretroviral treatment transformed the weakness of international human rights law on whether and how the right to health responded to this key health and human rights imperative. The current looming vaccine apartheid between high and low and middle-income countries suggests that the rhetoric of affordable medicines in international law and global health policies like the "Sustainable Development Goals" is little more than rhetoric. This is a weakness that unaddressed will deeply delegitimize the decade of legal and policy evolution on access to affordable medicines and global health equity that HIV and AIDS helped provoke.

HUMAN RIGHTS AND THE INTERNATIONAL HEALTH REGULATIONS

Outside of international human rights law, state duties to respond to pandemics are contained in the WHO's IHR adopted in 2005. The IHR were revised in 2005 to better protect against the global spread of disease and to preserve international travel and trade during outbreaks (Wilson 2020).[6] The IHR became binding on all WHO member states in 2007, creating a range of state duties, including developing minimum core public health capacities to respond to pandemics, requiring states to notify WHO of events that may constitute a public health emergency of international concern (PHEIC) and authorizing WHO to issue temporary recommendations during a PHEIC. These revisions sought to incorporate lessons from epidemics like Ebola, Zika and swine-flu to more effectively address the international spread of disease (Fidler and Gostin 2006, 85; Tonti 2020). Yet before COVID-19, no WHO member state had completely developed these core capacities (Tonti 2020), and during COVID-19, states have ignored IHR duties to report public health threats (*Financial Times* 2020) and requiring protective measures like travel bans to be based on scientific evidence and WHO guidance (Habibi, Burci, de Campos, et al. 2020).[7]

That compliance with the IHR during a global health crisis has been so weak is extremely damaging to the legitimacy of this body of law. Yet reform of the IHR is not currently planned: Neither a WHO committee which reviewed the function of the IHR during COVID-19 (WHO Executive Board 2021) nor the Independent Panel for Pandemic Preparedness and Response (IPPPR) appointed by the UN Secretary General reviewing the WHO's response to COVID-19 including through the IHR have suggested reforming the IHR (Independent Panel for Pandemic Preparedness and Response 2021). Instead, the WHO committee suggested improved implementation of the current IHR (WHO Executive Board 2021), and the IPPPR recommended instead moving towards a Pandemic Treaty that would complement the IHR and fill its gaps (IPPPR 2021).

Future implementation of the IHR will have to contend with the relative dearth of explicit guidance on human rights within the regulations. It will also need to more effectively link with existing human rights norms and procedures (Toebes, Forman, and Bartolini 2020; Taylor, Habibi, Burci, et al. 2020; Habibi, Burci, de Campos, et al. 2020). The IHR say little about human rights, save for scant and general requirements (Zidar 2015, 506) that health measures be implemented with respect for "the dignity, human rights and fundamental freedoms" of all people, including travellers, and be guided by the *Charter of the United Nations* and the *Constitution of the WHO* (WHO 2005, Articles 3.1 and 3.2). Moreover, the IHR's limited human rights provisions focus less on the right to health than on how public health interventions impact civil and political rights like freedom of movement (Zidar 2015, 511). Nor has international law scholarship extensively explored this relationship beyond acknowledging that state duties under the IHR are closely connected to the right to health (Zidar 2015, 511; Bogdandy and Villarreal 2020, 20).

Research is required to clarify two key aspects of this fragmented relationship: First, the extent to which the right to health can be restricted under the IHR, since this right (like certain other rights) can be limited for public health reasons.[8] The paradox in this regard is that during a public health crisis like COVID-19, state duties to provide health care become more important, not less. Evidence from the Ebola epidemic in West Africa underscores that measures like quarantine can weaken health systems and restrict rights to essential health care such as basic maternal services (Shannon, Horace-Kwemi, Najjemba, et al. 2017, S88), shelter, food, and water (Meier, Evans, and Phelan 2020). Similar impacts are playing out during COVID-19 in Uganda (Center for Health, Human Rights, and Development [CEHURD] 2020), Kenya (Odhiambo 2020), and Nigeria (Adepoju 2020). Second, research is required to elaborate how IHR duties can complement the realization of the right to health. UHC research underscores that right to health principles have an important role in reinforcing equitable strengthening of health systems (Forman, Beiersmann, Brolan, et al. 2016; Ooms et al. 2014; Sridhar et al. 2015). COVID is starting to prompt scholarship to explore the relationship between these two areas of international law (Toebes,

Forman, and Bartolini 2020). These are domains of considerable importance for more equitable interpretation, implementation and reform of international law related to health.

There are also questions about ways to achieve coherent interpretation between two relatively fragmented areas of international law that have only partially overlapping objectives (Bogdandy and Villarreal 2020, 16).[9] It is notable in this regard that a 2006 International Law Commission (ILC)[10] report on fragmentation in international law argued for a principle of systemic integration to link different areas of international law "so that the common good of humankind [is] not reducible to the good of any particular institution or regime (International Law Commission [ILC] 2006, para. 480)." The right to health could feasibly achieve such integration. Indeed, prominent scholars in global health law (an emerging field that explores diverse international law regimes governing health) see the right to health acting as "a core, unifying standard" (Toebes 2018, 15) and "pillar" (Gostin 2014, xv) in international law related to health including interpretation of the IHR. Moving towards greater integration between the IHR and international human rights law will offer greater protection of the health and human rights of people affected, and the right to health could play a central role in this endeavour.

Movement towards systemic integration could be achieved through normative and institutional steps. Normative steps could include assuring greater coherence between the standards of the right to health and specific provisions of IHR (Toebes, Forman, and Bartolini 2020). For example, researchers (including the present author) have considered the overlap between core obligations under the right to health and core capacities under the IHR, suggesting the former offer important standards that could enrich the conceptual framework of the IHR, as well as enhance state accountability under the IHR (Toebes, Forman, and Bartolini 2020). This coherence could be similarly advanced by measures that aimed to practically link state compliance under the IHR with the UN human rights regime, including by linking state reporting processes under the ICESCR with those under the IHR.

CONCLUSION

The COVID-19 pandemic underscores that the indivisibility of health and a range of human rights is not just a theoretical proposition: effective public health measures rely on public trust and the existence of affordable and accessible testing and health care for those who need it (Forman 2020). Yet the pandemic has also illuminated the strengths and weaknesses of international law protections of human rights and domestic and global health, and testing almost to breaking point (as with the WHO's IHR), their fitness for purpose. If past is prologue and offers any guidance to our immediate future, we can assume that the pandemic will act as a shock capable of prompting major reforms within international law both in the ways contemplated in this chapter and beyond. Yet in looking to the reformative potential of COVID-19 we should also heed Hilary Charlesworth's concern that "[t]hrough regarding 'crises' as its bread and butter and the engine of progressive development of international law, international law becomes simply a source of justification for the status quo" (Charlesworth 2002, 391). Charlesworth argues that instead we should "refocus international law on issues of structural justice that underpin everyday life" (Charlesworth 2002, 391).

This is an imperative partially embedded within the nascent scholarship of "decolonizing" the invisible inequities that frame academic enterprises including in relation to global health and human rights (Abimbola 2019; Barreto 2013). The imperative to refocus international law on everyday issues of structural justice is an idea fundamental to the legal protection of a right to health which has at its normative centre that idea that every person in the world has the right to the highest attainable standard of health and that this entitlement includes access to essential life-saving health care and to the social determinants of health. COVID pushes us to reconceive the scope and scale of these entitlements and duties and to take them more seriously when it comes to emerging major ethical and human rights breaches such as the stark disparity in access to COVID vaccines. Yet we should not forget in our efforts to reform international law that these are problems that have long existed and that COVID does not so much create new problems as amplify long standing inequities. In this respect, COVID highlights an uncomfortable truth about what it takes for even a system as dedicated to human wellbeing as international human rights law to consider daily misery, deprivation, and inequity as a "crisis" worthy of large-scale intervention and innovation.

NOTES

1. On this point, see also the chapter in this book entitled "A Stress Test for the World Health Organization (WHO) in a Pandemic World: What Can We Hope for the Future?" by Catherine Régis, Jean-Louis Denis, Pierre Larouche, Miriam Cohen, Stéphanie B.M. Cadeddu, and Gaëlle Foucault.
2. See for example, WHO 2005, 1.
3. See Forman and Kohler 2020; Public Health Ontario 2020; Human Rights Watch India 2020; Kwalimwa 2020; Morales and Joseph 2020; Alindogan 2020.
4. "Public health may be invoked as a ground for limiting certain rights in order to allow a State to take measures dealing with a serious threat to the health of the population or individual members of the population. These measures must be specifically aimed at preventing disease or injury or providing care for the sick and injured" (WHO 2005, 25).
5. This is specifically required in article 2.1 of the ISESCR (UN Commission on Human Rights 1966).
6. Article 2 of the IHR states that their purpose and scope are to "prevent, protect against, control and provide a public health response to the international spread of disease in ways that are commensurate with and restricted to public health risks, and which avoid unnecessary interference with international traffic and trade" (World Health Organization 2005).
7. On this point, see also the chapter in this book entitled "A Stress Test for the World Health Organization (WHO) in a Pandemic World: What Can We Hope for the Future?" by Catherine Régis, Jean-Louis Denis, Pierre Larouche, Miriam Cohen, Stéphanie B.M. Cadeddu, and Gaëlle Foucault.
8. Some rights can be temporarily suspended or derogated: See UN Human Rights Committee 2001.
9. These objectives are to, on the one hand, protect public health with the least restrictions to public trade, on the other, to create conditions where every person can enjoy the highest attainable standard of health.
10. The ILC is an independent organization established by the UN General Assembly to progressively develop international law.

REFERENCES

Abimbola, Seye. 2019. "The Foreign Gaze: Authorship in Academic Global Health." *BMJ Global Health* 4, no. 5: http://dx.doi.org/10.1136/bmjgh-2019-002068.

Adepoju, Paul. 2020. "Tuberculosis and HIV Responses Threatened by COVID-19." *The Lancet* 7, no. 3: E319-20.

Alonso-Zaldivar, Ricardo. 2020. "US Faces 'Truly Daunting' Challenges on Needed COVID Tests." *Associated Press*, 7 May 2020. https://www.ctvnews.ca/health/coronavirus/u-s-faces-truly-daunting-challenges-on-needed-covid-tests-1.4929649.

Barreto, José-Manuel. 2013. *Human Rights from a Third World Perspective: Critique, History and International Law*. Cambridge: Cambridge Scholars Publishing.

Birn, Anne-Emanuelle. 2020. "Perspectivizing Pandemics: (How) do Epidemic Histories Criss Cross Contexts?" *Journal of Global History* 15, no. 3: 336–59.

Bogdandy, Armin von, and Pedro A. Villarreal. 2020. "International Law on Pandemic Response: A First Stocktaking in Light of the Coronavirus Crisis." *Max Planck Institute for Comparative Public Law and International Law* MPIL Research Paper Series, no. 2020-07.

Center for Health, Human Rights, and Development (CEHURD). 2020. "Sexual Reproductive Health And Covid-19 In Uganda: Avoiding The Pitfalls of Unintended Consequences For Maternal, Newborn, Child, Adolescent, And Nutrition Health In The National Response." https://www.jasprogramme.ug/publication/sexual-reproductive-health-and-covid-19-in-uganda-avoiding-the-pitfalls-of-unintended-consequences.

Charlesworth, Hilary. 2002. "International Law: A Discipline of Crisis." *Modern Law Review* 65, no. 3: 377–392.

Cousins, Ben. 2020. "Lack of Resources Led to Limited COVID-19 Testing, But New Options are On the Way." *CTV News*, 9 April 2020. https://www.ctvnews.ca/health/coronavirus/lack-of-resources-led-to-limited-covid-19-testing-but-new-options-are-on-the-way-1.4891161.

Cohen, Jon. 2020. "Unveiling 'Warp Speed,' the White House's America-First Push for a Coronavirus Vaccine." *Science*, 12 May 2020. https://www.sciencemag.org/news/2020/05/unveiling-warp-speed-white-house-s-america-first-push-coronavirus-vaccine.

Fidler, David P., and Lawrence O. Gostin. 2006. "The New International Health Regulations: An Historical Development for International Law and Public Health." *Journal of Law, Medicine and Ethics*: 85–94.

Forman, Lisa. 2008. "'Rights' and Wrongs: What Utility for the Right to Health in Reforming Trade Rules on Medicines?" *Health and Human Rights: An International Journal* 10, no. 2: 37–52.

– 2020. "Reflections on the Evolution of the Right to Health in the Shadow of COVID-19." 2020. *Harvard Health and Human Rights*

Journal 22, no. 1: 375–8. https://www.hhrjournal.org/2020/04/the-evolution-of-the-right-to-health-in-the-shadow-of-covid-19/.

Forman, Lisa, Claudia Beiersmann, Claire E. Brolan, Martin McKee, Rachel Hammonds, and Gorik Ooms. 2016. "What Do Core Obligations Under the Right to Health Bring to Universal Health Coverage?" *Health and Human Rights Journal* 18, no. 2: 23–34.

Forman, Lisa, and Jillian Kohler. 2020. "Global Health and Human Rights in the Time of COVID-19: Response, Restrictions, and Legitimacy." *Journal of Human Rights* 19, no. 5: 1–10.

Frankema, Ewout, and Heidi Tworek. 2020. "Pandemics that Changed the World: Historical Reflections on COVID-19." *Journal of Global History* 15, no. 3: 333–5.

Freedom House. 2019. "Freedom in the World 2019: Democracy in Retreat."https://freedomhouse.org/report/freedom-world/freedom-world-2019/democracy-in-retreat.

Gostin, Lawrence. 2014. *Global Health Law*. Cambridge: Harvard University Press.

Gostin, Lawrence O., and Rebecca Katz. 2016. "The International Health Regulations: The Governing Framework for Global Health Security." *The Milbank Quarterly* 94, no. 2: 264–313.

Habibi, Roojin, Gian Luca Burci, Thana C. de Campos, Danwood Chirwa, Margherita Cinà, Stéphanie Dagron, Mark Eccleston-Turner, et al. 2020. "Do Not Violate the International Health Regulations During the COVID-19 Outbreak." *The Lancet* 395, no. 10225 (13 February 2020): 664–6. https://doi.org/10.1016/S0140-6736(20)30373-1.

Hale, Thomas, Thomas Boby, Noam Angrist, Emily Cameron-Blake, Laura Hallas, Beatriz Kira, Saptarshi Majumdar, et al. 2021. "Variation in Government Responses to COVID-19." *Blavatnik School of Government* Working Paper Version 11.0 (March). www.bsg.ox.ac.uk/covidtracker.

Hathaway, Oona. 2002. "Do Human Rights Treaties Make a Difference?" *The Yale Law Journal* 111, no. 8: 1935–2042.

Human Rights Watch India. 2020. "COVID-19 Lockdown Puts Poor at Risk." *Human Rights Watch*, 27 March 2020. https://www.hrw.org/news/2020/03/27/india-covid-19-lockdown-puts-poor-risk.

Human Rights Watch Uganda. 2020. "Uganda: Authorities Weaponize COVID-19 for Repression." *Human Rights Watch*, 20 November 2020. https://www.hrw.org/news/2020/11/20/uganda-authorities-weaponize-covid-19-repression.

Independent Panel for Pandemic Preparedness and Response (IPPPR). 2021. "COVID-19: Make it the Last Pandemic by The Independent

Panel for Pandemic Preparedness & Response." May 2021. https://theindependentpanel.org/wp-content/uploads/2021/05/COVID-19-Make-it-the-Last-Pandemic_final.pdf.

— 2021. "Second Report on Progress Prepared by the Independent Panel for Pandemic Preparedness and Response for the WHO Executive Board." January 2021. https://theindependentpanel.org/wp-content/uploads/2021/01/Independent-Panel_Second-Report-on-Progress_Final-15-Jan-2021.pdf

International Institute for Democracy and Electoral Assistance (IDEA). 2020. "The Global State of Democracy in Focus: Taking Stock of Global Democratic Trends Before and During the COVID-19 Pandemic." 9 December 2020. https://www.idea.int/sites/default/files/publications/global-democratic-trends-before-and-during-covid-19-pandemic.pdf.

International Law Commission. 2006. "Fragmentation of International Law: Difficulties Arising from the Diversification and Expansion of International Law: Report of the Study Group of the International Law Commission." U.N. Doc. A/CN.4/L.682. 13 April 2006.

Kwalimwa, David. 2020. "Uganda: Police Shoot Two on Bodaboda for Defying Museveni COVID-19 Order." *allafrica,* 27 March 2020. https://allafrica.com/stories/202003300087.html.

Kyrili, Katerina, and Matthew Martin. 2010. "The Impact of the Global Economic Crisis on the Budgets of Low-Income Countries." *Oxfam Research Report.* 29 July 2010.

Mann, Jonathan, Sofia Gruskin, Michael A. Grodin, and George J. Annas. 1999. "Introduction." In *Health and Human Rights: A Reader*, edited by Jonathan Mann, Sofia Gruskin, Michael A. Grodin, and George J. Annas, 1–34. New York: Routledge.

Meier, Benjamin Mason, Dabney P. Evans, and Alexandra Phelan. 2020. "Rights-Based Approaches to Preventing, Detecting and Responding to Infectious Disease Outbreaks." In *Infectious Diseases in the New Millennium: Legal and Ethical Challenges*, edited by Mark Eccleston-Turner and Iain Brassington.

Morales, Mark, and Elizabeth Joseph. 2020. "Blacks and Latinos are Overwhelmingly Ticketed by NYPD for Social Distancing Violations." CNN *Online*, 9 May 2020. https://www.cnn.com/2020/05/08/us/social-distancing-stats-nyc/index.html.

Nolan, Aoife. 2014. "Introduction." In *Economic and Social Rights After the Global Financial Crisis*, edited by Aoife Nolan. Cambridge: Cambridge University Press.

Odhiambo, Agnes. 2020. "Tackling Kenya's Domestic Violence Amid

Covid-19 Crisis." *Human Rights Watch*, 8 April 2020. https://www.hrw.org/news/2020/04/08/tackling-kenyas-domestic-violence-amid-covid-19-crisis.

Ooms, Gorik, Laila A Latif, Attiya Waris, Claire E Brolan, Rachel Hammonds, Eric A. Friedman, Moses Mulumba, and Lisa Forman. 2014. "Is Universal Health Coverage the Practical Expression of the Right to Health Care?" BMC *International Health and Human Rights* 14, no. 3: 1–7.

Ortiz, Isabel, and Matthew Cummins. 2013. "The Age of Austerity: A Review of Public Expenditures and Adjustment Measures in 181 Countries." *Isabel Initiative for Policy Dialogue and the South Centre Working Paper* [2013] (March).

Public Health Ontario. 2020. "COVID-19 – What We Know So Far About ... Social Determinants of Health." SYNOPSIS, 24 May 2020. https://www.publichealthontario.ca/-/media/documents/ncov/covid-wwksf/2020/05/what-we-know-social-determinants-health.pdf?la=en.

Quinn, Colm. 2020. "Hungary's Orban Given Power to Rule By Decree With No End Date." *Foreign Policy*, 31 March 2020. https://foreignpolicy.com/2020/03/31/hungarys-orban-given-power-to-rule-by-decree-with-no-end-date/.

Rabson, Mia. 2021. "Canada Seeking Reassurance as Europe Mulls Export Controls on COVID-19 Vaccines." CTV *News*, 26 January 2021. https://www.ctvnews.ca/health/coronavirus/canada-seeking-reassurance-as-europe-mulls-export-controls-on-covid-19-vaccines-1.5282454.

RTL *News*. 2020. "Judge Forbids Abortion Pill by Mail Despite Corona Crisis." RTL *News*, 12 April 2020. https://www.rtlnieuws.nl/nieuws/nederland/artikel/5088361/corona-maatregelen-quarantaine-abortus-pil-post-rechter.

Sekalala, Sharifah, Lisa Forman, Roojin Habibi, and Benjamin Meier. 2020. "Health and Human Rights are Inextricably Linked in the COVID-19 Response." BMJ *Global Health* 5, no. 9: 1–7.

Toebes, Brigit, Lisa Forman, and Giulio Bartolini. 2020. "Towards Human Rights Consistent Responses to Health Emergencies: What is the Overlap Between Core Right to Health Obligations and Core International Health Regulation Capacities?" *Harvard Health and Human Rights Journal*: 1–16.

Shannon, F. Q. II, E. Horace-Kwemi, Robinah Najjemba, Phillip Owiti, Jeffrey K. Edwards, Kalpita S. Shringarpure, P. Shivarama Bhat, F. N. Kateh. 2017. "Effects of the 2014 Ebola Outbreak on Antenatal Care and Delivery Outcomes in Liberia: A Nationwide Analysis." *International Union Against Tuberculosis and Lung Disease* 7, no. 1: S88-93.

Sridhar, Devi, Martin McKee, Gorik Ooms, Claudia Beiersmann, Eric Friedman, Hebe Gouda, Peter Hill, and Albrecht Jahn. 2015. "Universal Health Coverage and the Right to Health: From Legal Principle to Post-2015 Indicators." *International Journal of Health Services* 45, no. 3: 495–506.

Taylor, Allyn L., Roojin Habibi, Gian Luca Burci, Stephanie Dagron, Mark Eccleston-Turner, Lawrence O. Gostin, Benjamin Mason Meier, et al. 2020. "Solidarity in the Wake of COVID-19: Reimagining the International Health Regulations." *Lancet* 396: 82–3.

Toebes, Brigit. 2018. "Global Health Law: Defining the Field." In *Research Handbook on Global Health Law*, edited by Gian Luca Burci and Brigit Toebes, 2–23. Cheltenham: Edward Elgar Publishing.

Tonti, Lauren. 2020. "The International Health Regulations: The Past and the Present, but What Future?" *Harvard International Law Journal Blog*, April 2020. https://harvardilj.org/2020/04/the-international-health-regulations-the-past-and-the-present-but-what-future/.

UN Commission on Human Rights. 1966. "International Covenant on Economic, Social and Cultural Rights." 2200A (XXI). (16 December 1966; entry into force 3 January 1976). https://www.ohchr.org/EN/ProfessionalInterest/Pages/CESCR.aspx.

– 1984. "The Siracusa Principles: On the Limitation and Derogation Provisions in the International Covenant on Civil and Political Rights." E/CN.4/1985/4 (28 September 1984). https://www.refworld.org/docid/4672bc122.html.

UN Committee on Economic, Social and Cultural Rights (UNCESCR). 2000. "General Comment No. 14: The Right to the Highest Attainable Standard of Health." E/C.12/2000/4 (11 August 2000). https://www.refworld.org/pdfid/4538838do.pdf.

UN Human Rights Committee (HRC). 2001. *CCPR General Comment No. 29: Article 4: Derogations during a State of Emergency.* CCPR/C/21/Rev.1/Add.11 (31 August 2001). https://www.refworld.org/docid/453883fd1f.html.

Wilson, Kumanan. 2020. "Populism and Pandemics: The IHR was Meant to Address Outbreaks Like COVID-19, but Nations Have Ignored it." *CBC News*, 18 March 2020. https://www.cbc.ca/news/opinion/opinion-international-health-regulations-who-covid-1.5500166.

World Health Organization (WHO). 2005. *International Health Regulations*. 3rd Ed.

World Health Organization (WHO) Europe. 2020. "COVID-19: Responding Quickly to the Wave of Domestic Violence." (8 May 2020). https://unric.org/nl/covid-19-snel-reageren-op-de-golf-van-huiselijk-geweld-who-europa/ access date.

World Health Organization (WHO) Executive Board, "Report of the Review Committee on the Functioning of the International Health Regulations (2005) during the COVID-19 response," A74/9, 30 April 2021.

– 2005. "Strengthening Preparedness for Health Emergencies: Implementation of the International Health Regulations." *Interim Progress Report of the Review Committee on the Function of the International Health Regulations During the COVID-19 Response*. Report by the Director-General. EB148/19 (12 January 2021).

Yang, Yuan, and Nian Liu. "China Accused of Under-reporting Coronavirus Outbreak." 2020. *Financial Times*, 12 February 2020. https://www.ft.com/content/bb73bd9c-4d92-11ea-95a0-43d18ec715f5.

Zidar, Andraz. 2015. "WHO International Health Regulations and Human Rights: From Allusions to Inclusion." *The International Journal of Human Rights* 19, no. 4: 505–26.

16

A Stress Test for the World Health Organization (WHO) in a Pandemic World: What Can We Hope for the Future?

*Catherine Régis, Miriam Cohen, Pierre Larouche,
Jean-Louis Denis, Stéphanie B.M. Cadeddu and Gaëlle Foucault*

> "The world was not prepared, and must do better."
> The Independent Panel for Pandemic Preparedness
> and Response for the WHO 2021

INTRODUCTION

The COVID-19 crisis has drawn the world's attention to the unique role played by the World Health Organization (WHO). Part of the broader United Nations system, the WHO is the sole intergovernmental international organization entirely dedicated to health matters, with the ambitious objective of providing the "highest possible level of health" to all (Constitution of the World Health Organization 1946, Article 1). Furthermore, it is responsible for coordinating worldwide anti-pandemic efforts, relying mostly, yet not exclusively, on its *International Health Regulations* (IHR 2005), a binding international legal instrument. The COVID-19 pandemic provides a context for the global community, under WHO leadership, to rally around a common and pressing objective: combatting the SARS-COV-2 virus that affects all countries, individuals, health systems, and economies. The current pandemic clearly reveals that global health is not a "zero-sum game": countries depend on each other to ultimately protect the health of their own population (Alvarez 2020, 578).

Yet, while there was hope for global coordination and solidarity at the beginning of the pandemic, a year later it is clear that the story unfolded quite differently. As stated recently by the WHO Independent Panel for Pandemic Preparedness and Response: "We have failed in our collective capacity to come together in solidarity to create a protective web of human security" (The Independent Panel for Pandemic Preparedness and Response 2021). China has been denounced for not acting transparently and swiftly enough in divulging key information regarding the SARS-COV-2 virus that led to the pandemic, and the WHO has been criticized for placating China (Horton 2020) and waiting too long to declare a Public Health Emergency of International Concern (PHEIC; Colton 2020; Fidler 2020; Peters et al. 2020). Furthermore, many States chose not to comply with WHO recommendations at different stages of the pandemic (Von Tigerstrom and Wilson 2020). Instead, they engaged in protectionist and unilateral measures that not only damaged the global collaboration covenant, but also challenged the very legitimacy of the WHO, which relies on "persuasive power" as a key element of its normative leadership (Régis and Kastler 2018; Saxena 2021). The WHO's dependence on collaboration from States emphasizes that global health governance is not a long train where the WHO is the engine pulling States along, but rather a horse-drawn carriage where the WHO, with a loose set of reins, attempts to encourage States to do their part and pull in the same direction.

The COVID-19 pandemic forced the WHO to acknowledge more patently than before that global health governance is a highly political game it is ill prepared (structurally, culturally and resource-wise) to play. The decision of then President Trump to withdraw United States financial support from the WHO in the midst of the crisis made that reality crystal clear (Régis and Denis 2020).

In this chapter, we step back from the immediate context to better understand the challenges the WHO faces in becoming better prepared and equipped for the reality of pandemic societies. We start by exploring leadership capacities of the WHO displayed during the COVID-19 pandemic, focusing on the legal framework that defines these capacities. We then look at the actual implementation of this legal framework based on a synthesized chronology of WHO actions. This timeline, drawn from detailed data collection of measures introduced since the beginning of the pandemic, provides a first-level characterization of the current leadership role of the WHO with respect to its ability to elaborate and implement – or ensure implementation of – norms. After these preliminary steps, we then explore how the governance capacities of the WHO might be renewed in a pandemic world. We investigate two complementary paths: one that seeks to increase global accountability for the WHO and Member States, and another focused on the expansion of public health expertise networks in global health governance.

1. THE NORMATIVE LEADERSHIP CAPACITIES OF THE WHO IN A PANDEMIC WORLD

To fulfill its mandate, the WHO was endowed with norm-setting powers (Constitution of the World Health Organization 1946). These norms can be binding on States (forcing action) or non-binding (encouraging action). More specifically, norm-setting powers are found in Articles 2 (functions), 19 (conventions and agreements), 21 (regulations) and 23 (recommendations). By way of illustration, the WHO can "propose conventions, agreements and regulations, and make recommendations with respect to international health matters" (Article 2 (k)), develop international standards with respect to biological and pharmaceutical products (2 (u)), and, more broadly, "take all necessary action to attain the objective of the Organization" (2 (v)). Based on such broad powers, the WHO has adopted normative instruments to regulate a variety of health issues, such as *The WHO Framework Convention on Tobacco Control* (2005), its only convention thus far; *The WHO Global Code of Practice on the International Recruitment of Health Personnel* (2010), a non-binding instrument; and the *International Health Regulations* (IHR 2005) a legally binding instrument that we explore in greater detail below.

Over the years, the WHO has been criticized for underusing its normative powers, especially when it comes to issuing legally binding norms (Gostin 2014; Gostin et al. 2015). This reluctance can be explained by different factors, including the demanding process required to adopt a binding instrument and the WHO's historical tendency to focus on scientific over legal leadership (Saxena 2021; Régis and Kastler 2018). Yet, as mentioned by Dr Tedros Adhanom Ghebreyesus, WHO Director General: "Strong legal frameworks are critical for national COVID-19 responses," and they "should be aligned with international commitments to respond to current and emerging public health risks" (O'Neill 2020). That said, binding norms are not a silver bullet if the WHO (or an international court, for that matter) lacks the authority to impose sanctions on countries for non-compliance.

a. Analysis of the WHO Legal Framework: The International Health Regulations (IHR)

While the WHO holds normative powers to engage in different actions during a pandemic, including those mentioned in its Constitution (Burci 2020), the IHR serve as a point of reference. The IHR were created to prevent and manage international public health threats like SARS-COV-2. After the severe acute respiratory syndrome (SARS) epidemic of 2003 (the first global public health emergency of the twenty-first century), the IHR were revised to better address the contemporary reality of public health hazards (IHR Foreword 1). The 2005 version of the IHR, now in force, provides an internationally agreed framework – legally binding on 196 States – that defines the rights and obligations of States during public health events that have the potential to cross borders. Their binding nature means that Member States have to respect the IHR, yet these are a mix of norms that sometimes impose and other times recommend actions to be taken by States (see below).

At the outset, Article 2 introduces a counterbalancing objective that is fundamental to the interpretation and implementation of the IHR: public health responses must avoid unnecessary interference with international traffic and trade.[1] This balance is paramount in WHO decisions. The main usefulness of the IHR lies in providing a global assessment of border measures required to prevent the spread of disease, which enables States to align their respective measures and preserve international traffic and trade as best as possible (Resolution WHA48.7 of the World Health Assembly). Article 3 compels the WHO and States to conduct a further balancing act between public health requirements and the dignity, human rights, and fundamental freedoms of persons (see also IHR Articles 17(d) and 42), such as respect for informed consent and non-discrimination when applying health measures under the IHR.

As regards their "normative force," the duties created by the IHR can be split into three types: "*legally binding* obligations, ... *authoritative advice agreed by State Parties* concerning appropriate actions under the IHR ... *and provisions indicating discretion or authorization of State Parties* to take certain steps under the Regulations ..." (WHO 2009, our emphasis). This typology is relevant in assessing whether the WHO is truly able to act in certain circumstances and whether countries have an obligation to comply – as opposed to a mere invitation to comply – with WHO positions.

The IHR also define one of the most important powers of the WHO during a pandemic, namely the power held by the director general to declare a PHEIC. A PHEIC is defined as an extraordinary event that may constitute a public health risk across countries through the international spread of disease and may require a coordinated international response (Articles 1, 12 and the following). A PHEIC declaration formally and strongly alerts the international community. COVID-19 is the sixth PHEIC since the adoption of the new IHR in 2005. When determining whether a health event constitutes a PHEIC, the director general must weigh elements such as the information provided by the State in which the event first occurs (China in the case of COVID-19), the advice of an expert Emergency Committee (with equitable geographical representation), scientific principles and evidence, as well as risks to human health, international spread of disease, and interference with international traffic (Article 12 (4)).

The WHO is also tasked with coordinating the fight against the PHEIC. It is required to "provide appropriate guidance and assistance [to States] affected or threatened" by a PHEIC when requested to do so (Article 13(6)). When a PHEIC is officially declared, the director general is bound to issue Temporary Recommendations to guide countries with respect to appropriate health measures (Article 15). Temporary recommendations typically involve border measures. Such measures are defined as "time-limited" and "non-binding advice" (Article 1) and can relate to persons, baggage, cargo, containers, conveyances, goods, and postal parcels. For example, the WHO can recommend that States require medical examinations or vaccination, implement quarantine, trace contacts of affected persons, and refuse entry of goods or affected persons (Article 18). The IHR also allow the WHO to recommend that States take no specific measures, for instance that they do not close their borders (which has been recommended for several PHEIC). The IHR thus provide a framework for the WHO's norm-setting activities during a PHEIC by making the WHO responsible for adopting recommendations or other forms of assistance requested by States.

In return, States are expected to develop and maintain adequate response capacity to deal with a PHEIC (Article 13), and are bound to adopt health measures without delay (Article 42). However, given that WHO recommendations are non-binding, State health measures may or may not adhere to them. Article 43 establishes a framework to govern cases in which States wish to adopt measures that differ from the recommendations (so-called "additional measures"): these measures must afford a level of public health protection at least equal to the recommendation, while not restricting traffic or human rights more than available alternatives (Article 43(1)). Additional measures must be based on criteria such as scientific principles, available scientific evidence, and any specific guidance or advice from the WHO (Article 2; Hoffman and Fafard 2020). The purpose of these criteria is to emphasize the importance of grounding State decisions in science rather than factors such as politics, protectionism, discrimination, and so on. The current context, where science is increasingly attacked in public debate, poses a threat to this criterion, weakening international consensus on the value of science in global health decision-making. States must notify the WHO of "Additional Measures," and the WHO, in turn, shares this information with other States (Article 43(3)). The WHO may request that a State reconsider its divergent health measure (Article 43 (4)), potentially triggering diplomatic backlash when the deviant State's behaviour runs counter to that of most other States or to leading States.

b. WHO Actions During the Pandemic: A Legal Framework in Motion

We now turn to the specific actions and health measures recommended by the WHO during the COVID-19 pandemic. This "empirical incursion" reveals challenges confronting the WHO when it seeks to issue prescriptions for States and to monitor compliance.

EVENTS AND DECISIONS LEADING TO THE PHEIC DECLARATION
After receiving notification from China of a cluster of pneumonia cases on 31 December 2019 (WHO 2021), the WHO undertook various actions to understand and try to contain the emerging pandemic. It first requested more information from the Chinese authorities and set up an Incident Management Support Team (1 January 2020). Following this initial response, it informed Global Outbreak Alert

and Response Network partners (3 January) of the outbreak, issued its first disease outbreak news report (5 January), adopted advice related to travel, laboratory testing, risk communication, infection prevention and control (10 January), set up daily situation reports (21 January), and created an emergency committee (22 January) which met twice (23 and 30 January; WHO 2021). On 30 January, the WHO officially declared a PHEIC (WHO 2020f).

INTERNATIONAL TRAFFIC

One of the first WHO actions regarding COVID-19 concerned international traffic (10 January). Based on the IHR, its "[a]dvice for international travel and trade in relation to the outbreak of pneumonia caused by a new coronavirus in China" recommended that international traffic not be restricted, i.e. that States not take health measures for travelers (WHO 2020a). The WHO maintained this position in a subsequent declaration (23 January) and in two advisory updates – issued on 24 January (WHO 2020c) and 27 January (WHO 2020d) – recommending (WHO 2020b) "against the application of any restrictions of international traffic based on the information currently available on this event." On 30 January, the WHO issued a temporary recommendation (in connection with the PHEIC declaration) which still did not recommend restricting trade or travel, providing no further reasons for this recommendation. Despite its reluctance to restrict international traffic, the WHO nevertheless proposed health measures (IHR 2005, art. 2) for travelers in international and domestic airports and ports (24 January) such as exit temperature screening in countries with ongoing transmission of SARS-COV-2 and entry temperature screening in countries without such transmission.

After the PHEIC declaration, the WHO continued to advise against travel restrictions; however, on 4 February, it nuanced this position by publicly acknowledging, in its "Strategic preparedness and response plan" (SPRP), that restrictive measures could be "temporarily useful" under specific circumstances and after applying "risk and cost-benefit analyses"(WHO 2020h, 10). On 11 February, the WHO issued "Advice" on "[k]ey considerations for repatriation and quarantine of travelers," reiterating that interfering with international traffic for longer than a day "may have a public health rationale at the beginning of the containment phase" (WHO 2020i, 1). However the "Advice" stated that such measures should also respond to three other conditions: they "need to be short in duration, proportionate to the public health risks, and be reconsidered regularly as the situation evolves" (WHO 2020i, 1). Under this "Advice," States could "put arriving passengers, those not displaying symptoms, in a quarantine facility" under certain conditions (WHO 2020i, 3). On 27 February, the WHO published a "Joint Statement on Tourism and COVID-19 – UNWTO and WHO Call for Responsibility and Coordination" in collaboration with the World Tourism Organization (UNWTO) to advise the travel and tourism sectors. It restated that States should minimize unnecessary interference with international traffic and trade (WHO and UNWTO 2020).

On 14 April, the WHO updated its SPRP without, this time, recommending against travel restrictions. It advised that States' restrictions on non-essential domestic and international travel should be "appropriate and proportionate" (WHO 2020k, 5). The WHO did not define "appropriate and proportionate" or "non-essential," thereby leaving room for interpretations that varied by national context. The SPRP also detailed that, where community transmission was established, or at risk of increasing, States "must immediately adopt ... limits on national and international travel, enhanced screening and quarantine" (WHO 2020k, 9). Finally, on 1 May, in a new temporary recommendation (WHO 2020l), the WHO articulated a more flexible approach to travel restrictions by attaching just two conditions: restrictions must be "appropriate ...with consideration of their public health benefits, including ... quarantine" and must be reconsidered based on "risk assessments, transmission patterns ... cost-benefit analyses" and other circumstances. These recurrent modifications arguably made WHO instructions difficult to follow and somewhat arbitrary for States. For example, terms like "proportionate" and "appropriate" were used interchangeably; the WHO also overlooked the importance of providing clear definitions for "non-essential travel," among others. On the other hand, WHO guidance was nuanced and evolutive, and reflected important trade-offs between health (and evolving evidence) and other considerations.

WEARING OF MASKS

In addition to international traffic, the WHO provided norms on topics such as masks. The WHO published interim guidance on the subject every one to two months. On 29 January 2020, the WHO adopted the first interim guidance advising on "the use of medical masks in communities, at home and at health care facilities" (WHO 2020e). This guide stated that symptom-free individuals should use neither medical nor non-medical masks, except where this was local custom. On 6 April, the WHO adopted a more comprehensive interim guidance that maintained this position but, for the first time, acknowledged that States could require mask wearing, provided two conditions were fulfilled. First, considering that "the wide use of masks by healthy people in the community setting is not supported by current evidence and carries uncertainties and critical risk" (WHO 2020j, 2), the WHO advised decision-makers to apply "a risk-based approach" (WHO 2020j, 2). Second, "[w]hatever approach is taken, it is important to develop a strong communication strategy to explain to the population the circumstances, criteria, and reasons for decisions" (WHO 2020j, 2). The WHO also remained non-committal about a growing worldwide trend to wear non-medical masks. While finding "no current evidence to make a recommendation for or against their use in ... [the community] setting" (WHO 2020j, 2.), it proposed that if "decision makers may be moving ahead with advising the use of non-medical masks ... [certain] features related to non-medical masks should be taken into consideration" (WHO 2020j, 3). This position evolved on 5 June, as the WHO recommended the widespread use of masks, including non-medical masks, for States or localities facing community transmission (WHO 2020m). Compared to the approach taken for the closure of borders, the conditions attached to WHO guidance for masks were less ambiguous. These conditions, calling on States to employ a risk-based approach and develop a communication strategy, were clearly defined across the various interim guides published throughout the pandemic. However, the WHO's normative action here appears to conflict with emerging insights of scientific communities who were suggesting (however, non-unanimously) that States take a precautionary approach and promote the use of masks among the general population (Chu et al. 2020; Howard et al. 2021; UNCOVER 2020).

Along with specific actions and health measures, WHO situation reports present the daily epidemiological evolution of the pandemic and highlight instruments adopted for its management. Beyond their informative purpose, they often consolidate WHO normative statements and provide further explanations and clarifications. For example, Situation Report No. 138 (6 June 2020) clarifies the WHO's guidance on gatherings issued on 29 May 2020, and

Situation Report No. 172 (10 July 2020) explains the Scientific Brief published on 9 July. Situation reports also provide information on the implementation of IHR, particularly with respect to additional health measures that States adopt under Article 43. For example, Situation Report No. 18 (7 February 2020) indicates that seventy-two member States adopted health measures that significantly interfered with international traffic, but only twenty-three (or 32 per cent) sent an official report to the WHO justifying these measures (WHO 2020, 1). In subsequent reports, the WHO only included the number of Member States officially reporting additional health measures, without mention of whether justification was provided (e.g., Report No. 67, on 27 March 2020, 136 States; Report No. 88, on 17 April 2020, 167 States). On 31 July, WHO Report No. 193 included a brief assessment of States' compliance with Article 43, underlining that only one third of the 198 State Parties had provided a public health rationale for these measures. It also stated that "only a few countries conduct and communicate regular risk assessment and reviews measures" (who 2020n, 2). The Situation Reports provide ready evidence of the WHO's struggle to ensure compliance with specific guidance, such as the obligation to provide a rationale for constraining measures and justify their duration.

LESSONS LEARNED

A few conclusions can be drawn from these empirical observations of the WHO's normative action. First, the WHO actively used its norm-setting powers to guide countries during the pandemic (strategic plans, interim guidance, statements, advice, guidance, handbooks, etc.); norms on topics other than international traffic and masks were also produced. While the norms relating to masks were issued outside the framework of the IHR, norms relating to international traffic would fall squarely within the scope of the IHR. Nonetheless, the IHR was not used as a legal basis for all norms relating to international traffic: once the PHEIC was declared, the WHO used its temporary recommendation power sparingly, with the remainder of its normative action relating to international traffic taking place in the shadow of the formalized channel provided by the IHR. Secondly, the terminology employed in the WHO measures varied significantly, which may have created some misunderstanding or uncertainty around the WHO's expectations. A good example is the successive iterations of the test for justifying State restrictions on cross-border traffic. Finally, in line with previous literature, issues appeared around State compliance with the WHO's normative action – something we would need more data to fully explore (WHO 2017; Gostin and Wetter 2020). Various States did not comply with WHO measures – binding or not – at different times in the pandemic (Davies and Wenham 2020; Gebrekidan 2020). For instance, some States refused to follow the WHO opinion against imposing travel restrictions (Von Tigerstrom and Wilson 2020; Hoffman and Fafard 2020). Many States failed to comply with the obligation to communicate and justify additional health measures affecting international traffic, for example, Situation Report No. 193 (Gebrekidan 2020; Kiernan and DeVita 2020). The WHO did not seem to put pressure on deviant States by using public "blaming and shaming" tactics (Alvarez 2020, 583).

2. RENEWING THE NORMATIVE LEADERSHIP CAPACITIES OF THE WHO IN A PANDEMIC WORLD

a. Reducing the Accountability Gap

The WHO is an organization with a fundamental mandate in global health and vast normative capacities; however, it remains challenging for the organization to elaborate across-the-board norms, deal with ambiguous situations or evidence, and ensure that norms are respected. In combination with other factors, this leads to a lack of accountability in global health governance, with far-reaching consequences on current and future capacities to manage pandemics. Understanding the causes of this accountability conundrum is an important step to overcoming it. In this section, we focus on two causes in particular.

First, the actual structure of the organization makes it vulnerable to geopolitical crossfire, a situation that undermines its normative centre of gravity established around scientific principles and evidence (Gostin and Wetter 2020). For instance, the WHO still strongly relies on countries' willingness to provide information and allow investigations on their territory before declaring a PHEIC. Considering the major political and financial consequences that such a declaration entails, a country (and even the director general of the WHO) may resist doing so as long as possible, despite the fact that time is of the essence in public health threats. The WHO is also constrained by its "state-centered roots" (Alvarez 2020, 582): States, and therefore political leaders and their delegates, are its formal interlocutors and they bring political considerations (reputation, electoral dynamic and agendas, national interests, etc.) into the mix. This also means that the WHO cannot directly involve nonstate actors, such as airlines, under its governance even when they might impede adoption of WHO recommendations (Alvarez 2020, 582). In reality, global health governance involves more than the WHO and States; private actors exert a strong influence on this ecosystem, the Bill and Melinda Gates Foundation being a prime example (Gostin 2014).

A second cause for the lack of accountability is that WHO authority ultimately rests on its own legitimacy (persuasive power) and on States' willingness to comply with its recommendations and with international health law more broadly. International health law is a highly interdependent and collaborative enterprise, where a sufficient number of States need to follow the rules for the system to work. If States agree to respect the rules but come to see international health law as a "buffet"[2] where they can pick and choose what rules they want to apply in a given situation, they undermine the collaborative nature of global health governance. Why play fair when nobody else does, especially when there is a cost for doing so? Thus starts a vicious circle where less compliance leads to less legitimacy, and less legitimacy leads to even less compliance ... But this is a short-term vision of global health governance that disregards a reality COVID-19 has made plain: States depend on each other to protect the health of their own population.

A number of factors have contributed to weakening the WHO's authority in recent years. The organization has been increasingly underfunded, which has impacted its capacity to effectively accomplish its mission (Gostin and Wetter 2020). The WHO's biennial budget is presently $6 billion, in order to coordinate all global health efforts;[3] in comparison, the Centers for Disease Control and Prevention in the United States have an annual budget of $11 billion (Régis and Denis 2020). Importantly, the WHO has also become more dependent on "voluntary contributions" and less so on assessed contributions (i.e, countries' membership dues), which allows (mostly richer) States to influence the WHO's global health agenda by determining which projects to finance and prioritize (The Independent Panel for Pandemic Preparedness and Response 2021;

Sridhar, 2012).[4] Assuring that the WHO is adequately funded is a first condition for enabling it to accomplish its vast mission (Gostin and Wetter 2020), including providing normative leadership, in a credible and impactful way. As Benson mentions: "Money and authority are interrelated in that there is a generalized expectation of balance or correlation between the two. Authority to conduct activities is generally assumed to imply a claim upon money adequate to performance in the prescribed sphere" (Benson 1975).

Second, contrary to some other international organizations, the WHO does not have an effective dispute resolution mechanism to adjudicate conflicts about the interpretation and application of its normative instruments and impose decisions. This makes it difficult to resolve fundamental conflicts of interest that may exist among States or between States and the WHO. Only the IHR contains a dispute resolution process and it is ultimately predicated on Member State consent to compulsory arbitration (Article 56); arguably, China's consent to dispute resolution would have been very unlikely at the start of the pandemic (Tzeng 2020). In fact, the process has never been used (Fidler 2020). Consequently, there is no effective mechanism to hold Member States accountable in the event that they fall short of fulfilling their obligations under the WHO's constitutive instruments. Member States lack accountability vis-à-vis the WHO and the international community. Furthermore, establishing Member State responsibility for failing to comply with IHR obligations (e.g. timely notification, sharing information) raises the question of reparations for harm caused. The IHR includes no provision to provide reparations. However, under the international law on State responsibility, a State that violates international law has "an obligation to make full reparation for the injury caused by the internationally wrongful act" (ILC Articles, art. 31). One possibility for strengthening the WHO's ability to monitor and enforce compliance (Benvenisti 2020) would be to reform this dispute mechanism procedure (Hoffman 2014) in order to make it more enforceable and less reliant on States' willingness to participate in dispute resolution.

More broadly, establishing State responsibility in international law for contributing to the outbreak of a pandemic – which has been discussed for China (Tzeng 2020) – is not a straightforward endeavour. There are issues relating to: proof of violations (e.g. lack of cooperation of the potentially wrongful State may hinder access to elements that prove failure of timely notification, for example); potential defences for failing to comply with obligations under global health instruments (i.e. IHR, WHO Constitution); and the fora where such disputes could be adjudicated (Francisco-José Quintana and Justina Uriburu 2020). The International Court of Justice (ICJ) in The Hague, which deals with disputes among States concerning alleged violations of international law, has been identified as a potential venue to hold States accountable for failing in their global health obligations (Huremagić and Kainz). The ICJ, however, is not an international court open to each and every case of alleged violations of international law. The Court can adjudicate disputes if a jurisdictional basis is present. In the case of accountability in pandemics such as SARS-COV-2, the basis would likely come from binding global health instruments. For example, Article 75 of the WHO Constitution provides that "[a]ny question or dispute concerning the interpretation or application of this Constitution which is not settled by negotiation or by the Health Assembly shall be referred to the International Court of Justice ...." (Tzeng 2020). The provision of a jurisdictional basis is not, in and of itself, sufficient to mount a case against a State before the ICJ for evading its responsibility with regard to a pandemic. Proof that an obligation under the WHO Constitution or the IHR has been violated, as well as causation, would still be necessary (Tzeng 2020). While the ICJ has never had to adjudicate on disputes relating to violations of global health law, as one scholar put it: "faced with few alternative mechanisms, it is incumbent upon us to examine all possible devices for realising more effective enforcement of public health obligations for when the next virus hits." (Videler 2021). That said, adjudication before an international court remains a final recourse; a pandemic cannot be managed through such fora. The ideal approach would see collaboration among States increase so that pandemics do not occur in the first place.

b. Strengthening Collaborative Governance in an Evolving Global Health Reality

In addition to legal avenues, bolstering the WHO's legitimacy and normative leadership requires strengthening its leverage as a hub of scientific expertise within a global network. Like other international organizations, the WHO is evolving in a global environment that has changed significantly over the last thirty years. These changes have impacted the organization and functioning of international organizations, a phenomenon that has been chronicled and theorized in new branches of literature such as transnational governance and global administrative law (Slaughter and Hale 2010; Hooghe and Marks 2010; Abbott and Snidal 2009; von Bogdandy and Dann 2008). Interestingly, case studies in this scholarship rarely involve the WHO, and those that do have not focused specifically on the IHR (OECD 2014).

A number of useful lessons could be drawn by comparing WHO governance of public health emergencies with reasonably similar cases in other international institutions.

Firstly, the IHR places the WHO in the difficult position of having to reconcile global public health with the free flow of goods and persons and with fundamental rights. As the current pandemic reveals, when public health concerns reach existential levels, this reconciliation becomes a highly political balancing act, which plays out at cabinet level with the personal involvement of the head of government. In the current international context, it is not realistic to expect national governments to simply heed the WHO on such matters. Indeed, Article 43 of the IHR allows States to take measures that go beyond WHO recommendations. Article 43 also provides a legal framework for the conditions under which such measures may be taken, for the notification of such measures to the WHO and for their review. Yet, when setting norms for travel restrictions, the WHO incorporated an approximative version of the conditions of the Article 43 exception directly within its own documents, thereby creating a second path for States to enjoy leeway and discretion in how they respond to a recommendation. This probably added to the confusion around travel restrictions in the early stages of the pandemic.

As a complementary approach to providing legal constraints and boundaries on political decision-making at State level, the WHO could seek inspiration from other international bodies set up as global centres of expertise. Its main contribution would then be to foster and publicize the consensus view of experts on a given subject. When State decision-makers rule on matters such as necessity, appropriateness and reasonably available alternatives, they would do so on the basis of the same expert information and recommendations. By the same token, the WHO could shore up the credibility of domestic experts, enabling them to participate in national political processes with added legitimacy coming from the WHO.

Secondly, taking this one step further, national political processes are bound to result, on occasion, in diverging decisions and potentially in disputes. As mentioned above, the WHO is vulnerable to political crossfire between States. The events of the current pandemic reveal that the WHO is ill-suited to win a dispute with a State when that dispute is framed as a matter of political decision-making, that is, who is best discharging a political duty towards a polity. Here as well, existing literature suggests a number of avenues the WHO could take to avoid being drawn into destructive and disruptive battles, and instead reframe them as inter-state disputes. The IHR already provides mechanisms for States to exchange information and report to the WHO on how they implement IHR recommendations and other measures. These often include notions of proportionality, which are the natural vehicle by which apparently "untouchable" political decisions can be unwound and opened for discussion. A strengthening of reporting obligations – maybe even going towards a robust "comply or explain" mechanism – coupled with greater circulation of information towards the public and transparency, could position the WHO as an impartial party that helps to understand, potentially defuse, or at least structure, disputes between States regarding their respective public health measures (see also WHO 2016).

CONCLUSION

Undoubtedly, the year 2020 will be marked on all calendars for a long time. The WHO was put on the front line of global health efforts to combat the pandemic. While the organization had some weaknesses before this crisis, these were exacerbated and made visible to the entire world during COVID-19. It is now clear that the WHO is essential, but needs to better manage its normative leadership which, in turn, requires that sufficient legal, financial, and scientific means be given to the organization. The WHO's normative leadership is a key component of efficient global health governance and indispensable to the social justice pact Member States agreed to when joining the WHO. Preventing and managing pandemics entails a complex international effort and strong international determination. International engagement may ebb and flow, but global public health threats will remain. COVID-19 struck precisely when geopolitical tensions in the world were high (Guterres 2020). COVID-19 provided us an unwelcome reminder of our interconnected fate, but also offers a unique opportunity to reengage the international community on important discussions about the future of the WHO, State commitments to the organization, and, most of all, about how to prevent the occurrence of pandemic societies. There is hope: no one today can say that public health and the WHO do not warrant support.

NOTES

1 Article 2: "The purpose and scope of these Regulations are to prevent, protect against, control and provide a public health response to the international spread of disease in ways that are commensurate with and restricted to public health risks, and which avoid unnecessary interference with the international traffic and trade."
2 We would like to thank professor Steven Hoffman for this point.
3 See http://open.who.int/2018-19/budget-and-financing/gpw-overview.
4 See also the WHO's website to have a full picture of the financing situation of the organization, including the proportion of voluntary contribution: https://www.who.int/about/funding.

REFERENCES

Abbott, Kenneth W., and Duncan Snidal. 2009. "The Governance Triangle: Regulatory Standards Institutions and The Shadow of the State." *The Politics of Global Regulation*, edited by Walter Mattli and Ngaire Woods, 44–88. Princeton: Princeton University Press.

Alvarez, José E. 2020. "The WHO in the Age of the Coronavirus." *The American Journal of International Law* 114, no. 4: 578–87.

Benson, J. Kenneth. 1975. "The Interorganizational Network as a Political Economy." *Administrative Science Quarterly* 20: 229–49.

Bogdandy, Armin von and Philipp Dann. 2008. "International Composite Administration: Conceptualizing Multi-Level and Network Aspects in the Exercise of International Public Authority." *German Law Journal* 9, no. 11: 2013–39.

Burci, Gina Luca. 2020. "The Legal Response to Pandemics: The Strengths and Weaknesses of the International Health Regulations." *Journal of International Humanitarian Legal Studies* 112: 204–17. https://doi.org/10.1163/18781527-01102003.

Chu, Derek K., Elie A. Akl, Stephanie Duda, Karla Solo, Sally Yaacoub, and Holger J Schünemann. 2020. "Physical Distancing, Face Masks, and Eye Protection to Prevent Person-to-Person Transmission of

SARS-COV-2 and COVID-19: A Systematic Review and Meta-Analysis." *The Lancet* 395, no. 10242: 1973–87. https://doi.org/10.1016/S0140-6736(20)31142-9.

Colton, Emma. 2020. "Japanese Deputy Prime Minister Says WHO Should be Renamed China Health Organization." *Washington Examiner*, 2 April 2020. https://www.washingtonexaminer.com/news/japanese-deputy-prime-minister-says-who-should-be-renamed-china-health-organization.

Davies, Sara. E., and Clare Wenham. 2020. "Why the COVID-19 Response Needs International Relations." *International Affairs* 96, no. 5: 1227–51. https://doi.org/10.1093/ia/iiaa135

Fidler, David P. 2020. "The World Health Organization and Pandemic Politics." *Think Global Health*, 10 April 2020. https://www.thinkglobalhealth.org/article/world-health-organization-and-pandemic-politics.

Gebrekidan, Selam. 2020. "The World Has a Plan to Fight Coronavirus. Most Countries Are Not Using it." *The New York Times*, 12 March 2020. https://www.nytimes.com/2020/03/12/world/coronavirus-world-health-organization.html.

Gostin, Lawrence O. 2014. *Global Health Law*. Cambridge: Harvard University Press.

Gostin, Lawrence O., Devi Sridhar, and Daniel Hougendobler. 2015. "The Normative Authority of the World Health Organization." *Public Health* 129, no. 7: 854–63.

Gostin, Lawrence O. and Sarah Wetter. 2020. "Using Covid-19 to Strengthen the WHO: Promoting Health and Science Above Politics." *Milbank Quarterly Opinion* (6 May 2020). https://doi.org/10.1599/mqop.2020.0506.

Government of Russia. 2020. "Briefing with Deputy Prime Minister Tatyana Golikova and Head of the Federal Service for Supervision of Consumer Protection and Welfare Anna Popova Following the Meeting of the Emergency Response Centre to Prevent the Spread of the New Coronavirus in Russia." *Government of Russia*. 31 January 2020. http://government.ru/en/news/38893/.

Government of Singapore. 2020. "How is Singapore Limiting the Spread of Coronavirus Disease 2019?" *Government of Singapore*. 29 January 2020. http://www.gov.sg/article/how-is-singapore-limiting-the-spread-of-covid-19.

Hoffman, Steven J., and Patrick Fafard. 2020. "Border Closures: A Pandemic of Symbolic Acts in the Time of Covid-19." In *Vulnerable:*

The Law, Policy and Ethics of COVID-19, edited by Jane Philpott, Vanessa MacDonnell, Sophie Thériault, Sridhar Venkatapuram, and Colleen M. Flood, 555–70. Ottawa: University of Ottawa Press.

Hoffman, Steven J. 2014. "Making the International Health Regulations Matter: Promoting Compliance through Effective Dispute Resolution." In *The Routledge Handbook on Global Health Security*, edited by Simon Rushton and Jeremy Youde, 239–51. Oxford: Routledge.

Hooghe, Liesbet, and Gary Marks. 2010. "Types of Multi-Level Governance." In *Handbook on Multi-level Governance*, edited by. Henrik Enderlein, Sonja Wälti, and Michael Zürn, 17–31. Northampton: Edward Elgar.

Horton, Richard. 2020. *The Covid-19 Catastrophe: What's Gone Wrong and How to Stop it Happening Again.* Cambridge: Polity Press.

Howard, Jeremy, Austin Huang, Zhiyuan Li, Zeynep Tufeci, Vladimir Zdimal, Helene-Mari van der Weshuizen, Arne von Delft, et al. 2021. "An Evidence Review of Face Masks Against COVID-19." *Proceedings of the National Academy of Sciences* 118, no. 4: 1–12. https://doi.org/10.1073/pnas.2014564118.

Independent Panel for Pandemic Preparedness & Response. 2021. "Second Report on Progress, Report Prepared for the WHO Executive Board." *Independent Panel for Pandemic Preparedness & Response.* January 2021. https://theindependentpanel.org/wp-content/uploads/2021/01/Independent-Panel_Second-Report-on-Progress_Final-15-Jan-2021.pdf.

Italian Civil Aviation Authority. 2020. "Coronavirus: Sospesi tutti i collegamenti aerei tra Italia e Cina." *Italian Civil Aviation Authority.* 31 January 2020. https://www.enac.gov.it/news/coronavirus-sospesi-tutti-collegamenti-aerei-tra-italia-cina

Kiernan, Samantha and Madeleine DeVita. 2020. "Travel Restrictions on China due to COVID-19." *ThinkGlobal Health,* 6 April 2020. https://www.thinkglobalhealth.org/article/travel-restrictions-china-due-covid-19.

OECD. 2014. *International Regulatory Co-operation and International Organisations: The Cases of the* OECD *and the* IMO. Paris: OECD Publishing. https://doi.org/10.1787/9789264225756-en.

O'Neill Institute. 2020. "Press Release." *O'Neill Institute,* 22 July 2020. https://oneill.law.georgetown.edu/news/new-covid-19-legal-database/.

Peters, Michael A., Stephanie Hollings, Benjamin Green, and Moses Oladele Ogunniran. 2020. "The WHO, the Global Governance of

Health and Pandemic Politics." *Educational Philosophy and Theory.* 1–10. https://doi.org/10.1080/00131857.2020.1806187.

Régis Catherine and Jean-Louis. Denis. 2020. «L'OMS survivra-t-elle à la pandémie... et aux attaques de Trump?» *The Conversation,* 12 May 2020. https://theconversation.com/loms-survivra-t-elle-a-la-pandemie-et-aux-attaques-de-trump-138170

Régis, Catherine and Florian Kastler. 2018. "Improving the World Health Organization's Normative Strategy: What Should We Aim For?" *Revue Belge de droit international* 138: 138–151.

Guterres, António. 2020. "Secretary-General's Statement to the Press." *United Nations:Secretary-General.* 6 January 2020. https://www.un.org/sg/en/content/sg/press-encounter/2020-01-06/secretary-generals-statement-the-press

Teplin, Linda A., Gary M. McClelland, Karen M. Abram, and Jason J. Washburn. 2005. "Early Violent Death in Delinquent Youth: A Prospective Longitudinal Study." Paper presented at the Annual Meeting of the American Psychology-Law Society, La Jolla, CA, March 2005.

Shekhar Saxena. 2021. "World Health Organization: Redefining its Role in a Rapidly Changing World." Paper presented at *Les organisations internationals en transformation,* Université de Montréal, Montréal, 21 January 2021.

Slaughter, Anne-Marie. and Thomas N. Hale. 2010. "Transgovernmental Networks and Multi-Level Governance." In *Handbook on Multi-level Governance,* edited by Henrik Enderlein, Sonja Wälti, and Michael Zürn, 358–369. Northampton: Edward Elgar.

Sridhar, Devi. 2012. "Who Sets the Global Health Research Agenda? The Challenge of Multi-Bi Financing." *PLoS Med* 9, no. 9: e1001312. https://doi.org/10.1371/journal.pmed.1001312.

Tigerstrom, Barbara von and Kumanan Wilson. 2020. "COVID-19 Travel Restrictions and the International Health Regulations (2005)." *BMJ Global Health* 5: e002629. https://doi:10.1136/bmjgh-2020-002629

Tzeng, Peter. 2020. "Taking China to the International Court of Justice Over Covid-19." *EJIL: TALK! Blog for the European Journal of International Law,* 2 April 2020. https://www.ejiltalk.org/taking-china-to-the-international-court-of-justice-over-covid-19/.

UNCOVER. 2020. "Does the Use of Face Masks in the General Population Make a Difference to Spread of Infection?" *Government of the United Kingdom.* 7 April 2020. https://www.gov.uk/government/publications/does-the-use-of-face-masks-in-the-general-population-make-a-difference-to-spread-of-infection-7-april-2020

World Health Organization. 2005. *International Health Regulations, Third Edition*. France: WHO). https://www.who.int/publications-detail-redirect/9789241580496
— 2016. "Implementation of the IHR (2005) – Report of the Review Committee on the Role of the IHR (2005) in the Ebola Outbreak and Response." WHO. 13 May 2016: Doc. A69/21.
— 2017. "Evaluation of WHO's Normative Function, volume 1." WHO. July 2017.
— 2020a. "WHO Advice for International Travel and Trade in Relation to the Outbreak of Pneumonia Caused by a New Coronavirus in China." WHO. 10 January 2020. https://www.who.int/news-room/articles-detail/who-advice-for-international-travel-and-trade-in-relation-to-the-outbreak-of-pneumonia-caused-by-a-new-coronavirus-in-china.
— 2020b. "Statement on the Meeting of the International Health Regulations (2005) Emergency Committee Regarding the Outbreak of Novel Coronavirus 2019 (n-COV) on 23 January 2020." WHO. 23 January 2020. https://www.who.int/news/item/23-01-2020-statement-on-the-meeting-of-the-international-health-regulations-2005)-emergency-committee-regarding-the-outbreak-of-novel-coronavirus-2019-ncov).
— 2020c. "WHO advice for International Traffic in Relation to the Outbreak of the Novel Coronavirus 2019-nCOV (Updated)." WHO. 24 January 2020. https://www.who.int/news-room/articles-detail/updated-who-advice-for-international-traffic-in-relation-to-the-outbreak-of-the-novel-coronavirus-2019-ncov-24-jan.
— 2020d. "WHO Advice for International Traffic in Relation to the Outbreak of the Novel Coronavirus 2019-nCOV (Updated)." WHO. 27 January 2020. https://www.who.int/news-room/articles-detail/updated-who-advice-for-international-traffic-in-relation-to-the-outbreak-of-the-novel-coronavirus-2019-ncov.
— 2020e. "Interim Guidance. Advice on the Use of Masks in the Community, During Home Care and in Health Care Settings in the Context of the Novel Coronavirus (2019-nCOV) Outbreak." WHO. 29 January 2020. https://apps.who.int/iris/handle/10665/330987.
— 2020f. "Statement on the Second Meeting of the International Health Regulations (2005) Emergency Committee Regarding the Outbreak of Novel Coronavirus 2019-nCOV." WHO. 30 January 2020. https://www.who.int/news/item/30-01-2020-statement-on-the-second-meeting-of-the-international-health-regulations-2005)-emergency-committee-regarding-the-outbreak-of-novel-coronavirus-2019-ncov).

— 2020g. "Situation Report 11 – Annex 1." WHO. 31 January 2020. https://www.who.int/docs/default-source/coronavirus/situation-reports/20200131-sitrep-11-ncov.pdf?sfvrsn=de7c0f7_4.

— 2020h. "Strategic Preparedness and Response PLAN (SPRP)." WHO. 4 February 2020. https://www.who.int/docs/default-source/coronaviruse/srp-04022020.pdf.

— 2020i. "Interim Guidance, 'considerations for quarantine of individuals in the context of containment for coronavirus disease (COVID-19)'." WHO. 11 February 2020.

— 2020j. "Interim Guidance, 'Advice on the Use of Masks in the Context of COVID-19'." WHO. 6 April 2020.

— 2020k. "COVID 19 Strategy Update." WHO. 14 April 2020. https://www.who.int/publications-detail-redirect/covid-19-strategy-update---14-april-2020.

— 2020l. "Statement on the Third Meeting of the IHR (2005) Emergency Committee Regarding the Outbreak of Coronavirus Disease (COVID-19)." WHO. 1 May 2020. https://www.who.int/news/item/01-05-2020-statement-on-the-third-meeting-of-the-international-health-regulations-2005)-emergency-committee-regarding-the-outbreak-of-coronavirus-disease-(covid-19).

— 2020m. "Interim Guidance, 'Advice on the Use of Masks in the Context of COVID-19'" WHO. 5 June 2020. https://apps.who.int/iris/handle/10665/332293.

— 2020n. "Situation Report 193." WHO. 3 August 2020. https://www.who.int/docs/default-source/coronaviruse/situation-reports/20200731-covid-19-sitrep-193.pdf?sfvrsn=42a0221d_4.

— 2021. "Timeline: WHO's COVID-19 Response." WHO. https://www.who.int/emergencies/diseases/novel-coronavirus-2019/interactive-timeline.

WHO and UNWTO. 2020. "A Joint Statement on Tourism and COVID-19 – UNWTO and WHO Call for Responsibility and Coordination." WHO and UNWTO. 27 February 2020. https://www.who.int/news/item/27-02-2020-a-joint-statement-on-tourism-and-covid-19---unwto-and-who-call-for-responsibility-and-coordination.

Fortress World: Refugee Protection during (and after) the COVID-19 Pandemic

Y.Y. Brandon Chen

1. INTRODUCTION

International travel restrictions have long been employed by countries to combat disease outbreaks. They have become even more prevalent in the wake of the COVID-19 pandemic. By the end of April 2020, every country and territory in the world has imposed some form of border closures, flight bans, or additional conditions for border entry such as mandatory medical screening and quarantine as a part of their pandemic responses (UN World Tourism Organization 2020).

The effectiveness of entry prohibitions and flight suspensions in curtailing the spread of diseases, however, remains contested. Studies of past epidemics have shown that due to the porosity of borders and gaps in policy implementation, travel restrictions at best delay, rather than prevent, the propagation of diseases (Hoffman and Fafard 2020, 555, 558). Modelling data concerning the current COVID-19 pandemic have reached a similar conclusion, affirming the short-lived effects of travel restrictions on delaying the spread of the virus (Grépin et al. 2020). Once the local epidemic starts to unfold exponentially, the benefit of entry restrictions as an infection control tool greatly diminishes (Russell et al. 2020).

At the same time, international travel restrictions are known to come with serious social and economic consequences (Tejpar and Hoffman 2016). Among other things, these measures are prone to be coopted to serve xenophobic purposes. Especially when they are adopted by countries with high local incidence of concerned diseases, travel restrictions do little more than reinforce the stereotype of migrants as a public health threat and allow politicians to "externalize the responsibility for the [diseases'] spread" (Bieber 2020, 6). Such stigmatization of migrants fuels discrimination against individuals that appear "foreign," which in turn undermines public health by deterring the service access of people who fear being discriminated against (Gover 2020).[1]

Besides these stigmatizing effects, large-scale and prolonged travel restrictions instituted in response to the COVID-19 pandemic have wreaked havoc on the global refugee protection system. International refugee law guarantees everyone "the right to seek and to enjoy in other countries asylum from persecution,"[2] and the right not to be expelled or returned "to the frontiers of territories where [their] life or freedom would be threatened."[3] By limiting people's ability to flee their countries of residence in the first place, measures like border closures and flight suspensions significantly attenuate the realization of these fundamental human rights. Moreover, travel restrictions slow the resettlement of refugees from their initial countries of asylum to another state that is better resourced and more removed from the conflict or natural disaster that causes them to migrate. In a world where 85% of refugees are hosted by lower- and middle-income countries ("LMICs"), disruptions in resettlement efforts necessarily raise concern about the deepening of global injustice (Global Trends Report 2019).

In this chapter, I take a closer look at such impact of COVID-19 related travel restrictions on international refugee protection, with a focus on the availability of asylum and resettlement in high-income countries. I begin by providing a bird's-eye view of the global situation before zeroing on the Canadian context. I show that as the global demand for asylum persists, travel restrictions either trap asylum seekers and refugees in precarious circumstances or force them to attempt more dangerous routes to arrive at intended destinations. Leaning on international law as well as Thomas Pogge's theory of global justice, I argue that affluent countries have a duty to ameliorate these harms perpetrated against one of the world's most vulnerable populations. The fulfilment of this duty will require governments of high-income countries to recalibrate the balance between public health concerns and refugee protection. Inter alia, some exemptions from travel restrictions should be extended to asylum seekers; resettlement programs must be ramped up from their current level; and adequate aid must be provided to support refugees now stranded in LMICs.

2. EFFECTS OF TRAVEL RESTRICTIONS ON INTERNATIONAL REFUGEE PROTECTION

Broadly speaking, individuals may receive refugee protection in high-income countries via one of two ways. They may travel to these countries, apply for asylum, and hope to have their applications approved. Or, they may be identified as refugees in the initial country of asylum and subsequently resettled to a high-income country. Both of these mechanisms have come under threat in recent times.

Over the last several decades, affluent countries have introduced an array of *non-entrée* policies to limit the arrival of asylum seekers (Gammeltoft-Hansen and Hathaway 2015, 241). Some of them have erected physical barriers along their borders while others have routinely conducted maritime interception to deter asylum seekers and other unauthorized migrants from entering by land or by sea (Ghezelbash and Tan 2020, 3–4). Strict visa policies coupled with the requirement that carriers deny boarding to passengers without proper entry documents further stamp out the arrival of many asylum seekers from LMICs by air (Rodenhäuser 2014). In the event that these *non-entrée* practices fail to fully keep asylum seekers at bay, high-income countries have further adopted safe third country policies to send asylum seekers who made it onto their territories to another country deemed capable of offering protection (Ghezelbash and Tan 2019, 4–5). The *Canada-US Safe Third Country Agreement*, for example, allows both countries, with some narrow exceptions, to return asylum seekers who arrive at their respective border crossings via the other country.[4] Between 2016 and 2020, more than 4,400 asylum seekers were turned away by Canada under this agreement (Harris 2020a).

Meanwhile, the commitment of some affluent countries to refugee resettlement has also been on the wane. Whereas governments under international law have binding obligations toward asylum seekers who have reached their territories, their participation in refugee resettlement is completely voluntary, leaving the vigour of resettlement programs highly sensitive to political calculus. Take the United States (US) as an example. The number of refugees it resettles annually has generally trended downward over the past four decades, dropping from more than two hundred thousand refugees admitted in 1980 to below twenty thousand in 2020 (Migration Policy Institute 2020). Commentators have pointed to rising anti-migrant sentiment, Islamophobia, and racial politics as some of the contributors to this decline (Barkdull et al. 2012; Darrow and Scholl 2020). Likewise, in Canada, immigration policies that once emphasized a balance between economic immigrants, family-class immigrants, and refugees now prioritize the first over the other groups (Challinor 2011). The number of refugees resettled to the country relative to the total number of foreign nationals admitted each year as permanent residents has decreased from an average of 18% in the 1980s to an average of 12% during the 2010s (Government of Canada 2018 and 2020c).

Travel restrictions adopted by countries during the COVID-19 pandemic have continued these recent trends and exerted further pressure on the international refugee protection system. According to the United Nations Refugee Agency (UNHCR), over half of the countries that sealed off their borders during the pandemic made no exceptions for asylum seekers (UNHCR 2020a). Among them are high-income countries like Australia, New Zealand, Canada, and a handful of European countries (Ghezelbash and Tan 2020, 5–8; New Zealand Immigration 2020). In the US, an order issued by the Centers for Disease Control and Prevention in March 2020 led to similar results. The order required virtually all unauthorized migrants arriving at the land borders to be returned "as rapidly as possible" (US Centers for Disease Control and Prevention 2020). Between April and December 2020, over 390,000 migrants were removed under this expedited mechanism (US Customs and Border Patrol 2020, 2021). Some of these migrants were reportedly deported within hours of their arrival, which made it almost impossible for them to file for asylum (Lakhani 2020).

Some countries have gone further to actively impede asylum seekers from even reaching their ports of entry. In April 2020, Italy took the unprecedented step of declaring all its seaports "unsafe" for the entire duration of the country's public health emergency, effectively blocking the disembarkation of asylum seekers that have been rescued from the Mediterranean Sea (Tondo 2020). Malta followed suit soon after (Human Rights Watch 2020). The country, along with Cyprus, has also been accused of intercepting and pushing back migrant boats in the name of pandemic response (European Union

Agency for Fundamental Rights 2020). Partly due to such deterrence and *non-entrée* measures, the number of asylum applications received by European countries in April 2020 plummeted by 87% when compared with the figure from January (Huet 2020).

On the refugee resettlement front, pandemic-related travel restrictions have had devastating impact as well. Most countries that partake in refugee resettlement rely on the UNHCR and the International Organization for Migration (IOM) to help them identify eligible refugees and facilitate these refugees' movements. Between 2010 and 2019, of the 1.1 million refugees that were resettled, 70% were through the assistance of the UNHCR (Global Trends Report 2019, 4). In March 2020, however, disruptions to international travel caused the UNHCR and the IOM to temporarily suspend all resettlement departures (UNHCR 2020b). Despite the gradual resumption of resettlement operations a few months later, the number of refugees resettled in 2020 is expected to be the lowest in recent years. As of September 2020, less than 15,500 refugees globally were resettled, compared to over fifty thousand during the same period in the year before (UNHCR 2020e).

The drop in resettlement numbers has heightened existing concerns about the arbitrariness embedded in refugee selection. As governments enjoy considerable lattitude in designing their resettlement programs, they have been criticized for cherry picking refugees based on immigration objectives as opposed to refugees' actual need for protection (de Boer and Zieck 2020). This worry has persisted during the pandemic, as a number of resettlement countries now seek to prioritize the most urgent cases. While such prioritization is not per se problematic, the criteria used by countries to identify refugees in need of emergency protection are not always clear (Garnier 2020). At times, it appears that some of the refugees that were identified for emergency resettlement could have been admitted into the receiving countries through alternative immigration channels such as family reunification programs (Garnier 2020). This raises the spectre that, insofar as resettlement has persevered during the pandemic, it may not be reaching the most vulnerable refugees.

Notwithstanding the diminishing availability of asylum and resettlement, the demand for refugee protection has remained high. The number of asylum applications lodged with European countries in the first two months of 2020 were up by 16% when compared with the same time in the previous year (European Asylum Support

Office 2020). Even when COVID-19 related restrictions have since slowed international movements, with pre-existing conflicts waging on and new ones emerging, the UNHCR has projected the number of refugees worldwide to reach 26.4 million in 2020, slightly higher than the 26 million recorded in 2019 (UNHCR 2020d). Indeed, the pandemic and its related socioeconomic impact could by themselves constitute a driver of displacement. For example, as the pandemic causes more people to be confined to their homes, a rise in domestic and gender-based violence incidents has been reported around the world (Taub 2020; UNHCR 2020f). It is not unthinkable that such violence may drive some people to seek asylum in another country or, in cases involving refugees, flee their current country of asylum.

The result of travel restrictions in the face of such persistent demand for refugee protection is what some have dubbed the "crisis of immobility" (Piccoli 2020). Numerous asylum seekers and refugees are now stranded in their countries of origin, unable to escape active conflicts or persecution. For many refugees that live in LMICs, the COVID-19 pandemic and its economic fallout have stoked discrimination against them and jeopardized their livelihoods and food security (Dempster 2020), while their prospect for resettlement dwindles. As a case in point, a survey conducted by the UNHCR found that 65% of Syrian refugees living in Jordan had permanently lost their jobs because of the pandemic (Alemi et al. 2020). The circumstances are equally dire inside refugee camps and settlements. Not only is the living condition of these camps often overcrowded and not conducive to protective measures against COVID-19, but many residents have also been pushed to the brink of severe food shortage as pandemic-related restrictions aggravate longstanding financial woes (International Organization for Migration 2020). Even refugees who have been selected for resettlement may find themselves suddenly thrust into limbo. As some had left their jobs or sold all their belongings in preparation for their departure, delays in resettlement now leave them with little to fall back on (Bulman 2020).

Because of these challenges, some asylum seekers and refugees have decided to push forward with their migration journeys. But in order to bypass the array of travel restrictions, they are now pressed to attempt routes that are more dangerous. Between January and July 2020, the number of migrants risking the deadly trip across the Mediterranean to reach Europe was up by 91% in comparison with the same period the year before (France 24 2020). More than

1,150 migrants lost their lives doing so in 2020 (Missing Migrants Project 2020). Likewise, there has been a surge in the number of migrants who travelled from the West African coast to the Canary Islands. Whereas fewer than 2,700 people arrived in the Spanish archipelago by boat in the entire 2019, as of the start of December 2020, almost twenty thousand migrants have already done so and close to six hundred people have perished on their journey (Shryock 2020). Interviews conducted with refugees and other migrants in Guatemala and Mexico have uncovered the same trend: since the onset of the COVID-19 pandemic, smugglers have relied on more dangerous routes to facilitate people's movement inside and across countries (Mixed Migration Centre 2020, 3–4).

3. REFUGEE PROTECTION IN CANADA DURING THE COVID-19 PANDEMIC

Having considered the effects of pandemic-related travel restrictions on refugee protection globally, in this section, I turn my gaze to Canada specifically and examine the state of its refugee system in the advent of COVID-19.

In accordance with international law, Canada offers protection to three groups of people: those who qualify as refugees under the *Convention Relating to the Status of Refugees*; people who fled their countries to escape civil war, armed conflict, or massive violation of human rights; and individuals at risk of torture or cruel and unusual treatment or punishment if returned to their countries of origin.[5] Foreign nationals that are deemed eligible can apply for asylum upon reaching a Canadian port of entry or, if they are already inside Canada, at an inland immigration or border services office. Their applications will then be reviewed by an administrative tribunal to determine whether they indeed come within one of the groups that are entitled to protection. In 2019, nearly 58,400 eligible asylum claims were lodged in Canada (Immigration and Refugee Board of Canada 2020).

One reason that migrants may be prevented from claiming asylum in Canada, as mentioned earlier, is if they arrive by land via the US and do not qualify for the narrow exceptions under the *Canada-US Safe Third Country Agreement* (STCA). Some of these exceptions include unaccompanied minors, those with a close family member who is lawfully in Canada, and holders of a valid admission document issued by Canada.[6] But because the STCA only applies to individuals who attempt to enter the country through an official port of entry, some asylum seekers have managed to circumvent it by crossing the Canada-US border at points between these ports. In recent years, the possibility of applying for asylum in Canada following such irregular border crossing provided much needed escape to an increased number of foreign nationals in the US that faced a hostile, anti-migrant environment under the Trump administration (Mercier and Rehaag 2021).

A series of emergency orders introduced by Canada's federal government in the wake of the COVID-19 pandemic, however, has drastically limited foreign nationals' ability to arrive in the country to claim asylum. On 18 March 2020, an Order in Council (OIC) made under the authority of the *Quarantine Act* barred all foreign nationals from entering Canada by air unless they meet certain exceptions.[7] Asylum seekers were not expressly exempted. This ban was buttressed by a subsequent OIC that amended the *Immigration and Refugee Protection Regulations* to require private transportation companies such as airlines to not carry to Canada any foreign national whose entry into the country is forbidden by the *Quarantine Act*.[8]

The scope of entry restrictions prescribed by the OIC issued on 18 March has since been revised on multiple occasions. Among other things, the Canadian government has decided to distinguish between foreign nationals that are seeking to enter Canada from the US and those from all other countries. With respect to the latter, entry prohibition now applies to virtually everyone regardless of the mode of transportation used, unless the foreign national in question is a close family member of a Canadian citizen or permanent resident, possesses a valid authorization to work or study in Canada, or qualifies for certain compassionate grounds.[9] Again, the intention to claim asylum does not by itself exempt a person from this entry ban.

In contrast, since the end of April 2020, asylum application has been allowed to resume for foreign nationals seeking to enter Canada from the US by land, albeit in a much curtailed fashion than before the COVID-19 pandemic. Pursuant to an OIC issued on 22 April, foreign nationals may enter Canada via the US for the purpose of claiming asylum if they cross the border at designated ports of entry, provided that they also meet the exceptions set out in the STCA or are either citizens or stateless habitual residents of the US.[10] The entry of asylum seekers from the US through locations between land ports of entry remains prohibited, meaning that irregular border crossings that were permitted previously under the STCA is now outlawed. Anyone found to contravene this entry ban is to be directed back to the US, a procedure that was in the past reserved for "exceptional circumstances" when dealing with asylum seekers (Mercier and Rehaag 2021). Under such a direct-back order, those who fail to comply or try to enter Canada again while their entry is still prohibited will be excluded from Canada for one year.[11]

The combined effect of these OICs is that, since the COVID-19 pandemic started, it has been exceedingly difficult for foreign nationals to arrive in Canada to claim asylum. For the calendar year of 2020, Canadian immigration and border authorities received just 23,880 asylum applications, representing a decline of more than 60% when compared with the year before (Government of Canada 2021). And over two-thirds of the asylum claims made in 2020 were filed at inland offices by people already inside Canada, whereas the figure from 2019 was 55% (Government of Canada 2021).

Not only do Canada's border restrictions contribute to the global crisis of immobility, they also pose a genuine threat to asylum seekers' human rights. In July 2020, Canada's Federal Court ruled that the STCA in its pre-pandemic form was unconstitutional for having unduly violated asylum seekers' rights to liberty and security of the person (Immigration, Refugees and Citizenship 2020). Among the Court's findings was the fact that some asylum seekers caught by the STCA were immediately detained by US authorities upon being returned by Canadian border officials (Immigration, Refugees and Citizenship 2020, para. 97). While in detention, some of them were placed in solitary confinement and denied access to such basic necessities as culturally-appropriate food, baths, blankets, and adequate medical care (Immigration, Refugees and Citizenship 2020 paras. 110–12). The Court also found that due to trouble accessing legal assistance when being detained, which hurt their chances of establishing an asylum claim in the US, some of the asylum seekers sent back by Canadian officials were in danger of being deported to their former countries of residence where they faced persecution or violence (Immigration, Refugees and Citizenship 2020 paras. 106–09). Barring a sudden change to the US asylum system, one would expect these human rights breaches to continue, if not worsen, during the pandemic as Canada's border restrictions have further increased the chances of asylum seekers being turned back to the US.

Like the asylum process, Canada's resettlement program has suffered as a result of pandemic-related travel restrictions. Between 2010 and 2019, the Canadian government along with private organizations and community groups resettled more than 210,000 refugees to Canada for permanent residence, accounting for one-fifth of all refugee resettlement carried out globally during the decade (Global Trends Report 2019, 52). Since 2018, Canada has led the world in the number of refugees resettled, whereas the previous leader, the US, has cut its annual resettlement ceiling to the lowest level since 1980 (Radford and Connor 2019; Krogstad 2019). Against this backdrop, the reduction of Canada's resettlement efforts during the pandemic arguably has a significant impact on the state of international refugee protection.

At the time of writing, a pair of programs that allow the Canadian government to resettle refugees in partnership with private sponsors (i.e. the Blended Visa Office-Referred Program and the Joint Assistance Sponsorship Program) have been temporarily suspended owing to pandemic-related operational disruptions (Government of Canada 2020d). Other resettlement processes, while continuing, have incurred notable delays. Canada is presently issuing travel documents only to refugees whose resettlement application was approved on or before 18 March 2020, when the country's entry prohibition against foreign nationals was initiated (Government of Canada 2020d). The arrival of refugees whose resettlement was accepted after 18 March has been put on hold until further notice. The only exception to this travel ban is if the approved refugees have immediate family members in Canada or if they qualify for the Urgent Protection Program, which provides rapid resettlement to UNHCR-referred refugees that require emergency protection (Government of Canada 2020d). But even if refugees meet one of these exemptions, their departure for Canada still may be impeded by travel restrictions in their current country of residence, delay in obtaining exit permits, airport closures, or flight suspensions (Harris 2020b).

For all these reasons, the level of resettlement to Canada has fallen sharply during the pandemic. While over 2,700 privately sponsored refugees arrived in Canada between 1 January and 17 March 2020, only 316 did between 18 March and 2 July of that year (Swan 2020). By mid-November, the total number of refugees resettled in Canada for the calendar year was still under six thousand, making it highly unlikely that the government would fulfil its pre-pandemic target of admitting 31,700 refugees in 2020 (Harris 2020b). To make up for this shortfall, the government has raised its resettlement targets for 2021 and 2022 from 31,950 and 32,450 respectively to thirty-six thousand (Government of Canada 2020a and 2020b). These increases, however, even assuming that they can be achieved, do not appear sufficiently large to fully make up for the deficit in 2020.

As seen, such contraction of resettlement opportunities leaves many refugees, including those already approved for relocation to Canada, in precarious situations in LMICs, which have been exacerbated by the global pandemic and its associated economic challenges (Dayal 2020). What is more, reduction in resettlement numbers today could have a knock-on effect on how long it takes refugees to be resettled in the future, as it adds to the backlog of resettlement applications needing to be processed by Canadian immigration officials (Swan 2020). It stands to reason that the longer refugees must wait to be resettled, the greater the toll such wait will have on their wellbeing (see generally Mzayek 2019, 369).

4. INJUSTICE OF FORCED IMMOBILITY

In light of its human cost, the disruption to the global refugee system precipitated by pandemic-related travel restrictions raises both legal and ethical ramifications. And such concerns cannot be overcome by simply acknowledging the purported public health rationale behind the travel restrictions. In this section, I develop these claims further before identifying the responsibilities of high-income countries vis-à-vis asylum seekers and refugees during the pandemic.

Legally, countries are prima facie in breach of international law when they institute travel restrictions that prevent individuals from seeking asylum in their territories. Article 14(1) of the *Universal Declaration of Human Rights*, which is considered part of the customary international law (Boed 1994, 6), recognizes that everyone "has the right to seek and to enjoy in other countries asylum from persecution."[12] It is generally accepted that the right to seek asylum encompasses at minimum a right for individuals who have arrived in a foreign country to apply for refugee protection therein (Worster 2014, 477). This right to accessing asylum proceedings is also tacitly guaranteed in the *Convention Relating to the Status of Refugees*, which requires signatory states to not penalize refugees who "enter or are present in their territory without authorization, provided they present themselves without delay to the authorities."[13] An array of regional human rights instruments further entrenches the right to seek asylum in international law, including Article 18 of the *Charter of Fundamental Rights of the European Union*.[14] When countries outright deny foreign nationals' ability to apply for asylum by physically blocking their arrival, such as by closing their ports of entry, they are certainly acting in contravention of the spirit, if not the substance, of these binding rules.

Additionally, international law prohibits states from expelling or returning refugees to another country where they may suffer such irreparable harm as persecution, torture, ill-treatment, or other serious human rights violations (UNHRC 2007). Indeed, an emerging consensus suggests that this principle of non-refoulement has crystalized into a peremptory norm of the international community and is not subject to any derogation (UNHRC 2007; see also Allain 2001, 533). Thus, even on the pretext of combating the pandemic, the forcible return of asylum seekers by such countries as the US, Malta, and Cyprus to places with questionable human rights records is legally suspect (Dickerson 2020; Amnesty International 2020; and Lyritsas 2020). So, too, is the expansion of safe third country policies during the pandemic, as seen in Canada. To the extent that asylum seekers sent to the supposedly safe countries may lack adequate access to asylum proceedings and are at risk of being deported to danger, as found by Canada's Federal Court in regard to asylum seekers returned to the US, introduction or expansion of safe third country policies as a pandemic response sparks concern about "indirect refoulement." The prohibition against refoulement under international law extends not only to situations where a person may face irreparable harm "in the country to which removal is to be effected," but also when they could incur such risks "in any country to which [they] may subsequently be removed" (UNHRC 2004, 13, para. 12).

Questions about illegality aside, the current upheaval in the international refugee protection regime raises a more fundamental ethical problem. Affluent nations, according to Thomas Pogge, have at least a negative duty to refrain from "imposing on [others] an institutional order that foreseeably produces avoidable human rights deficits" (Pogge 2005, 61). By way of illustration, Pogge argued that this duty to do no harm obliges rich countries to eradicate severe poverty found in parts of the world, seeing as radical inequality and its human costs are a foreseeable and avertable outcome of the prevailing international economic system, which is heavily biased against the global poor (Pogge 2017, 721). In other words, high-income countries as architects of the global order are morally responsible for institutional harms that they "both caused and benefit from" (Parekh 2017, 108).

Pogge's account of global justice illuminates the iniquity of the current immobility crisis. As described, pandemic-related travel restrictions have caused many asylum seekers and refugees to be stranded, most likely in LMICs, where they face persecution, violence, discrimination, and dangerously deteriorating socioeconomic conditions. Many have also been pressed to attempt riskier migration routes to circumvent travel restrictions, with deadly consequences. To quote Pogge, forced immobility has resulted in human rights deficits in asylum seekers and refugees by depriving them of "basic goods [that] are important for both the ethical and the personal value of human life" (Pogge 2008, 55). All the while, the pandemic has seemingly granted high-income states a free pass from refugee protection. This is morally wrong.

As much as governments around the world have defended the necessity of travel restrictions for controlling the spread of covid-19,[15] best available evidence suggests otherwise. As noted at the outset of this chapter, it remains unsettled whether some of the more drastic measures like prolonged, blanket border closures are effective as an infection control tool. To the extent that strict travel restrictions have not completely halted international movements but rather driven desperate migrants to irregular migration channels, they may actually complicate screening and contact tracing efforts and undermine public health objectives (UNHCR 2020d, 2).

As such, the UNHCR has recommended a more balanced approach to regulating asylum seekers' arrival during the pandemic. It urges countries to explicitly exempt asylum seekers from entry bans and to manage travel-related public health risks by way of medical screening and mandatory quarantine (UNHCR 2020d, 2). To the extent that these strategies have been adopted by some European countries without any known detriment to their pandemic responses, they arguably present a workable alternative to the harsher travel restrictions adopted by other high-income countries. Not to mention, in some of the countries that have prohibited the entry of asylum seekers, like Canada, exemptions to entry bans have in fact been provided to other foreign nationals, including migrant workers and international students.[16] There is no reason why asylum seekers should be treated differently.

Equally avoidable is the foreseeable harm flowing from high-income countries' suspension or scaling back of refugee resettlement for reasons of pandemic control. As Pogge explained, this harm demands remedy. To that end, high-income countries must immediately step up their resettlement efforts. Again, most public health risks can be mitigated by admitting refugees on condition that they undergo screening and quarantine. And insofar as resettlement during the pandemic may be hampered by legitimate operational challenges, thus causing countries to fall short of their targets, two sets of responsibility follow for high-income receiving countries. They must provide adequate aid to refugee-hosting LMICs as well as refugee-assisting organizations to help refugees cope with the mischief of forced immobility. They must also significantly boost the level of resettlement post-pandemic to make up for the disruptions in previous years and to clear the accruing backlogs of resettlement applications.

CONCLUSION

The COVID-19 pandemic has laid bare the fragility of the international refugee protection system. It turns out that on account of public health concerns, many countries, Canada included, are quick to abandon their legal duties with respect to the right of asylum and non-refoulement, as well as their commitment to responsibility sharing in the context of refugee resettlement. This has led to an immobility crisis among asylum seekers and refugees, exacting a heavy toll on this already-marginalized group.

Although governments would like us to believe that the status quo is exceptional and the travel restrictions implemented temporary, there are good reasons to worry that the troubling state of international refugee protection at present may well extend into the post-pandemic world. For one thing, even before the COVID-19 pandemic, affluent countries had taken considerable steps to fortify their borders and limit the arrival of asylum seekers. Likewise, their solidarity with refugees was checkered at best. The onset of the pandemic, in many ways, appears to have simply hastened these trends. This may help explain why a good number of countries continue to insist on broad-based entry prohibitions and border closures during the pandemic, despite the clear availability of, and repeated pleas from organizations like the UNHCR for, less harmful alternatives.

To push back against these anti-refugee policies and their potential entrenchment beyond the pandemic, countries must be held accountable for failing to strike a more proportionate balance between safeguarding public health and protecting refugees. Justice, and indeed the very survival of the international refugee protection system, demands nothing less.

NOTES

1. See also Chapter 10 in this book: "Borders and the Global Pandemic of COVID-19" by Élisabeth Vallet, Mathilde Bourgeon, Laurence Brassard, Gabrielle Gagnon, and Julie Renaud.
2. *Universal Declaration of Human Rights*, GA Res 217A (III), UNGAOR, 3rd Sess, Supp No 13, UN Doc A/810 (1948) 71 art 14(1).
3. *Convention Relating to the Status of Refugees*, 28 July 1951, 189 UNTS 137 art 33(1) (entered into force 22 April 1954).
4. *Agreement between the Government of Canada and the Government of the United States of America for cooperation in the examination of refugee status claims from nationals of third countries*, 5 December 2020, Can TS 2004 No 2 (entered into force 29 December 2004) [STCA].
5. *Immigration and Refugee Protection Act (2001)*.
6. *Agreement between the Government of Canada and the Government of the United States of America for cooperation in the examination of refugee status claims from nationals of third countries*, 5 December 2020, Can TS 2004 No 2 (entered into force 29 December 2004) [STCA], 4.
7. *Minimizing the Risk of Exposure to COVID-19 Coronavirus Disease in Canada Order (Prohibition of Entry into Canada)*, PC 2020-0157.
8. *Regulations Amending the Immigration and Refugee Protection Regulations*, PC 2020-160, (2020) C Gaz II, 552 [OIC 2020-160].
9. *Minimizing the Risk of Exposure to COVID-19 in Canada Order (Prohibition of Entry into Canada from any Country other than the United States)*, PC 2021-0010 [OIC 2021-0010].
10. *Minimizing the Risk of Exposure to COVID-19 in Canada Order (Prohibition of Entry into Canada from the United States)*, PC 2020-0263.
11. *Regulations Amending the Immigration and Refugee Protection Regulations*, PC 2020-160, (2020) C Gaz II, 552 [OIC 2020-160].

12 *Universal Declaration of Human Rights*, GA Res 217A (III), UNGAOR, 3rd Sess, Supp No 13, UN Doc A/810 (1948) 71 art 14(1).
13 *Convention Relating to the Status of Refugees*, 28 July 1951, 189 UNTS 137 art 33(1) (entered into force 22 April 1954). Article 31(1).
14 18 December 2000, [2012] OJ, C 326/02. For other regional instruments that guarantee the right to asylum, see, for example, *American Convention on Human Rights*, 22 November 1969, 1144 UNTS 123, art 22(7) (entered into force 18 July 1978); *African Charter on Human and Peoples' Rights*, 27 June 1981, 1520 UNTS 217, art 12(3) (entered into force 21 October 1986).
15 See, for example, OIC 2021-0010 (the preamble indicates that the Canadian federal government is of the view that "no reasonable alternative to prevent the introduction or spread of [COVID-19] are available").
16 OIC 2021-0010.

REFERENCES

Alemi, Qais, Carl Stempel, Hafifa Siddiq, and Eunice Kim. 2020. "Refugees and COVID-19: Achieving a Comprehensive Public Health Response." *Bulletin of the World Health Organization* 98: 510–510A.

Allain, Jean. 2001. "The *Jus Cogens* Nature of *Non-refoulement*." *International Journal of Refugee Law* 13, no. 4: 533–58.

Amnesty International. 2020. "Malta: Illegal tactics Mar Another Year of Suffering in Central Mediterranean." *The Amnesty International report*, 8 September 2020. amnesty.org/en/latest/news/2020/09/malta-illegal-tactics-mar-another-year-of-suffering-in-central-mediterranean/.

Barkdull, Carenlee, Bret Weber, Amy Swart, and Amy Phillips. 2012. "The Changing Context of Refugee Resettlement Policy and Programs in the United States." *Journal of International Social Issues* 1, no. 1: 107–119.

Bieber, Florian. 2020. "Global Nationalism in Times of the COVID-19 Pandemic." *Nationalities Papers*, 1–13. doi:10.1017/nps.2020.35.

Boed, Roman. 1994. "The State of the Right of Asylum in International Law." *Duke Journal of Comparative and International Law* 5, no. 1: 1–34.

Bulman, May. 2020. "'It's Killing Us': These Syrian Refugees Were Set for a New Life in the UK – Then Coronavirus Struck." *The Independent*, 7 October 2020. independent.co.uk/news/uk/home-news/refugees-coronavirus-uk-migrants-resettlement-covid-syria-lebanon-b806953.html.

Canadian Council for Refugees v Canada (Immigration, Refugees & Citizenship), 2020 FC 770.

Challinor, A.E. 2011. "Canada's Immigration Policy: A Focus on Human Capital." *Migration Policy Institute*. migrationpolicy.org/article/canadas-immigration-policy-focus-human-capital.

Chang, Felicia, Helen Prytherch, Robin C Nesbitt, and Annelies Wilder-Smith. 2013. "HIV-Related Travel Restrictions: Trends and Country Characteristics." *Global Health Action* 6, no. 1. doi.org/10.3402/gha.v6i0.20472.

Darrow, Jessica H., and Jess Howsam Scholl. 2020. "Chaos and Confusion: Impacts of the Trump Administration Executive Orders on the US Refugee Resettlement System." *Human Service Organizations: Management, Leadership & Governance* 44, no. 4: 362–80.

Dayal, Pratyush. 2020. "For Amir and Many Refugees, the Pandemic Clouds Dreams of Canada." *The Tyee*, 6 November 2020. thetyee.ca/News/2020/11/06/Refugees-Pandemic-Clouds-Dreams-Canada/.

de Boer, Tom, and Marjoleine Zieck. 2020. "The Legal Abyss of Discretion in the Resettlement of Refugees: Cherry-Picking and the Lack of Due Process in the EU." *International Journal of Refugee Law* 32, no. 1: 54–85.

Dempster, Helen, Thomas Ginn, Jimmy Graham, Martha Guerrero Ble, Daphne Jayasinghe, and Barri Shorey. 2020. "Locked Down and Left Behind: The Impact of COVID-19 on Refugees' Economic Inclusion." *Refugees International*. 8 July 2020. https://www.refugeesinternational.org/reports/2020/7/6/locked-down-and-left-behind-the-impact-of-covid-19-on-refugees-economic-inclusion.

Dickerson, Caitlin. 2020. "10 Years Old, Tearful and Confused After a Sudden Deportation." *New York Times*, 21 October 2020. nytimes.com/2020/05/20/us/coronavirus-migrant-children-unaccompanied-minors.html.

European Asylum Support Office. 2020. "COVID-19: Asylum Applications Down by 43% in March." *European Asylum Support Office*. 30 April 2020. easo.europa.eu/news-events/covid-19-asylum-applications-down-march.

European Union Agency For Fundamental Rights. 2020. "Migration: Key Fundamental Rights Concerns – Quarterly Bulletin 2 – 2020." *European Union Agency For Fundamental Rights*. 27 May 2020. fra.europa.eu/en/publication/2020/migration-key-fundamental-rights-concerns-quarterly-bulletin-2-2020.

Gammeltoft-Hansen, Thomas, and James C. Hathaway. 2015. "*Non-Refoulement* in a World of Cooperative Deterrence." *Columbia Journal of Transnational Law* 53, no. 2: 235–84.

Garnier, Adèle. 2020. "The COVID-19 Resettlement Suspension: Impact, Exemptions and the Road Ahead." *FluchtforschungsBlog*, 16 June 2020. blog.fluchtforschung.net/the-covid-19-resettlement-suspension/.

Ghezelbash, Daniel, and Nikolas Feith Tan. 2020. "The End of the Right to Seek Asylum? COVID-19 and the Future of Refugee Protection." *European University Institute* Working Paper: 1–10.

Gover, Angela R., Shannon B. Harper, and Lynn Langton. 2020. "Anti-Asian Hate Crime During the COVID-19 Pandemic: Exploring the Reproduction of Inequality." *American Journal of Criminal Justice* 45: 647–67.

Government of Canada. 2018. "Permanent Residents – Ad Hoc IRCC (Specialized Datasets)." *Government of Canada*. 20 March 2018. open.canada.ca/data/en/dataset/ad975a26-df23-456a-8ada-756191a23695.

—. 2020a. "Notice – Supplementary Information for 2020–2022 Immigration Levels Plan." *Government of Canada*. 12 March 2020. canada.ca/en/immigration-refugees-citizenship/news/notices/supplementary-immigration-levels-2020.html.

—. 2020b. "Notice – Supplementary Information for 2021–2022 Immigration Levels Plan." *Government of Canada*. 30 October 2020. canada.ca/en/immigration-refugees-citizenship/news/notices/supplementary-immigration-levels-2021-2023.html.

—. 2020c. "Permanent Residents – Monthly IRCC Updates." *Government of Canada*. 11 December 2020. open.canada.ca/data/en/dataset/f7e5498e-0ad8-4417-85c9-9b8aff9b9eda.

—. 2020d. "Resettlement: COVID-19 Program Delivery." *Government of Canada*. 22 September 2020. canada.ca/en/immigration-refugees-citizenship/corporate/publications-manuals/operational-bulletins-manuals/service-delivery/coronavirus/resettlement.html.

—. 2021. "Asylum Claims by Year – 2020." *Government of Canada*. 14 January 2021. canada.ca/en/immigration-refugees-citizenship/services/refugees/asylum-claims/asylum-claims-2020.html.

Grépin, Karen A., Tsi Lok Ho, Zhihan Liu, Summer Marion, Julianne Piper, Catherine Z. Worsnop, and Kelley Lee. 2020. "Evidence of the Effectiveness of Travel-Related Measures During the Early Phase of the COVID-19 Pandemic: A Rapid Systematic Review." *medRxiv*. https://doi.org/10.1101/2020.11.23.20236703

Harris, Kathleen. 2020a. "Canada Has Turned Back 4,400 Asylum Seekers in 5 Years." *CBC*, 24 November 2020. cbc.ca/news/politics/asylum-seekers-canada-us-trump-pandemic-1.5813211.

—. 2020b. "Refugee Advocates Say Canada Must Step Up Resettlement

Efforts Despite Pandemic." *CBC News,* 12 November 2020. cbc.ca/news/politics/refugees-canada-pandemic-mendicino-1.5797361.

Hoffman, Steven J., and Patrick Fafard. 2020. "Border Closures: A Pandemic of Symbolic Acts in the Time of COVID-19." In *Vulnerable: The Law, Policy and Ethics of COVID-19,* edited by Jane Philpott, Vanessa MacDonnell, Sophie Thériault, Sridhar Venkatapuram, and Colleen M. Flood. Ottawa: University of Ottawa Press, 2020.

Huet, Natalie. 2020. "EU Asylum Claims Drop to Lowest Level in 12 Years Amid COVID-19 Border Closures." *EuroNews,* 12 June 2020. euronews.com/2020/06/12/eu-asylum-claims-drop-to-lowest-level-in-12-years-amid-covid-19-border-closures.

Human Rights Watch. 2020. "Malta: Disembark Rescued People." *Human Rights Watch,* 22 May 2020. hrw.org/news/2020/05/22/malta-disembark-rescued-people.

Immigration and Refugee Board of Canada. 2020. "Refugee Protection Claims (New System) by Country of Alleged Persecution – 2019." *Immigration and Refugee Board of Canada.* 22 September 2020. irb-cisr.gc.ca/en/statistics/protection/Pages/RPDStat2019.aspx.

Krogstad, Jens Manuel. 2019. "Key Facts about Refugees to the US" *Pew Research Center,* 7 October 2019. pewresearch.org/fact-tank/2019/10/07/key-facts-about-refugees-to-the-u-s/.

Lakhani, Nina. 2020. "US Using Coronavirus Pandemic to Unlawfully Expel Asylum Seekers, Says UN." *The Guardian,* 17 April 2020. theguardian.com/world/2020/apr/17/us-asylum-seekers-coronavirus-law-un.

Lyritsas, Loukianos. 2020. "Refugee Pushbacks by Cyprus Draw Attention from EU, UN." DW, 16 September 2020. dw.com/en/refugee-pushbacks-by-cyprus-draw-attention-from-eu-un/a-54908678.

Mercier, Elise and Sean Rehaag. 2020. "The Right to Seek Asylum in Canada (During a Global Pandemic)." *Osgoode Hall Law Journal* 57, no. 3: 705–738.

Migration Policy Institute. 2020. "US Annual Refugee Resettlement Ceilings and Number of Refugees Admitted, 1980–Present." *Migration Policy Institute.* migrationpolicy.org/programs/data-hub/charts/us-annual-refugee-resettlement-ceilings-and-number-refugees-admitted-united.

Missing Migrants Project. 2020. "Spotlight on the Mediterranean." *Missing Migrants Project.* 29 December 2020. missingmigrants.iom.int/region/mediterranean.

Mixed Migration Centre. 2020. "Refugees and Migrants in Guatemala and Mexico: A Focus on Smuggling During the COVID-19 Pandemic."

Mixed Migration Centre: 1–4. mixedmigration.org/wp-content/uploads/2020/12/155_covid_snapshot_smuggling_LAC.pdf.

Mzayek, May. 2019. "Understanding Waiting and Wellbeing Through Liminal Experiences of Syrian Refugees." *Migration Letters* 16, no. 3: 369–77.

News Wires. 2020. "Boat Carrying Nearly 370 Migrants Reaches Italy's Lampedusa." France 24, 30 August 2020. france24.com/en/20200830-boat-carrying-nearly-370-migrants-reaches-italy-s-lampedusa.

New Zealand Immigration. 2020. "Border Restrictions: How to Enter New Zealand or Request to Travel." *New Zealand Immigration*. immigration.govt.nz/about-us/covid-19/border-closures-and-exceptions.

Parekh, Serena. 2017. *Refugees and the Ethics of Forced Displacement*. New York: Routledge.

Pogge, Thomas. 2005. "Severe Poverty as a Violation of Negative Duties." *Ethics and International Affairs* 19, no. 1: 55–83.

– 2008. *World Poverty and Human Rights*, 2nd ed. Cambridge, UK: Polity Press.

– 2017. "Severe Poverty as a Human Rights Violation." In *Challenges in International Human Rights Law*, vol 3, edited by Menno T Kamminga. London: Taylor & Francis.

Piccoli, Lorenzo. 2020. "Coronavirus Restrictions on Movement May Jeopardize the Lives of the Most Vulnerable." *Washington Post*, 5 April 2020. washingtonpost.com/politics/2020/04/05/coronavirus-restrictions-movement-may-jeopardize-lives-most-vulnerable/.

Radford, Jynnah and Phillip Connor. 2019. "Canada Now Leads the World in Refugee Resettlement, Surpassing the US" *Pew Research Center*, 19 June 2019. pewresearch.org/fact-tank/2019/06/19/canada-now-leads-the-world-in-refugee-resettlement-surpassing-the-u-s/.

Rodenhäuser, TIlman. 2014. "Another Brick in the Wall: Carrier Sanctions and the Privatization of Immigration Control." *International Journal of Refugee Law* 26, no. 2: 223–47.

Russell, Timothy W., Joseph T. Wu, Sam Clifford, W. John Edmunds, Adam J. Kucharski, and Mark Jit. 2020. "Effect of Internationally Imported Cases on Internal Spread of COVID-19: A Mathematical Modelling Study." *The Lancet* 6, no. 1. doi.org/10.1016/S2468-2667(20)30263-2.

Shryock, Ricci. 2020. "What's Driving the Deadly Migrant Surge from Senegal to the Canary Islands?" *The New Humanitarian*, 7 December 2020. thenewhumanitarian.org/news-feature/2020/12/7/senegal-canary-islands-migration-overfishing-coronavirus-restrictions.

Swan, Michael. "COVID-19 Crisis Could Increase Refugee Backlog Say Canadian Advocates." *Catholic Saskatoon News*, 15 July 2020. news.rcdos.ca/2020/07/15/covid-19-crisis-could-increase-refugee-backlog/.

Taub, Amanda. 2020. "A New Covid-19 Crisis: Domestic Abuse Rises Worldwide." *New York Times*, 6 April 2020. nytimes.com/2020/04/06/world/coronavirus-domestic-violence.html.

Tejpar, Ali, and Steven J Hoffman. 2016. "Canada's Violation of International Law During the 2014–2016 Ebola Outbreak." *Canadian Yearbook of International Law/Annuaire Canadien De Droit International* 54: 366–383.

Tondo, Lorenzo. 2020. "Italy Declares Own Ports 'Unsafe' to Stop Migrants Arriving." *The Guardian*, 8 April 2020. theguardian.com/world/2020/apr/08/italy-declares-own-ports-unsafe-to-stop-migrants-disembarking.

US Centers for Disease Control. 2020. "Order Suspending Introduction of Certain Persons from Countries Where a Communicable Disease Exists." *US Centers for Disease Control*. 13 October 2020.cdc.gov/quarantine/pdf/CDC-Order-Prohibiting-Introduction-of-Persons_Final_3-20-20_3-p.pdf.

US Customs and Border Protection. 2020. "FY 2020 Nationwide Enforcement Encounters: Title 8 Enforcement Actions and Title 42 Expulsions." *US Customs and Border Protection*. 20 November 2020. cbp.gov/newsroom/stats/cbp-enforcement-statistics/title-8-and-title-42-statistics-fy2020.

– 2021. "Nationwide Enforcement Encounters: Title 8 Enforcement Actions and Title 42 Expulsions." *US Customs and Border Protection*. 10 February 2021. cbp.gov/newsroom/stats/cbp-enforcement-statistics/title-8-and-title-42-statistics.

UNHCR. 2019. "Global Trends: Forced Displacement in 2019." UNHCR. https://www.unhcr.org/globaltrends2019/#:~:text=One%20per%20cent%20of%20the,people%20%E2%80%93%20is%20now%20forcibly%20displaced.&text=During%202019%2C%20an%20estimated%2011.0,the%20borders%20of%20their%20countries.

– 2020a. "COVID-19 Crisis Underlines Need for Refugee Solidarity and Inclusion." UNHCR, 7 October 2020. unhcr.org/news/latest/2020/10/5f7dfbc24/covid-19-crisis-underlines-need-refugee-solidarity-inclusion.html.

– 2020b. "IOM, UNHCR Announce Temporary Suspension of Resettlement Travel for Refugees." UNHCR, 17 March 2020. unhcr.org/news/

press/2020/3/5e7103034/iom-unhcr-announce-temporary-suspension-resettlement-travel-refugees.html.
- 2020c. "Mid-Year Trends." UNHCR. https://www.unhcr.org/5fc504d44.pdf.
- 2020d. "Practical Recommendations and Good Practice to Address Protection Concerns in the Context of the COVID-19 Pandemic." UNHCR. unhcr.org/cy/wp-content/uploads/sites/41/2020/04/Practical-Recommendations-and-Good-Practice-to-Address-Protection-Concerns-in-the-COVID-19-Context-April-2020.pdf
- 2020e. "UNHCR Warns 2020 Risks Lowest Resettlement Levels in Recent History." UNHCR, 19 November 2020. unhcr.org/news/press/2020/11/5fb4e6f24/unhcr-warns-2020-risks-lowest-resettlement-levels-recent-history.html.
- 2020f. "UNHCR Warns Second Wave of COVID Pandemic Driving Further Violence against Refugee Women and Girls." UNHCR, 25 November 2020. unhcr.org/news/press/2020/11/5fbe0f394/unhcr-warns-second-wave-covid-pandemic-driving-further-violence-against.html.

UNHRC. 2004. *General Comment No. 31: The Nature of the General Legal Obligation Imposed on State Parties to the Covenant, 80th Session*, adopted 26 May 2004, UN Doc CCPR/C/21/Rev.1/Add. 13, para. 12. https://www.refworld.org/docid/478b26ae2.html
- 2007. "Advisory Opinion on the Extraterritorial Application of *Non-Refoulement* Obligations under the 1951 Convention Relating to the Status of Refugees and its 1967 Protocol." UNHRC, 26 January 2007. https://www.refworld.org/docid/45f17a1a4.html.

World Food Program. 2020. "Population at Risk: Implications of COVID-19 for Hunger, Migration and Displacement." *World Food Program*, 9 November 2020. https://www.wfp.org/publications/populations-risk-implications-covid-19-hunger-migration-displacement-2020.

World Tourism Organization. 2020. "100% of Global Destinations Now Have COVID-19 Travel Restrictions, UNWTO reports." *World Tourism Organization*, 28 April 2020. unwto.org/news/covid-19-travel-restrictions.

Worster, William Thomas. 2014. "The Contemporary International Law Status of the Right to Receive Asylum." *International Journal of Refugee Law* 26, no. 4: 477–99.

Contributors

HASSANE ALAMI holds a bachelor's degree in biology (Sorbonne University – UPMC/Paris VI), a master's degree in public health and biomedical informatics (Faculty of Medicine of Rennes), a master's degree in administration of public health policies (School of Advanced Studies in Public Health and Rennes Institute of Political Studies) and a PhD in community health (Laval University, Quebec). He is a postdoctoral fellow with the In Fieri research program on Responsible Innovation in Health (RIH) at the Public Health Research Center (CRESP) of the University of Montreal. His research focuses on the challenges raised by the integration of innovative technologies into health systems, in particular artificial intelligence and digital solutions.

MATHILDE BOURGEON is a PhD student in political science at the University of Quebec in Montreal and researcher at the Raoul-Dandurand Chair in Strategic and Diplomatic Studies within the Center of Geopolitics and the Center for United States Studies. Her research focuses on security studies, borders, immigration and climate change politics, and undocumented migration in North America.

LAURENCE BRASSARD is a master's student in political science at the University of Quebec in Montreal and Fellow Researcher at the Raoul-Dandurand Chair in Strategic and Diplomatic Studies within the Center of Geopolitics and the Center for United States Studies. Her research focuses on seasonal workers, borders, and immigration with a feminist perspective.

GAËLLE CACHAT-ROSSET is a member of the BMO Chair in Diversity and Governance, School of Industrial Relations at the University of Montreal. She holds a PhD in management sciences (Toulouse Business School). Her research interests include the development of skills in digital work environments and diversity and inclusion management practices in organizations.

STÉPHANIE B.M. CADEDDU received her doctorate in the management of frugal innovation in start-ups at Swinburne University of Technology (Australia) in 2018. She is now a post-doctoral researcher at the Health Hub: Politics, Organizations, and Law (Canada) since September 2019 and focuses on the WHO's normative leadership; on "bottom-up" innovations in health organizations; on responsible, digital, and frugal innovation; and on equity in healthcare systems. She has also collaborated with practitioners and academics in the assistive technology (AT) sector and the WHO to integrate frugal innovation with AT equipment.

KEVIN CARILLO is associate professor in data science and information systems at Toulouse Business School (France). He is the director of the Master of Science in Big Data, Marketing, and Management. His current research interests include artificial intelligence, big data and data-driven business, free and open source software communities, online communities, and peer production.

CHRISTOS CARRAS read philosophy at Cambridge University and then at the Sorbonne where he earned his PhD. Since 2000, he has been working in the cultural sector, initially as the project manager of the EU funded MediMuses network. In 2009, he joined the Onassis Foundation as the executive director of the Onassis Cultural Centre. He is responsible for the music program and other interdisciplinary projects, developing European networks and the overall coordination of the Centre. He regularly writes on themes related to the aesthetics and sociology of sonic art and cultural policy.

CLARA CHAMPAGNE holds a joint degree in civil and common law (BCL/JD) from McGill University and an MSc from the University of Montreal. She is a PhD student in communication at the University of Montreal. Her doctoral research focuses on the science of science communication.

Y.Y. BRANDON CHEN is an assistant professor at the University of Ottawa's Faculty of Law (Common Law Section). He holds a doctor of juridical science, juris doctor, and master's of social work from University of Toronto. His current research leverages socio-legal studies, action research, and community engagement to critically examine health inequities facing noncitizens and racialized minorities. His published work has touched on such topics as migrant health care, the right to health, law as a social determinant of health, and health care solidarity.

MIRIAM COHEN is an assistant professor of international law and human rights at Université de Montréal. She is the author of *Realizing Reparative Justice for International Crimes* (Cambridge University Press). She holds a PhD in international law from Leiden University, and a master's of law from Harvard Law School and from the University of Cambridge. Prior to her academic career, she practiced international law at the International Court of Justice (United Nations) and the International Criminal Court. She is a barrister and solicitor with the Quebec Bar and has appeared as Counsel before the International Tribunal for the Law of the Sea.

JEAN-LOUIS DENIS is a full professor in health policy and management at the School of Public Health, Université de Montréal – CRCHUM. He holds the Canada Research Chair on design and adaptation of health systems and is the co-founder of the Health Hub: Politics, Organizations, and Law (H-POD). His research program is located at the intersection of applied health services research, organizational studies and policy research. Dr Denis is a member of the Academy of Social Sciences of the Royal Society of Canada (2002), fellow of the Canadian Academy of Health Sciences (2009), and fellow of the UK Academy of Social Sciences (2019). His work has been published in top health policy, public sector, and management journals like *BMC Health Services Research*, *Journal of Health Politics, Policy and Law*, *Human Relations*, *Organization Science*, *Academy of Management Annals*, and *Journal of Public Administration Research and Theory*.

Since 2016, he has been co-editor of the Organizational Behaviour in Healthcare series at Palgrave.

LISA FORMAN is the Canada Research Chair in Human Rights and Global Health Equity (Tier 2), and an associate professor at the Dalla Lana School of Public Health (University of Toronto). She is an international human rights law scholar whose research explores how the right to health may contribute to reducing global health inequities. Professor Forman qualified as an attorney of the High Court of South Africa, with a BA and LLB from the University of the Witwatersrand. Her graduate studies include a master's in human rights studies from Columbia University and a doctorate in juridical science from the University of Toronto's Faculty of Law.

GAËLLE FOUCAULT holds a master's degree in international law at the University of Lyon III, and is now a PhD candidate in law at the University of Montreal. Her research is mainly focused on public international law, international organizations, international criminal law, and human rights.

GABRIELLE GAGNON is a master's student in political science at the University of Quebec in Montreal and fellow researcher at the Raoul-Dandurand Chair in Strategic and Diplomatic Studies within the Center of Geopolitics. Her researches focus on borders and migratory flows in North Africa and the Middle East.

PHIL JAMES is professor of employment relations at Middlesex University in London. He has researched and published widely in the fields of both employment relations and occupational health and safety through both books and published papers. Areas of recent research have encompassed the employment implications of the personalization of social care services, the impact on staff recruitment and retention of introducing a living wage for care workers, the occupational health and safety dynamics within both domestic and global supply chains, and, most recently, regulatory responses to the workplace risks of COVID-19.

NICHOLAS KING is an associate professor in the Biomedical Ethics Unit and associate member in the Institute for Health and Social

Policy, and the Department of Epidemiology, Biostatistics, and Occupational Health at McGill University. He directs the Policy and Data Science program and is a board member of the Center for Social and Cultural Data Sciences at McGill. Dr King studies the ways that "black boxes" of all sorts – from seemingly objective measures of health and health inequalities, to complex algorithms – are shaped by human interests and hidden value judgments, which in turn shape individual decisions, collective behaviours, and public policies. He has published in the *Milbank Quarterly*, *Annals of Internal Medicine*, BMJ, PLOS *Medicine*, the *American Journal of Public Health*, and the *Bulletin of the World Health Organization*.

ALAIN KLARSFELD is senior professor at TBS Business School in Toulouse (France). He has been doing research on skill-based management, corporate social responsibility, international human resource management and equality, diversity, and inclusion. His present research includes talent management, gendered careers, gender pay gap, comparative equality and diversity management, the management of religious diversity, diversity climate, and remote work.

QUILL R KUKLA is professor of philosophy and senior research scholar in the Kennedy Institute of Ethics at Georgetown University, as well as a Humboldt Research scholar at Leibniz Universität Hannover. They are the editor-in-chief of the *Kennedy Institute of Ethics Journal*. In addition to holding a PhD in philosophy from the University of Pittsburgh, Kukla completed a postdoctoral fellowship at Johns Hopkins School of Public Health and an MA in urban geography at CUNY, and is currently completing a master's degree in urban planning at Georgetown University. Their latest book, forthcoming from Oxford University Press, is entitled *City Living: How Urban Spaces and Urban Dwellers Make One Another*. Kukla is also an amateur competitive boxer and powerlifter.

ETIENNE LALÉ is an associate professor in the department of economics at the University of Quebec in Montreal. He received his PhD in economics at Sciences Po Paris in 2013. His research focuses on macroeconomics and labour economics, with a special interest in understanding cyclical and secular fluctuations in labour markets. His work has been published in the best academic journals of his field, such as *American Economic Journal: Macroeconomics*. His current research on the labour market impacts of the COVID-19 pandemic crisis has been discussed regularly in the *Wall Street Journal*.

PIERRE LAROUCHE holds the chair of Law and Innovation at the University of Montreal, where he is associate dean for curriculum development, and quality, and director of the new PhD program on Innovation, Science, Technology, and Law. He is a graduate of McGill University, Bonn University, and Maastricht University, and he was a law clerk at the Supreme Court of Canada. Larouche was professor of competition law at Tilburg University (Netherlands) from 2002 to 2017, where he founded and directed the Tilburg Law and Economics Center (TILEC), one of the largest research centres on economic governance. His research centres around economic governance, and in particular how law and regulation struggle to deal with complex phenomena such as innovation. His works have been cited by the European Court of Justice and the UK Supreme Court, and have influenced EU policy on electronic communications and competition. He currently teaches competition law, economic regulation, tort law, as well as patents and trademarks.

PASCALE LEHOUX is professor with the Department of Health Management, Evaluation and Policy at the School of Public Health of the University of Montreal. Her research seeks to improve our understanding of and ability to govern technological change in health. She published around 150 scientific papers on computerized medical records, telemedicine, science and policy networks, home care equipment used by patients, mobile and satellite dialysis units, and the impact of technology assessment on policy-making. The goal of her research program, In Fieri, is to generate knowledge on the design, financing, and commercialization of Responsible Innovation in Health (RIH). This seven-year research program focuses on the ways hybrid organizations such as social enterprises, impact investing, and alternative business models can lead to innovations that better address the needs and challenges of health systems.

ERIC LEWIS is a professor of philosophy and an associate member of the department of Music Research at McGill University. He is the author of: *Intents and Purposes: Philosophy and the Aesthetics of*

Improvisation; *The Video Art of Sylvia Safdie*; *Alexander of Aphrodisias on Bk. IV of Aristotle's Meterologica*; and co-editor of *Improvisation and Social Aesthetics*. He is the director of The Laboratory of Urban Culture (LUC), and former director of the Institute for the Public Life of Arts and Ideas (IPLAI). His research focuses on the philosophy of improvised art, including new digital art. He is a member of the new media art collective Medea Electronique and numerous improvising music ensembles where he performs on brass and electronics.

KATHERINE LIPPEL, LLL, LLM, FRSC, is a full professor of law at the Faculty of Law (Civil Law Section) of the University of Ottawa and distinguished research chair in Occupational Health and Safety Law. The focus of her research is on legal issues relating to occupational health and safety, workers' compensation, and return to work after work injury and includes, in particular, an interest in health effects of compensation systems, regulatory challenges related to precarious employment and globalisation, and health and safety issues related to gender. Research awards received include the Prize for Excellence in Research, from the University of Ottawa and the Award for Academic Excellence of the Canadian Association of Law Teachers. A fellow of the Royal Society of Canada (2010), in 2017 she received the Council's highest award: the Social Sciences and Humanities Research Council Gold Medal.

JOSIANNE MARSAN is vice dean of research and innovation, full professor in information systems (IS), and head of the Centre de recherche en technologies de l'information et affaires (CERTIA) at the Faculty of Business Administration at Université Laval (Quebec). She holds a PhD in business administration with a focus on IS and information technology (IT) from HEC Montreal.

BARBARA NEIS, PhD, FRSC, CM, is John Lewis Paton Distinguished University Professor in the Department of Sociology, Memorial University of Newfoundland. Professor Neis received her PhD in sociology from the University of Toronto in 1988. She is a past president of the Canadian Association for Research on Work and Health. Professor Neis has worked for more than two decades in multi-disciplinary teams carrying out research in marine and coastal contexts including on social and environmental change, occupational health and safety, and mobile work. She is currently project director on an eight-year SSHRC-funded partnership grant entitled *On the Move: Employment-Related Geographical Mobility in the Canadian Context*. She is also the former co-director of the SafetyNet Centre for Occupational Health and Safety Research, a member of the Order of Canada, and a fellow of the Royal Society of Canada.

SOPHIE OSOTIMEHIN is an associate professor of Economics at the University of Québec at Montreal. She studies macroeconomic productivity, innovation, and firm growth. Before joining the University of Québec at Montreal in 2018, she was an assistant professor at the University of Virginia. She obtained her PhD in economics from the Paris School of Economics in 2011.

RENATA POZELLI SABIO holds a bachelor's degree in food sciences (University of São Paulo) and a master's degree in administration (Higher School of Advertising and Marketing). She is a PhD candidate and a research assistant with the In Fieri research program on Responsible Innovation in Health (RIH) at the Public Health Research Center of the University of Montreal (CRESP). Her thesis focuses on food systems transition, analyzing the emergence of responsible organizations and practices in food systems from different economic contexts.

ANDREW POTTER is associate professor at the Max Bell School of Public Policy at McGill University. He is the former editor-in-chief of the *Ottawa Citizen* and holds a PhD in philosophy from the University of Toronto.

CATHERINE RÉGIS is a full professor at the Faculty of Law of the University of Montreal and holds a Canada Research Chair in Health Law and Policy. She is the co-founder of the Health Hub: Politics, Organizations, and Law, as well as a researcher at the Centre de recherche en droit public (CRDP), Mila (a research institute in artificial intelligence), and the Centre de recherche du Centre hospitalier universitaire de l'Université de Montréal (CRCHUM). Her main areas of research are health law and policy, law and digital innovation (including artificial intelligence), collaborative governance in healthcare systems, and global health law. She has published numerous articles, book chapters, and books, and she collaborates to public policy debates in Quebec, Canada and internationally.

JESS REIA is currently appointed as Andrew W. Mellon postdoctoral researcher in the Department of Art History and Communication Studies at McGill University, and BMO postdoctoral fellow at the Centre for Interdisciplinary Research on Montreal (CIRM). They are a member of the Conseil de Nuit at MTL 24/24 (2020–2022). Reia's work appears in *Nocturnes: Popular Music and the Night* (Palgrave Macmillan, 2019), *Shadow Libraries: Access to Knowledge in Global Higher Education* (The MIT Press, 2018), and *Mapping Digital Media Brazil* (OSF/FGV, 2014).

JULIE RENAUD is a master's student in political science at the University of Quebec in Montreal and fellow researcher at the Raoul-Dandurand Chair in Strategic and Diplomatic Studies within the Center of Geopolitics. Her research focuses on borders, climate change, and migration.

FELIX RIGOLI is researcher and lecturer at Nucleo de Bioetica e Diplomacia em Saude (NETHIS-FIOCRUZ; Brazil). He has acted as council member and adviser in many organizations and is currently a member of the Outreach Project for Complexity and COVID-19 at the University of Sao Carlos. He is a guest lecturer and speaker at the Universidade de Sao Paulo, Universitey de Montreal, Universidade Federal de Rio de Janeiro, Universidade de Campinas, Universidad de la Republica, and many others. He holds a PhD in complex systems and healthcare from Universidade de Sao Paulo, an MD (Medical Doctor) from Universidad de la Republica Uruguay, and an MSc in Health Management from University of Montreal.

LYSANNE RIVARD holds a bachelor's degree in psychology, a master's degree in child studies and a PhD in educational studies from McGill University (Montreal). She is senior research adviser with the In Fieri research program on Responsible Innovation in Health (RIH) at the Public Health Research Center of the University of Montreal (CRESP). Health, gender equality, technology, and innovative practices that value and integrate participants' knowledge and priorities are at the heart of her research interests. With In Fieri, she conducts qualitative and participatory research with health innovators on the design and operationalization of RIH.

TANIA SABA is the founder and holder of the BMO Chair in Diversity and Governance and is a full professor at the School of Industrial Relations at the University de Montreal. Professor Saba has published extensively on issues of diversity management, workforce aging, intergenerational value differences, knowledge transfer, future skills, transformation of employment relations, and work organization. Her publications were awarded on many occasions. She collaborates on major research projects with public and private organizations on issues of employment integration and adaptation of disadvantaged groups. In addition to her academic career, Tania Saba has held several leadership positions at the University of Montreal; first female chair of the School of Industrial Relations (2008–2010); associate dean of Undergraduate Studies (2010–2012) and associate dean of Graduate Studies and External Affairs at the Faculty of Arts and Sciences (2012–2015). She acted as dean of the Faculty of Arts and Science from 2015 to 2017.

HUDSON P. SILVA holds a bachelor's degree in economics (State University of Campinas), a PhD in public health (University of São Paulo) and completed his postdoctoral studies in health innovation (University of Montreal). He is a senior research adviser with the In Fieri research program on Responsible Innovation in Health, based at the Public Health Research Center (CRESP) of the University of Montreal. He was previously a public policy and management professor at the State University of Campinas. He also worked as a technical adviser for the Brazilian Ministry of Health and as a research assistant at the Center for Public Policy Studies (University of Campinas) and at the Department of Social and Preventive Medicine (University of São Paulo).

WILL STRAW is James McGill professor of urban media studies at McGill University in Montreal, where he teaches within the Department of Art History and Communications Studies. He is the author of *Cyanide and Sin: Visualizing Crime in 50s America* (Andrew Roth Gallery, 2006) and co-editor of several volumes including

The Cambridge Companion to Rock and Pop (with Simon Frith and John Street, 2001), *Circulation and the City: Essays on Urban Culture* (with Alexandra Boutros, 2010), *Formes Urbaines* (with Anouk Bélanger and Annie Gérin, 2014), and *The Oxford Handbook of Canadian Cinema* (with Janine Marchessault, 2019).

TIM TENBENSEL is an associate professor in health policy at the School of Population Health, University of Auckland, New Zealand, where he has been based since 2005. Since the late 1990s he has researched and published extensively in the areas of health and public policy, comparative health policy, health policy implementation, and New Zealand health services research. His current research interests are focused on primary health care policy and performance management in New Zealand and in comparative contexts.

ÉLISABETH VALLET is currently associate professor in international studies at the RMCC-Saint Jean, director of the Center for Geopolitical Studies at the Raoul-Dandurand Chair – UQAM as well as Quebec research lead for the Borders in Globalization program (University of Victoria). Her current research focuses on borders and globalization, border governance and border fencing. She has published several books and scientific articles, both in French and English, the most recent of which are *Borders and Border Walls-In-Security, Symbolism, Vulnerabilities* (co-edited, Routledge 2020) and *Comment Trump a changé le monde* (co-authored, Éditions du CNRS 2020). She is also a regular chronicler for the Canadian National Network (Radio-Canada) as well as the newspaper *Le Devoir*. She was awarded the 2017 Richard Morrill Outreach Award. She is also a 2020–2022 Canadian International Council fellow.

JUSTIN WARING is professor of medical sociology and healthcare organization at the Heath Services Management Centre, University of Birmingham. Professor Waring's work focuses on the changing organization and governance of health care services. He is particularly interested in applying sociological theories on knowledge, power and practice to understand the dynamic processes of organizational change. Much of his research has focused on the role of professional groups in stimulating and stymying change processes. He has designed and carried out research on many significant policy reform agenda across the areas of patient safety and quality improvement, public-private partnerships, inter-organizational networks, major system change, and political leadership. His research has been published in journals such as *Sociology of Health and Illness*, *Social Science and Medicine*, *Sociology*, *Health and Social Behavior*, *Human Relations*, and *Organizational Studies*, and he has published four monographs.

DANIEL WEINSTOCK holds the Katharine A. Pearson chair in civil society and public policy in the Faculties of Law and Arts at McGill University (Montreal). His research focuses on the normative foundations of public policy across a wide range of policy fields including health, education, drugs, and immigration. He has published over 150 scholarly articles, and is a frequent contributor to public policy debates in Quebec and in Canada.